# Child-Centered Play Therapy

# Child-Centered Play Therapy

## A Practical Guide to Developing Therapeutic Relationships with Children

Nancy H. Cochran
William J. Nordling
Jeff L. Cochran

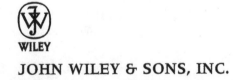

WILEY

JOHN WILEY & SONS, INC.

Published by John Wiley & Sons, Inc., Hoboken, New Jersey.
Published simultaneously in Canada.

*Library of Congress Cataloging-in-Publication Data:*

Cochran, Nancy H.
  Child-centered play therapy : a practical guide to developing therapeutic relationships with children / Nancy H. Cochran, William J. Nordling, Jeff L. Cochran.
    p. cm.
  Includes index.
  ISBN 978-0-470-44223-4 (cloth : acid-free paper); 978-0-470-63489-9 (ebk);
978-0-470-63490-5 (ebk); 978-0-470-63491-2 (ebk)
  1. Play therapy.  I. Nordling, William J.  II. Cochran, Jeff L.  III. Title.
  RJ505.P6C63 2010
  618.92'891653—dc22

                                                                    2009054222

Printed in the United States of America

SKY10025695_031721

To our son, Erzhan. Thank you for reminding us each day that we are lovable and capable of loving, and playful and able to play.
—NHC and JLC (Mommie and Papa)

To my wife, Claudia, who has made my life's work seem like play.
—WJN

And to all the courageous and amazing teachers, students, counselors, therapists, parents, and children—especially the children—who have taught us and continue teaching us so well. We thank you.

# Contents

# FOREWORD

In 1947, when Virginia Axline published the original edition of her now famous book, *Play Therapy*, she only could have hoped that it would still be the leading reference for the teaching of child play therapists more than 60 years later. The method she then espoused, known as nondirective play therapy, has continued to be practiced, virtually unchanged, and has proven to be empirically valid.

Axline's Eight Basic Principles are the foundation of her method and guide the therapeutic behavior of practitioners of child-centered play therapy (CCPT). However, because Axline expressed her system as eight discrete principles stated in general terms, her method is susceptible to misapplication. In fact, it is sometimes said that Axline's is the approach to child therapy most used and most misused.

One of the major challenges to the correct application of Axliness's approach is to fully grasp that her brilliant principles together comprise a complete, coherent system of therapy. Axline herself explained that the "principles are overlapping and interdependent . . . [for example] the therapist cannot be accepting without being permissive" (p. 91). When therapists use one principle or a few without the others, the effectiveness of the method is weakened, constituting a misuse.

Another major challenge therapists encounter is in distilling Axline's broad principles into specific therapeutic behaviors that can be consistently used by all therapists in their application of the method. It is not surprising that the proponents of Axline's approach have developed minor variations in translating the principles into practice. Interestingly, empirical evidence demonstrates that all these variations are equally effective. This suggests that essential adherence to the basic prescription of each principle outweighs any minor variations in their operationalization.

Since Axline's day, advances in teaching methodology have enabled proponents of her principles to establish greater uniformity in their application within each variation. Most notably, skills training has emerged as a very productive method of teaching and learning the operationalized behaviors derived from the principles. Each proponent's variation naturally leads to different levels of emphasis on particular skills.

These authors are advocates of my variation, having been associated with me at the National Institute of Relationship Enhancement (NIRE). I am especially pleased to see that they have emphasized in their book the skill of role-playing, which I greatly value. I believe that role-playing is one productive way to actualize Axline's third and fourth principles, respectively " . . . to [support] the child in expressing his feelings completely," and "to express them back to him in such a manner that helps him gain insight into his behavior." I have always found that, when skillfully used, therapist involvement in child-directed role-play allows children to give life to unexpressed conflicts they are experiencing and to play out positive attitudes and behaviors to which they aspire in real life.

These authors have included "all the things you need to know" about applying this skill, so that the method may be used to the best advantage for facilitating the child. They highlight common pitfalls such as overplaying and underplaying roles that children assign to the therapist, and failure to adhere to limits necessary to maintain the comfort of the child and therapist during the role-play. This is but one example of the authors' professionalism when writing on skills such as the use of CCPT in schools and in other nontherapeutic settings, which requires special sensitivity on the part of the therapist.

The authors' experience in skills training and especially in supervising play therapists is apparent throughout the book in the way they explain the subject matter and provide devices for reinforcing the material covered in the skills chapters. Their extensive experience is also evident in their delicacy with personal feeling issues that therapists might have when applying the method. Their suggestions for dealing with these issues will, I think, be very useful to therapists who have such concerns.

The breadth of coverage provided in this book would make it easier for a beginner in this variation to self-learn. However, the depth of insightful detail would also enrich those already experienced in the method. Of course, no book could take the place of workshop or classroom instruction, for which this book would be a very appropriate reference.

I am happy to be linked to this book by being given the opportunity to write this foreword. I thank the authors for providing this opportunity and for helping to make CCPT readily understandable to those who wish to take advantage of its long history of helping children overcome problems and grow emotionally to a level of maturity difficult to achieve by any other approach.

Louise F. Guerney, PhD, RPT-S
*Professor Emerita*, Pennsylvania State University
National Institute of Relationship Enhancement
Bethesda, Maryland
August 2009

# PREFACE

**W**e find child-centered play therapy (CCPT) to be a most powerful, versatile, and practical approach to helping children, families, schools, and communities, and this is well supported in the research, of course (e.g., Bratton, Ray, Rhine, & Jones, 2005; Guerney, 2001; Landreth, 2002; Landreth, Homeyer, Bratton, Kale, & Hilpl, 2000). It is an approach applicable across the helping professions and settings and with widely ranging child difficulties, from depression, conduct disorder, attachment problems, physical and sexual abuse, and other trauma to grief and other more normally occurring concerns. It can be extraordinarily helpful when applied singularly or within sets of services at schools, agencies, and private practices. It works well in clinics as well as residential and hospital settings, and it has been extensively and effectively applied in schools. CCPT empowers clinicians to help children, families, schools, and communities when clinicians have access to ideal sets of system interventions, and when clinicians have limited access and can simply devote an hour or less per week to the child for a period of weeks.

This being said, we don't believe CCPT is being used as frequently, extensively, or effectively as it could be. The purpose of this book is to help change that—to make clear the practicality, power, and efficiency of CCPT and to help ensure that practitioners apply CCPT with optimal effectiveness.

## A Deficit of Perception

One reason for a deficit in application may be a deficit in perception. It may be that for many, on first impression, CCPT does not *sound* very practical. For example, Virginia Axline (1947, 1969), the "mother of play therapy," described a *permissive* atmosphere as a key to the intervention. *Permissive* is not what many parents, teachers, and administrators want to hear about an intervention for children in dire need of help, often for children whose behavior is seemingly "out of control"!

The use of *play* in the title may not be entirely supportive to the credibility of the approach either, as many parents will report, "My child already knows how to play" and some teachers may complain,

"All he does in class is play!" In a way, at least politically, the approach is misnamed; for example, a speech therapist helps children *learn to speak well*, but a play therapist helps children heal emotionally and master the behavioral problems hindering growth and well-being. While children may increase their playfulness and creativity during the CCPT process, the goal is not to *learn to play well*. In play therapy, play is the medium of the work, not the object.

In addition, the term *nondirective*, as used in Axline's original works, is often misinterpreted to the impression that CCPT is a vague, unstructured method that is both passive and easily employed with little expertise. In fact, although children are allowed to take the lead in therapy and permitted to make many choices surrounding self-expression, there are very clear skills sets that the therapist employs, and the child-centered play therapist, though *not directing*, is very active in sessions. *Facilitating open self-expression, helping the child to self-direct and grow in self-responsibility* are key curative factors in CCPT, and are tasks requiring delicate balance and well thought out skill application.

Another possible reason for the deficit in utilizing CCPT is that this therapy is often incorrectly represented as a long-term, open-ended approach that does not work "fast enough" or can not be used in the short-term or brief therapy context. When a child is struggling with behavioral problems and hurting emotionally, we all feel pressure to hurry to fix the problem, or to "make it feel better." So, for many, the intuitive response is to take responsibility for the child, to teach or guide, or to actively try to solve the problem. When a child is grief stricken and painfully withdrawn, rarely is the intuitive response to provide a therapy for the child that allows for *more time* to find a way for opening up and relating—for self-expression in her own way and in her own time. When a child is full of defiance and acting out, rarely is the intuitive response to provide a therapy that allows for *more freedom to be*—to refuse, vent, and test limits—in his own way and in his own time. Yet our experience and research has taught us that when a child has significant behavioral and emotional difficulties, a child-centered approach *facilitating* change vs. an approach or intervention *directing* change is the only method to provide for significant, enduring change—change that *comes from within, and therefore belongs to* the child as she moves forward in life.

Additionally, because CCPT is focused on *therapeutic relationships with children* rather than *techniques to use with children*, there is the possibility that some potential learners and practitioners misunderstand the potential in the approach—viewing it as only theory and an abstract conceptualization rather than a therapeutic approach with clear, skill-based guidance for application. For this and other reasons, our book is highly skill based, making the potentially abstract child-centered approach highly accessible, concrete, teachable, and learner-ready for students and practicing clinicians. It follows in the tradition of breaking subtle relationship-building qualities into skill-teaching units, begun by Louise and Bernard Guerney, and developed by Bill Nordling and the National Institute for Relationship Enhancement (NIRE).

## Our Goals in Skill Development

To address the possible misconceptions of the CCPT model above, we set as our primary goal to make the approach cogent, practical, and applicable. The greater each reader and practitioner's mastery of CCPT skills, the more children, families, schools, and communities are helped. Therefore, the essential skills sets of the CCPT model are well defined in our book, and our goal is to systematically teach them in a way accessible to the practitioner new to the model, and to bring new insights into the method for those who already know it. In doing so, we do not ignore the richness of the theory underlying CCPT since it serves as the foundation from which the core therapist skills and attitudes spring forth.

Our secondary goal is to clarify for the reader the broader implications of the CCPT approach in their work. CCPT is not merely a series of techniques, but a wide-ranging philosophy that has implications for building relationships with parents and other caregivers to bring about a climate of change and growth. We intend to guide practitioners not only to do exceptional work counseling children, but also to carefully evaluate their work and their clients' progress, and to build the strong parent, teacher, administrator, and other community relationships that will support CCPT as powerful, curative, and essential in helping children in need of counseling.

Our final goal and hope for this book is to prepare practitioners to articulate the power and expediency of the CCPT approach to their communities and stake holders, so that more children can be helped, and so that their agencies, clinics, and practices will thrive.

## Key Themes of This Book

A theme or subtext of this book is to help graduate students and current practitioners learn to slow down, have faith in a child's ability to lead the way, and to realize that *haste* really does *make waste*. Expert child therapists and child-development specialists, from Virginia Axline to

Jean Jacques Rousseau to Jean Piaget, have warned against the temptation to hurry children's change processes, that doing so may prolong rather than shorten children's process and progress in development. This can be particularly true when a therapeutic intervention is needed; and, ironically, at just the time that we feel the most pressure to hurry. Our aim is for readers to see that the gentle, child-centered approach is not only highly practical, but is often optimally efficient.

Further, we want readers to learn to *articulate* CCPT as an efficient, practical approach. While helping readers and students learn the skills of CCPT, we also strive to help them see how it fits into practical, needed contexts. A theme throughout the book is helping readers understand not only *what* they are doing, but also *why*. Our aim is to empower readers to make understandable the practicality of CCPT—to be better able to explain what they do and why as a therapist/counselor who uses CCPT to help children in need.

While preparing readers to employ the skills of CCPT, we also maintain a strong focus on the development of the person of the therapist. Therefore, another of our objectives is to have each reader see that she is "the best toy" in the playroom. It is the therapeutic relationship with her that matters more than any toy or technique, and that if she is "broken" and unable to relate with the core conditions of deep empathy, genuineness, and unconditional positive regard, then therapy will not happen. To this aim, we strive to illustrate the truth of this, and guide readers to self-reflect and strive for self-development.

We have attempted to provide our goals and objectives in a form that is highly practical and skill-based. Each chapter begins with a scenario illustrating an application focus issue (AFI) to draw the reader into the core application issue of that chapter. Each AFI is followed by primary skill objectives to orient readers and establish the goals of that chapter in skill-based terms. Each chapter is filled with case examples, vignettes, and real world illustrations. The book includes ample opportunities for readers and students to practice and apply the skills as they study.

As a result, this book should serve equally well for graduate students who are studying with teachers and peers, as it should for current practitioners working on their own to understand and develop skills in CCPT. It is an advanced skill level text. While it could be used by a beginner in a mental health field, that reader would likely need to return to it again in his continued education, training, and supervision as a child therapist.

We believe each practitioner's work needs to be well grounded in theory. Therefore, while teaching skills, we help readers develop deep understanding of the theory base of Axline's and Rogers's work. Our explanations and backgrounds for understanding CCPT and change are also well-informed by cognitive, behavioral, existential, psychoanalytic/psychodynamic, and other approaches—yet our point of view always values the therapeutic relationship as the primary healing element, and thus constantly returns to that value and theme.

## Context for This Book

For over 25 years NIRE has taught and supervised CCPT in a highly skill-based manner, which we see as one of the major sources for objectifying, applying, and remaining true to Virginia Axline's original work. This book addresses unique aspects of Louise Guerney's and NIRE's approach to play therapy for the first time in book form and in a comprehensive way. These unique aspects to the approach include the rich opportunities for empathic connection developed through therapists' involvement in children's role-play; a highly concrete, subtle, and existential approach to limit setting; the use of identifiable stages in children's work in CCPT to monitor progress; as well as other aspects distinctive to the Guerney/NIRE approach to teaching CCPT skills.

We have also long been informed and inspired by the existing literature on play therapy, especially the work of Garry Landreth and his colleagues at the University of North Texas's Center for Play Therapy. As our work adds a comprehensive presentation of the approach developed by our mentor, Louise Guerney, our aim is to build upon the work of the great leaders in fields of play therapy, family therapy, and counseling across settings.

## Conclusion

We hope that this book will make a useful contribution to the training and education of mental health professionals as they work to become more aware of CCPT as a powerful, efficient, and skill-based approach to child counseling and therapy. We hope for each reader to become maximally effective in and empowered by CCPT in the care they provide for children, families, schools, and communities. We invite readers to study with us through our text, and then perhaps to join the family of child-centered play therapists worldwide who provide healing opportunities for the many children in need. Welcome. Please read on.

# ACKNOWLEDGMENTS

We'd first and foremost like to acknowledge Lisa Gebo for connecting us with our editor, Isabel Pratt, and for encouraging us in going forward with this written work together. You are a wonder to all who know you, Lisa, in your abilities to bring people together to do good work. We wish to thank all of our reviewers—Athena Drewes, Dee Ray, Paris Goodyear-Brown, and Jodi Crane—for their time, insight, and hard work in reviewing the proposal for this book.

Our thanks also to the following colleagues and friends—to Barb Higgins for your assistance with Chapter 2, and for sharing the great pictures from your private practice for use in our book as well. To Melinda Gibbons, also for your insights and the time taken to review Chapter 2. For the professional attention to detail from Lindsey Teague and Tinah Utsman—your willingness to help with graphs and tables went well beyond the call of duty. To Peggy Higgins for the pictures of the ideal playroom setting and toys, and to Steve Demanchick for the same. The pictures provided from your play therapy centers are a wonderful addition to our book. To Erzhan Cochran, Ruth Haldeman, and Hansol Haldeman; Aliya and Mark Alewine and daughter, Kayla; Shawn Spurgeon and sons, Maurice, Shane, and Michael; Melinda Gibbons and sons, Ben and Ryan; Christina Poles and Jaiden Rodriguez; great students and counselors, Ashley McIntyre, Lindy Cohen, and Christopher Ellison—thank you all for help with pictures, too.

And, of course, much thanks and love goes out to our families—for your patience, support, and encouragement. An extra special thanks to Erzhan for laughing at all of Bill's goofy jokes, and for mistakenly, but aptly, calling what we do and write about "child-centered play therabe." It is, after all, all about "a way of being."

Finally, but with full awareness of how far we have come, we want to acknowledge the profound influence that the work and writings of Carl Rogers and Virgina Axline have had on our formation, as well as that of Louise Guerney and Garry Landreth, who first systemized training in CCPT. We also wish to express our appreciation to Bernard

Guerney, Jr., who gave the world an incredible gift by developing the filial therapy model, which transformed CCPT into a family-based therapy model. We thank them for their commitment to the study, promotion, and practice of play therapy, but most of all for their inspiring love for children and families.

# Introduction: The Child-Centered Approach, Student and Practitioner Approaches to Learning, and Our Approach to Teaching

## 1

### Chapter

*Play therapy is based upon the fact that play is the child's natural medium of self expression. It is an opportunity which is given to the child to 'play out' his feelings and problems just as, in certain types of adult therapy, an individual 'talks out' his difficulties.*
*—Excerpt from the classic* Play Therapy *by Virginia Axline*

## Overview: The Core Application Focus Issues

Perhaps you are a student in the helping professions. You want to help children and you've heard of play therapy, but you don't know how and why it works, or how to do it. While you will additionally need supervision and instruction, this book is designed to take you as far as possible toward being ready to apply the skills needed to be a deeply healing therapeutic agent for the children you serve. When you complete your study, you should be well on your way to being able to do the work, as well as to acquiring a deep understanding of the "how and why" behind the skills. As you come to understand the work through your study, we encourage you to think of how you can explain what you are learning to others with interests in helping children, but who do not yet have the background and education to know how. Honing your skills in explaining to others the benefits of child-centered play therapy (CCPT)—what you do and why—will be an important addition to your overall proficiency as a play therapist.

Perhaps you are a practicing counselor or therapist, but learning play therapy and the child-centered approach is quite different from the work that you have been doing. This book is well designed for active learning and will provide you guidance in applying what you learn as you study. It is comprehensive in the skills you will need in addition to your graduate education in your particular discipline. Most of our chapters, especially the core or "essential skill sets" chapters, have "Common Problems Encountered" sections near the end. You may use these to prevent or troubleshoot common errors as you begin to apply your CCPT skills.

Perhaps you are a therapist or counselor who has long served adults and adolescents, but have limited experience providing direct counseling to children. Perhaps you have become discouraged by watching children continue to suffer, and dysfunction continue to cross generations, as some of your adult clients resist change. As Virginia Axline (1947, 1969) pointed out in the time-honored work *Play Therapy*, "while therapy (for children) might move ahead faster if the adults were also receiving therapy or counseling, it is not necessary for the adults to be helped in order to insure successful play therapy results (pg. 66)." We look forward to introducing you to the world of children and the child-centered approach to play therapy. In that world, change can come very quickly—if you are patient, almost anything is possible—and if you are open to it, the work can renew hope for children and parents, and be very gratifying.

In the coming pages we introduce child-centered play therapy and ourselves. Following this, we address some of the frequently asked questions that can be addressed in the beginning. In the following chapter, we address child-centered play therapy in the context of child and human development (Chapter 2), discuss ideal therapist qualities (Chapter 3), the underlying principles of play therapy, and the functions of play. In Part II, the essential skill sets, we guide you through preparing your contexts and each of the skills that you must master over time, from tracking with empathy (Chapter 6) to setting limits (Chapter 7), from role-play (Chapter 9) to understanding children's stages in child-centered play therapy (Chapter 10), from working with parents and teachers to evaluating progress and termination (Chapters 11 and 12). In Part III, we introduce you to wrap-around skills (Filial Therapy and Helping Children Capitalize on Gains Made in CCPT—Chapters 13 and 14) that grow from CCPT and are often helpful additions. And in Part IV we address CCPT in the context of governing principles of the helping professions such as ethical and professional issues and diversity issues in CCPT (Chapters 15 and 16).

Whatever your circumstances, theoretical base, or point of view in beginning your study, we encourage you to be an active learner. You may notice that each chapter begins with an application focus issue, intended to draw you into the core problem in helping children therapeutically that the chapter addresses. Following from this, each chapter continues with primary skill objectives that orient you to the goals of the chapter in skill-based terms. We encourage you to picture yourself in each of the case studies and illustrations. We encourage you to complete as many of the activities for further study as possible, in order to deepen your contemplation of CCPT and skill development.

While CCPT is a comprehensive skill set and we lay out a logical sequence of chapters and sections, as an engaged learner you may choose to jump to the chapters that seem to answer your most pressing questions first, coming to others as you follow the questions that come to your mind next. The book is designed to use as a reference, as well as an initial text. Our hope is that it will serve you in this time of your development, and also as a reference in your work in service to children for many years to come.

In concluding this introduction, may we say, "Welcome. Read on. We are optimistic for what you will learn. We are hopeful that our book will support you in the work you will do. There are many children in need of counseling, who are hurting and can use the help of a great new (or rejuvenated and renewed) child therapist or counselor. The better your skill development from this study of CCPT, the better our world will be."

## Primary Skill Objectives

The following Primary Skill Objectives are provided to guide you through this introductory chapter, and for reflection and review after the completion of the chapter. After reading, it is our hope that you will:

1. Gain a basic understanding of what CCPT is and orient yourself for further study.
2. Meet the authors and gain some knowledge of our backgrounds, especially how we came to be passionate about this work.
3. Consider the importance of and establish goals for your personal development related to CCPT.
4. Gain the answers to frequently asked questions that are generally on the minds of professionals or students beginning their study of CCPT.

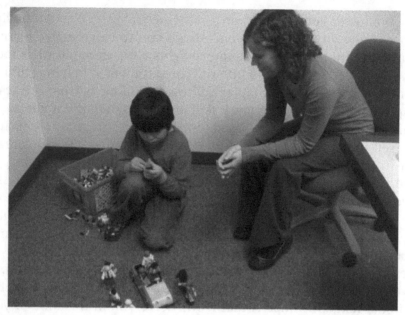

Figure 1.1

## What Is Child-Centered Play Therapy?

Child-centered play therapy is evolved from and true to the approach that Virginia Axline simply called *Play Therapy* (Axline, 1947). As can be noted in the quote that leads into this chapter, play in therapy is the child's mode of communication, for sharing his world, his inner thoughts and feelings, and the meanings that he makes of his experience of his world. It is the child's opportunity to communicate what he could not as easily put into words. Play in therapy is also child-to-self communication. This is quite similar to the way that many adults go over and over a topic that has been bothering them when working with their counselor—in ways that they will not when thinking about it alone, even if they are thinking about it "all the time." When troubled, many humans will think about a matter or topic to a point of anxiety. This anxiety causes interruption in the thought, and they will then stop thinking about it—most times without reaching resolution or new meaning from the experience. In adult therapy, the counselor's listening and empathic responses help the adult client work through this anxiety and gain insight. In CCPT, with the counselor's attentive tracking and empathic responses, children work all the way through such repetitive, unproductive loops to reach new understandings of their experience, and new decisions of who they want to be and how they want to behave. A skilled child-centered play therapist can facilitate this process for a child without the child having to do what may not be developmentally possible—that is, articulate in words such a complex and abstract process.

Please don't think that because the child need not articulate this process in words, and because it is child-centered (i.e., adult facilitated, but child led), that you cannot set practical goals, measure progress, and gain indications of a child's internal process from her play. Certainly you can, and as a rule should. We address these topics throughout the book, especially in Chapters 10–12.

Also, you may know that Virginia Axline and others referred to the approach in the early years as *nondirective*. We find this to be a misnomer. Being nondirective, attentive, and loving with a child is a very valuable and beautiful thing, but it does not approach the power and efficiency of a skilled child-centered approach when therapy or a significant counseling intervention is needed. We don't see child-centered play therapy as nondirective, even though it is child-centered. As playroom toys are carefully selected for child self-expression, it could be said that the playroom directs a child to self-express. However, it is important to also understand that children do not have to be directed to self-express. To facilitate a child's therapeutic self-expression, one only has to remove the impediments to self-expression. How to do this is addressed throughout the book, and through detailed descriptions and examples of the core skills of CCPT.

As the therapist attends to the child client's experience with empathic acceptance, the child is freed up and in a sense "directed" by being allowed to attend to his inner experience, his thoughts, feelings, reactions to his outer world, and his choices. As we explain in terms of child and human change theory in Chapter 2, a child does not need to be directed by his therapist to better behavior. This direction can come from his inner desire and drive to mature, once the child is open to it as opposed to defended against what he does not want to admit about himself or his experience. As the counselor attends to the child client's attempts at self-direction, facilitated through the structure and skills of CCPT, the child is directed to attend to his attempts at self-direction, self-responsibility, internal locus of control, and internal locus of evaluation.

CCPT is a different experience than everyday play for the child. In CCPT, the therapist utilizes a well defined set of skills in a consistent, predictable manner which creates a context which promotes children's

**Table 1.1** **Examples of Mechanisms of Change in CCPT**

- Developing the Ability to Self-Express & Finding the "Moral Compass"
- Experiencing Self-Regulation
- Evaluating and Changing Irrational Self-Talk
- Choosing New Life Directions

self-expression and self-direction; so the therapist in CCPT is active, disciplined, and predictable. Paradoxically, this allows the child to engage in self-expression that is not structured or predictable, in which the child communicates to self and therapist through play, much the way an adult may discuss his concerns in a counseling session, leading to new awareness, new life decisions, and more mature choices.

CCPT has applications for common childhood problems and normally occurring concerns as well as anxiety, depression, oppositional defiance, sexual and physical abuse trauma, grief, and adjustments to life events. CCPT cannot "cure" problems of a more organic or biological nature such as attention deficit/hyperactivity disorder (ADHD), obsessive-compulsive disorder, or biochemical depression, but nonetheless it can successfully be utilized as a highly effective intervention before diagnosis, for example, to rule out or determine if the child's symptoms are transient and due to adjustment problems or developmental delays. And for children with correct diagnoses of neurological, biological, or organic disorders, CCPT is a highly effective adjunctive treatment. It helps children overcome effects that *can be* within their control. Because children with such disorders also tend to have concurrent emotional problems, they benefit greatly from CCPT, which strengthens internal locus of control and self-regulation and promotes a sense of self-worth, self-responsibility, and self-efficacy.

## Mechanisms of Change in CCPT

It may help to introduce you to CCPT if we briefly introduce you to some of the many mechanisms of change within CCPT. Examples follow.

## Developing the Ability to Self-Express

A child thrives when given the opportunity to discover her own "voice" in CCPT. Becoming aware of one's beliefs, intentions, and desires can be difficult when constantly faced with the many expectations of others (not to mention the media) and the competitive environments of school and society. When a child is given the opportunity to experience himself as a thinking, feeling, autonomous being, he discovers that he can tap into internal resources to find a "moral compass" and that his thoughts and feelings can be experienced and expressed in an individual way. This "voice" may be found in art or music, in drama, movement, or words. It is a child's unique language that is listened to and understood by his therapist.

## Experiencing Self-Regulation

CCPT provides a structure in which a child can self-express and cannot fail. This does not mean that there are no limits or consequences—certainly there are. As you will see, carefully applied limits and consequences are applied as needed to anchor the child's work to reality *and to* facilitate self-expression. However, the structure directs a child to realize the mistake made, realize the consequences, and continue the self-expression that he is driven to do in an acceptable way. In this process, a child learns that she can express her deepest, darkest emotions, and she can *manage the monster*, so to speak. She learns that she can let intense emotions out, and still control her actions. The child learns to self-regulate—release the emotions and contain oneself as needed.

## Evaluating and Changing Irrational Self-Talk

Many children appear to change self-talk or their expectations for themselves in relation to their world in CCPT. If that self-talk happens to be irrational, it will not stand up to the clear light of examination through experience in the child-centered playroom. This leads to children's viewing themselves as good and lovable . . . and this leads to viewing others as good and approachable . . . and this leads to more secure attachment, approachability, and enhanced relationships with others.

## Choosing New Life Directions

Very often, a child's choices can be too abstract for him to discuss in words, but can appear quite obviously in play therapy. Children can often be seen to vacillate between "good" and "bad," alternating from characters that represent the worst of their thoughts and inclinations to those of their best. In such moments, children may be trying on the different personas as if to see how they feel, to see which feels like the person he wants to be. Fortunately, given the opportunity, a child will choose the best he can be. When a child is stuck in the "bad" or inhibited from choosing to be his best, CCPT provides the opportunity to get to that best self that he *is almost ready* to be, but has been defended and inhibited from being.

## Can the Process Really Be Child-Centered? Does a Child Really Know the Way?

Our answers to the questions in the section title are "yes" and "yes, given the necessary conditions." We find these questions very understandable. Trusting that the child knows the way—the true path to her healing—can be a difficult leap of faith. By socialization or intuition, we, like many adults, learn to take care of children, to teach and guide them. Obviously, there is much that children cannot do for themselves. That is the nature of being a child in contrast to being an adult.

But can a child really know the way to his own deep internal repairs, to the changes needed to guide his external behavior to a better way? Can he overcome his progress inhibiting factors if you don't teach and guide him toward wise behavior? We address this in more depth in Chapter 2 and following chapters, but for this introduction suffice it to answer: Yes, he can—if he is provided with the right therapeutic conditions and with a structure carefully built to facilitate his explorations, a structure where there is nothing else to do but master the awareness and self-learning that he needs in order to direct his path toward his best self. If his problem is a discreet surface concern, it would be best to simply teach the behavior. But if his problem approaches the deep and internal, akin to "facing the monster" inside himself, or visiting a scary place or vulnerable time in his development, he needs a skilled therapist to be *right there with him* and to accompany him into his inner world. Yes, he can find the way, in the context of CCPT, but he cannot go there alone. Empowered in the therapeutic relationship, he can find his way there with his counselor accompanying him, and he will come back better, stronger, clearer thinking, and ready to face the challenges of his life with all the wisdom and maturity appropriate for his age.

# Research Supporting CCPT

There is a significant research base supporting CCPT. In this section, we review one very helpful meta-analysis, a small sample of recent studies, and a small sample of older studies indicating the breadth of applications and results possible with CCPT.

## Meta-Analysis

In a recent meta-analysis of 93 studies from 1953 to 2000 regarding the effectiveness of play therapy, Bratton, Ray, Rhine, and Jones (2005) found good effect sizes for play therapy in general, led in volume of studies (78%) and effect size (significantly larger at $p < 0.03$) by studies that are child-centered or very similar to CCPT. It would be difficult to make an exact claim for the child-centered approach from within this analysis partly due to the varying ways that persons in the field refer to child-centered and other approaches. Currently, there are multiple approaches to play therapy, so the child-centered approach is now commonly designated "child-centered," but originally, following from Axline's work, all play therapy was child-centered but referred to simply as "play therapy." Bratton et al. concluded, "Play therapy can be considered effective regardless of therapeutic approach, with the humanistic [CCPT or closely related] interventions demonstrating a large effect size and the non-humanistic treatments [e.g., behavioral, cognitive, and directive play therapy interventions, such as board games] demonstrating a moderate effect size" (p. 380).

## Recent Studies

We provide a sample of recent studies representing the wide variety of successful results and applications of CCPT below. In a study of 36 elementary school children who are homeless, Baggerly and Jenkins (2009) found indications congruent with previous research of the effectiveness of CCPT with children who are homeless, demonstrating "improvement in homeless children's development related to classroom learning processes after receiving CCPT" (p. 51). Previously, in a study of child-centered group play therapy with 42 children who were homeless, Baggerly (2004) found significant improvements in self-esteem, anxiety, and depression.

Shen (2002) investigated the effectiveness of short-term child-centered group play therapy for 65 children in Taiwan who had experienced an earthquake. In support of previous studies of play therapy with American children, children in the experimental group demonstrated significantly lower anxiety and suicide risk than children in the control group.

In a study with 41 elementary school–age children assigned to CCPT treatment or wait list control group, Ray, Blanco, Sullivan, and Holliman (2009) found that children with CCPT decreased aggressive behaviors statistically significantly, while children from the control group did not. Ray et al. explained that CCPT is an "intervention that offers the child an environment in which aggression can be expressed and empathically responded to" (p. 162).

In a study of 60 elementary school–age children identified as symptomatic of attention deficit/hyperactivity disorder by *Diagnostic and Statistical Manual of Mental Disorders*, 4th edition, Text Revision (DSM-IV-TR) criteria (American Psychiatric Association [APA], 2000) randomly assigned to sixteen 30-minute weekly sessions of CCPT or reading mentoring, Ray, Schottelkorb, and Tsai (2007) found that both groups demonstrated improvement critical to the disorder and school success, with the CCPT group demonstrating significantly more improvement in measurement areas "indicating that children in [CCPT] were significantly less stressful to their teachers in personal characteristics, specifically emotional distress, anxiety, and withdrawal difficulties" (p. 107). Additionally, in a longer term study of 23 children identified as exhibiting behavioral and emotional difficulties, Muro, Ray, Schottelkorb, Smith, and Blanco (2006) took extensive measures after 16 and 32 sessions, finding significant global improvements across a variety of relevant scales after 32 sessions, with improvement being statistically steady over the full duration of therapy.

Danger and Landreth (2005) found a large practical significance in helping prekindergarten and kindergarten children with speech difficulties improve expressive and receptive language skills. Garza and Bratton (2005) examined the effects of CCPT compared to a curriculum-based small group intervention for 29 Hispanic children referred due to behavior problems, finding CCPT to show statistically significant decreases and large treatment effects in externalizing behavior problems compared to the curriculum-based treatment group, as well as moderate treatment effects on internalizing behavior problems.

Demanchick, N. H. Cochran, and J. L. Cochran (2003) presented two case studies indicating improvement in adults with developmental disabilities who were experiencing severe and persistent behavioral and emotional difficulties for which no other intervention had seemed effective. Demanchick et al. noted that "due to problems in communicating with psychologists, counselors, and other daily helpers, adults with developmental disabilities may experience a lifetime of daily routines that involve few if any opportunities for emotional expression, validation and growth" (p. 47).

Similarly, Ledyard (1999) presented three cases studies of CCPT with elderly nursing home residents. Observed changes include decreased depression, heightened self-esteem, and improved socialization skills.

## Older Research

Sampling from older research to exemplify the breadth of application and results, CCPT has been evidenced as effective with: alleviation of hair pulling (Barlow, Strother, & Landreth, 1985), amelioration of selective mutism (Barlow, Strother, & Landreth, 1986), increased emotional adjustment of sexually abused children and witnesses of domestic violence (Kot, Landreth, & Giordano, 1998), progress from poor reading performance (Axline, 1947; Bills, 1950; Bixler, 1945), improved academic success for children with learning disabilities (Axline, 1949; Guerney, 1983c), decreased speech problems (Axline & Rogers, 1945; Dupent, Landsman, & Valentine, 1953), improved social and emotional adjustment (Axline, 1948; 1964), and improved self-concept (Kot, Landreth, & Giordano, 1998) and self-efficacy (Fall, 1999).

# The Background of CCPT in Theories of Counseling and Psychotherapy and Links to Varied Theories

Virginia Axline was a student, and subsequently a colleague of, Carl Rogers. Child-centered play therapy is the person-centered approach applied to helping children. It carries the clear person-centered focus on the core conditions of therapeutic relationships, including psychological contact and conveyance of the therapist's empathy, unconditional positive regard, and congruence (Rogers, 1957). It values an individual's self-responsibility, with choices in self-direction facilitated through self-awareness or discovery of previously denied aspects of self. And it values the therapist's being involved with and affected by clients through deep and genuine empathic connections.

In addition to person-centered, we see the mechanisms of change within CCPT resonating with a wide range of approaches to counseling and psychotherapy. For example, in a cognitive-behavioral approach (Beck & Weishaar, 2008; Ellis, 2008), a counselor might readily teach an adult client to think about thinking, to evaluate her thoughts, her "shoulds and musts," in order to change thought patterns that create dysfunction. But *thinking about thinking* is a higher order thought process not available to most children. We find that for children to change dysfunctional thoughts, a greater awareness of experience is needed rather than a greater awareness of thought. In CCPT, children gain awareness of previously denied experiences, and dysfunctional thoughts appear to change as evidenced in behavior change.

That process of realizing previously denied experience also has a partial connection with psychoanalytic, psychodynamic, or object relations approaches (Luborsky, O'Reilly-Landry, & Arlow, 2008). CCPT shares with the approaches a focus on the therapist-client relationship and each client's apparent inner experience. The focus is often on what is going on between the therapist and client. But unlike these approaches, interpretation would not be a part of the work for the same reason that a child-centered play therapist would not attempt to direct a child to think about thinking—to make meaning of the therapist's interpretation requires a cognitive function not possible for most children.

In an additional difference with these theories, a child-centered play therapist would also not direct a child to think about thinking or interpret a child's behavior because of the tremendous power differential between adult and child when a child is in counseling. To do so would be disempowering the child when the child-centered play therapist's goal is to empower the child to more self-responsible decisions. Also, to do so would tend to limit or end the child's self-expression before the child achieves the new awareness necessary to engage a new path of more self-responsible decisions.

CCPT shares the values from existential (Mendelowitz & Schneider, 2008) and gestalt (Yontef & Jacobs, 2008) approaches of awareness of one's experience in the here and now, including the experience of the "I thou" relationship with the therapist (Friedman, 1995, 2001; based on Buber, 1955). It shares reality therapy's (Wubbolding, 2000) high value of self-responsibility, while making much greater use of the child's own ability to take responsibility for himself and his actions. It shares the solution-focused (de Shazer, 1988; Fish, 1996; Hawkes, Marsh, & Wilgosh, 1998) perspective of seeing persons as capable, seeing little need to focus on the problem or history, while providing a structure within which children choose to move in forward directions.

At times, it even shares key foci with behaviorism (Skinner, 1953). For example, limits are applied when necessary (see Chapter 7) to anchor the child's work to reality and to ensure a structure that facilitates self-expression. In such a situation, a child who has great difficulty tolerating limits (a common aspect of reasons for referral) learns the skill of tolerating limits. For such a child, the motivating reward in the CCPT structure may be continued time to self-express and the child-centered play therapist's continued empathy, unconditional positive regard, and genuine relating. For these naturally occurring rewards of the CCPT structure and therapeutic relationship, such a child becomes motivated to increase his tolerance of necessary limits in ways that he was not motivated in the structures of his other relationships.

## Who We Are

It occurs to us that you should want to know about us, some of the backgrounds from which we write this book, and some of how we came to be passionate about CCPT. We will admit that we are "child-centered nerds," that is to say that we enjoy talking with others "on end" about our work and life experiences in providing child counseling services and teaching CCPT. Our work on this book together has been gratifying. We contend that a "child-centered nerd" is a great (and fun) kind of nerd to be! In order that you may know us better, we introduce ourselves next.

### Nancy Cochran

Nancy's passion for CCPT seems an obvious outgrowth of her commitment to the care of and respect for children. She has long been a caregiver, observer, counselor, and passionate advocate of children. Nancy opens her CCPT classes and presentations remembering and sharing the play of her own childhood—and she likes to convey this time of childhood as being a time to be revered. From an early age she remembers her own free play and many creative opportunities. She also remembers the adults in her life who took the time to provide safety, caring attentiveness, and freedom as she explored the outdoors, painted and created, wrote, directed, and acted in plays she put on in her backyard. She has found that during discussions of "childhood memories," as her students reveal varied experiences, some have a very difficult time remembering childhood at all, or when they do, it is very painful, and they are unable to share with others for some time. In these cases, most of the students report "always feeling like a little grown-up" or "lack of time to play" or "I really don't remember playing" for a variety of reasons. In further sharing during the class, members soon unsurprisingly develop an understanding of the meaning and value of play in childhood. As they listen with empathy to the voices of those who remember childhood play—and those who don't—it becomes all too apparent that having time to play was especially meaningful and enlivening for those who were so fortunate. Those who remember childhoods of spontaneity, playful games, imaginary fun, and freedom to be tell stories that make everyone's eyes light up with joy; and there is communal laughter in remembering.

Nancy's early training and professional practice was as a school psychologist. She grew up with a younger sibling who, due to ADHD and emotional problems, constantly struggled in school and life. This had a profound effect on her. While she always knew she wanted to learn more about evaluation and assessment, her true aspiration was to help children who struggle with learning, behavioral, and emotional difficulties to feel valued as individuals, and not to become defined and painfully restricted by their difficulties and labels. She initially learned about and was supervised in CCPT and filial therapy from her school psychology professor at Appalachian State University, Eric J. Hatch, who was a former Penn State student of Bernard Guerney, Jr., and Louise Guerney. In working with families and children as a school psychologist, she naturally evolved to a focus on providing CCPT and filial therapy (Chapter 13) from a longing to be a more direct positive influence, and from a passion to help the child in need (and whole family) when possible. She met and was supervised by coauthor Bill Nordling when she was pulling a rolling duffle bag of toys from school to school as a "traveling play therapist" to provide play therapy to child victims of abuse. She subsequently became a frequent trainer/supervisor in CCPT for the National Institute for Relationship Enhancement (NIRE). Over the past 20 years, Nancy's counseling work has encompassed schools, public agencies, and a private practice. Specific areas of work interests have included attachment issues and foster/adoptive care, working with child victims of abuse, and diversity issues in CCPT. She has enjoyed working with many amazing and courageous children, parents, and therapists while focused on CCPT, filial therapy, CCPT training, and related services in a number of different states and on the island of Guam.

Nancy and coauthor and husband, Jeff, currently teach and write about CCPT together, and by 2009 they had taught 13 graduate sections of their CCPT course, including over 200 students, many of whom have gone on to do substantial work with CCPT in school settings (including Head Start and urban, rural, and suburban schools) as well as agency, hospital, and private practice settings. Their work has ranged from the direct applications with children to adapted applications, for example, with highly troubled youth (J. L. Cochran, Fauth, N. H. Cochran, Spurgeon, & Pierce, in press), the full range of youth concerns in middle and high schools, and adults with developmental disabilities (Demanchick, N. H. Cochran, & J. L. Cochran, 2003). Some of those completing CCPT study with Nancy and Jeff now teach their own CCPT courses in university and other settings.

Nancy also stays busy as a mother, writer, and as an adjunct faculty member at the University of Tennessee, Knoxville, in the Department of Educational Psychology and Counseling. She is also the coordinator for Building Resilient Youth and Families: The Child-Centered Outreach in Knoxville (the REACH Program—Relationship Enhancement and Child Harmony), a grant-funded project that provides CCPT, empathic communication for conflict resolution (J. L. Cochran, N. H. Cochran, & Hatch, 2002), the Parent Skills Training Program (Guerney, 1995), and filial therapy (Guerney, 2000; Chapter 13) at a large urban elementary school that serves high risk children and families from high poverty communities. She is president-elect of the Association for Filial and Relationship Enhancement Methods (AFREM). Her goal for the book is to add to the voices and excellent teachers who are working to value and revere childhood, and to improve through compassionate outreach and counseling the well-being of children, families, and communities in need.

### Bill Nordling

Many folks would say that Bill's interest in play therapy developed from the fact that he sees life in general as one grand personal therapeutic play experience, with the time he is most serious being when he is in the playroom with children, since in that special hour it is their turn to enter a grand therapeutic play experience. However, although he was interested in marital and family therapy from the time of his undergraduate days at the University of Dallas and throughout his master's degree training at Duquesne University, his interest in working with children began to develop when he took a job in a residential therapeutic wilderness program for emotionally disturbed children. There, he was able to see the important role that activity and creativity—not just "talking"—had for these children. Following this, Bill worked for two years as an online staff member at Lutheran Youth and Family Services, a more traditional residential treatment program for children and adolescents in New Brighton, Pennsylvania, prior to leaving to complete his doctoral studies at the University of Maryland, College Park.

During his doctoral training Bill was mentored by Robert Freeman, who ran Parent Consultation and Child Evaluation Service at the University of Maryland. Coursework and a supervised practicum under Dr. Freeman, in which Bill had practical experiences doing individual and group therapy with children and working with parents, produced a deep love for child therapy. In 1989, while at the University of Maryland, Bill experienced two life-changing events when he met Bernard Guerney, Jr., and Louise Guerney, who were professors at Penn State University. The Guerneys generously taught, supervised, and mentored him in relationship enhancement, marital/family therapy, child-centered play therapy, and filial therapy. Early in his career, Bill often said that 90% of everything that he learned about working with children, parents, and families came from the Guerneys. Although that percentage has decreased (slightly), still many of the most important things were learned from his relationship with them.

After graduation in 1992, Bill cofounded the National Institute of Relationship Enhancement (NIRE) with the Guerneys and served as the Clinical Director of NIRE's Center for Children and Families. He also served as Director of NIRE's Training and Certification Programs in child-centered play therapy and filial therapy—a position he continues to hold. Bill considers among his most treasured experiences the over-20-year professional and personal friendship with the Guerneys, with whom he has co-conducted well over 100 training workshops.

Bill left full-time employment at NIRE in 1999 to become Chair of the Department of Psychology at the Institute for the Psychological Sciences (IPS), a Catholic professional school of psychology in Arlington, Virginia. Bill teaches an average of three courses per year in the areas of play and filial therapy, as well as supervising students, presenting and publishing in these areas.

Bill is a firm believer in the importance of building strong professional organizations to support mental health professionals. He was a founding board member of the Maryland Association for Play Therapy.

He also served as a founding board member and as the first president of the Association for Filial and Relationship Enhancement Methods (AFREM), an organization formed to preserve and promote the methodologies developed by the Guerneys (which includes filial therapy). Bill also was a founding board member of the Catholic Psychotherapy Association, a board on which he continues to serve. Bill is currently finishing up his second term on the board of directors of the Association for Play Therapy (APT), and was elected to serve as the president of the APT for 2010. He was also recently elected to his 23rd-year term as "husband" by his wife and playmate, Claudia—the most important of his elective offices.

Bill considers the formation of mental health professionals a major reason he was put on this earth. He considers it a great privilege to have participated in the education and training of many hundreds of talented mental health professionals—many who serve children and who have gone on to become skilled clinicians, educators, and leaders in their communities.

### Jeff Cochran

Jeff's passion for CCPT can be said to have evolved from his interest in helping troubled adolescents who were "falling through the cracks" and for whom many had given up hope. Jeff began his professional career as a teacher at an alternative school program for troubled youth, and these youth were the focus of his early counseling interests. As a teacher, Jeff wanted to "change the world" by helping to create a better educated citizenry and to helping troubled youth increase their opportunities through education. When this progressed into his study of counseling, he had intended to counsel mainly adolescents and adults.

However, like "accidental magic," Jeff's eventual progression into a child-centered counselor and advocate seemed meant to be. Jeff and Nancy met in graduate school. As both were graduating and looking for work—Jeff in school counseling, and Nancy in school psychology—they found that one would have a good job prospect in one area, but not the other. When they learned that they could both interview with the Guam public schools and have the additional chance for travel and adventure, they interviewed and immediately accepted positions. Jeff's position was intended to be with middle school youth, in a setting related closely to his interests. But when the contract came in the mail, the counseling position assigned to him was at an elementary school. As he said to Nancy, "I don't know what to do with little kids; that's your talent—help!" He thought about trying to correct the error, but at the time, he and Nancy were too poor to make the long distance phone calls necessary to have the contract corrected—this was *way* before cell phones! So, Nancy loaned him her dog-eared copies of *Dibs in Search of Self* and *Play Therapy*, and he read Virginia Axline (1949, 1964) on the long plane trip to Guam!

His work in the school setting was relatively clinical, fitting with the needs of his setting. So, however poorly trained he may have been at the time, CCPT became a major and effective core of his work. He continued to practice CCPT off and on, while also developing other counseling interests, and grew to teach and do trainings in CCPT with Nancy and Bill, and eventually as a university faculty member to supervise many graduate interns applying CCPT skills in schools and agencies.

Jeff is currently an associate professor and the coordinator of the Mental Health Counseling Program in the Department of Educational Psychology and Counseling at the University of Tennessee in Knoxville. His counseling experience includes school and agency settings and clients throughout the life span and from a wide variety of back-grounds, and has taken place in a number of states as well as Guam. His research foci are by and large the effects of therapeutic relation-ships, but a significant part of his background of training and research are in rational emotive therapy (Ellis, 2008) and other cognitive behavioral approaches (Beck & Weishaar, 2008). You can likely see this influence in how we often conceptualize clients and CCPT, and in some of the ways we explain how CCPT works. Most recently, Jeff became the director, principal investigator, and cofounder with Nancy and Bob Kronick of the Building Resilient Youth and Families project, the grant-funded project utilizing CCPT and related wrap-around services to prevent juvenile delinquency among high-risk children and families.

When Jeff first began teaching CCPT in the course that Nancy and he designed, he opened by asking students to introduce themselves and tell others what brought them to the elective course and what they hoped to get out of it. Jeff's own answer, with a smile and a wink, was generally something like, "I want to change the world!" Then, he would add, with more seriousness, "As Nancy and I consult and observe the counseling and care of children, we are not at all contented with the level of effectiveness that we see. We know that a child in need of counseling—if given the opportunity—will look within for powerful resources of his very own for healing and growth. However, there are not enough counseling opportunities for each child in need to do this. We want to change this. We want to help you be optimally effective in helping the many child clients you encounter." And this, Jeff's customary answer to his CCPT class members, sums up his intention in helping with this book. He wants to change the world—one child-centered play therapist at a time!

## And Who Are You?

While we don't really have the chance to ask this of you as reader, it is an important question. Your study of CCPT can and ought to also be a study of yourself. The approach is counterintuitive for many, including some experienced therapists, and the study may require you to examine many of your established constructs and beliefs. The world of childhood has become fairly foreign to most adults. Entering that world requires treading gently as there is much more of a power differential between you and your child clients than you and your adult clients. It requires a keen awareness of who you are and the "baggage" you bring and forethought of who and how you want to be in your therapeutic relationships with children.

## Guidance for the Reader in Use of the Book

Generally, we encourage you to study slowly with this book, to take time to fully and deeply contemplate the skills presented, to put yourself in the place of the therapists or counselors in the many examples, and to work through as many of the practice and further learning activities as possible (many can be done independently, if you are studying alone). We encourage you to use the sequence of presentation that we provide. However, just as there are many ways to progress for children in CCPT, there can be many ways to learn with this book. For example, while most readers will benefit from the background, context, and overall understandings of CCPT provided in the early chapters, some may want to skip ahead to the most concrete skill chapters first, and return for depth of understanding later. It is also our hope and intent in design that in your many years of good work, you will return to this book as a reference, refresher, and to "troubleshoot" when faced with case situations that seem to stump you or impede the CCPT process.

## Frequently Asked Questions

In place of our "Common Problems" section that is supplied in most chapters (especially in the essential skill sets section), for this chapter we address some of the questions that are commonly on the minds of practitioners who are beginning a study of the child-centered approach. These are as follows:

1. **For what populations and what problems does CCPT work best?** The child-centered approach to play therapy works well for children ages 3–12 who are struggling with behavioral/emotional difficulties that affect a sense of well-being and ability to obtain optimum learning, growth, and health.

2. **How long do play sessions need to be, and how long does the therapy process usually last?** CCPT sessions typically last from 45 minutes to 60 minutes. While it is true that for each child, the therapy process is a unique journey, making it impossible to predict a number of sessions, in most cases 15–20 sessions are sufficient.

3. **Do I need to have a state-of-the-art playroom?** Certainly not. Therapeutic toys and art supplies are an important component in CCPT, but more important is the skilled child-centered play therapist who is able to provide the core conditions of empathy, genuineness, and unconditional positive regard in relationship to children. She is able to respond to the child in a way that facilitates self-generated activity and self-expression. Toys and art supplies do not need to be "over the top" in abundance or sensational—in fact, this can hinder progress. What is most important is that the child has a safe and confidential space to meet with a skilled child-centered play therapist, and that the toys and art supplies are sufficient to offer a variety of opportunities to self-express. It is preferable to have enough space in the meeting area for the child to move about (100 square feet at least). For more on providing CCPT with a "traveling play kit" and on how "you are the best toy in the playroom," see Chapter 5, Preparing Your Setting for Providing Child-Centered Play Therapy.

4. **How can I master and perfect the apparently complex skill sets of CCPT before I begin?** You cannot perfectly hone all the skill sets immediately, but, fortunately, CCPT is a very robust model. Although your work may be less efficient in the

beginning, most errors will not end therapeutic progress for the child. Supervised experience that involves watching taped sessions with an experienced and skilled child-centered play therapist trainer/supervisor is invaluable as you begin using CCPT. One of the most wonderful aspects of allowing each child to lead is that you will always be getting to know a unique being who is self-expressing in his own way. Indeed, much will be learned over a lifetime! That being said, with experience you will at some point start to notice a comfort and ease in CCPT sessions with all the children you help. You will no longer feel awkward with questions or preoccupied with "doing the right thing" or "making the right response" in limit-setting or role-play situations. You'll find that your CCPT skill sets are well honed and seem to come naturally. You'll find your qualities of empathy, genuineness, and unconditional positive regard working in synchronization with these skills.

## Notes on Terms Used

### School and Agency Settings

At times, we use *agency* to refer to all nonschool settings, including outpatient clinics, private practices, hospitals, and residential treatment centers. At other times, we specify agencies and private practices, since some of the most common nonschool settings for CCPT are outpatient public clinics and private practices. We also vary our examples between both school and agency settings, as the approach is commonly applied both in schools and nonschool agency settings.

### Counselor vs. Therapist

We alternate between referring to practitioners applying CCPT as *therapists* and *counselors*. In some settings, one term is preferred over another. CCPT is applied by persons from various degree backgrounds, including mental health counselors, school counselors, counseling psychologists, school psychologists, clinical psychologists, social workers, psychiatric nurses, and others in a wide variety of settings. Our aim is to be inclusive. We are much more concerned that each practitioner do good work than in what the practitioner is called.

## Activities to Solidify Study So Far and Prepare for Ongoing Learning

- *Activity A:* Work on your own or with a group of peers to define CCPT in your own words, but with as few words as possible. Design a series of bumper stickers to represent CCPT using words or graphics. As your understandings of CCPT could only have just begun from this book, allow yourself to speculate, to fill in the gaps in your definitions from what you expect to find in your continued study. Revisit and modify your words and designs regularly as you study.

- *Activity B:* Review Bratton, Ray, Rhine, and Jones's (2005) meta-analysis of the effectiveness of play therapy and review the literature on the effectiveness of CCPT, especially using the excellent resource of the *International Journal of Play Therapy.*

- *Activity C:* Speculate on parts of your personality that you know or anticipate will fit easily with the child-centered approach and those that you think will be challenged by the approach. Work to identify areas of growth and development that you can reconsider throughout your study.

# CCPT in Context: Key Concepts From Child Development and Principles of Human Change

*If I can provide a certain type of relationship, the other person will discover within himself the capacity to use that relationship for growth and change, and personal development will occur.*

*—Carl Rogers*

*Playing is how the child tries out his world and learns about his world, and it is therefore essential to his healthy development. For the child, play is serious, purposeful business through which he develops mentally, physically, and socially. Play is the child's form of self-therapy, through which confusions, anxieties, and conflicts are often worked through . . . play serves as a language for the child—a symbolism that substitutes for words.*

*—Violet Oaklander*

*Few things in life are more important to a person than rich human relationships . . . the attainment of good interpersonal relationships is a key factor in determining one's social-psychological adjustment.*

*—Eric J. Hatch and Bernard Guerney, Jr.*

*Whatever is important or necessary for children's growth already exists in children. The therapist's role or responsibility is not to reshape children's lives or make them change in some predetermined way but, rather, to respond in ways that facilitate release of creative potential that already exists in them.*

*—Garry Landreth*

## Application Focus Issue 1

"I have taught and taught that behavior and still he won't do it! Jimmy knows all the answers in the Good Behavior Game. We can even role-play the right thing to do. But when situations in real life call for the behavior, he always does the wrong thing [sighing with worried exasperation]."

We have often consulted with clinicians in school and agency settings regarding how to change seriously troubled behavior patterns such as conduct disorder or oppositional defiant disorder (American Psychiatric Association [APA], 1994) and have often heard frustrated reports similar to the quote above. The problem typically is that Jimmy does not apply the new behaviors because internal and external forces, which are stronger than the very well-meant skill teaching that his counselor has offered so far, keep him from it. He needs an internal change in order to act differently. He needs an internal change in order to *be different*, so that he will *naturally act differently on his own*. And he needs that internal change to be strong enough to withstand pressures to stay the same. In this chapter, we explore aspects of child development that inhibit children with aberrant behaviors from applying newly learned skills, and factors of child development that make it possible for child-centered play therapy (CCPT) to facilitate the needed internal change that results in new ways of being, which, in turn, results in new ways of behaving.

## Application Focus Issue 2

"[Stating an old axiom] You can't change the child if you can't change the family."

In our work with teachers, therapists, and other child helpers, we often encounter this mind-set. Due to the unfortunate and sometimes tragic conditions that some families are in, therapists and other child helpers can become disheartened and lose hope when it comes to making a difference for the children in these families. We know that the family is a child's foundation and is a powerful force in shaping his behaviors and way of being. But does that mean that a child whose family functions very poorly is destined for an unfortunate and unhappy life? No. Certainly not. While we would always work to change the family for the better if possible, child-centered play therapy gives us the opportunity to help even those children whose families are mired in dysfunction, unwilling or unable to change.

Consider that, while the odds are against it, some individuals do succeed to great mental health and life success out of tragic circumstances and miserable families. This reality brings to mind a key question: How do you tap into the mechanisms of change that allow children in need—those who have become hardened or heavily defended due to very poor functioning families—to become those surprisingly well functioning, mentally healthy exceptions? Those mechanisms of change in child development that empower the CCPT process for such children in great need are the focus of this chapter.

## Primary Skill Objectives

1. Explain the notion of "early maps of the world" in child development, including the implications for the change inhibiting factors in some children's development and the implications for the kind of intervention needed for change in troubled children's development.
2. Briefly explain the relationship of shaping behavior to child therapy.
3. Explain seven to eight aspects of child development that empower the child-centered approach.
4. Relate the thoughts of at least five major theorists to the child-centered approach.
5. Briefly explain why play is emphasized in the child-centered approach.
6. Briefly explain six aspects of human development from existential thought and the family of counseling theories that work as change mechanisms in CCPT.
7. Explain and provide three to four illustrations of how it can be that you can help a child under difficult circumstances and family problems to change and grow—even without changing his family system (even though, when possible, we prefer to also be his advocate and change agent within the family system).

## Introduction and Chapter Overview

This chapter addresses the counterintuitive (for many) notion of *child-directed* (adult facilitated, but child-centered) solutions to problems in children's development. For many adults, the natural inclination is to think of education, or teaching a new skill, as the answer to all significant developmental deficits in children. We see skill teaching as a practical solution for some problems in child development. When skill teaching will suffice in assisting the child with her developmental "stuck places" or behavioral and emotional difficulties, we see it as reasonable to help the parent or teacher facilitate the new skill acquisition, or perhaps to have the counselor teach the developmental skill in a classroom or other large-group setting. In such cases, a significant counseling intervention would not be warranted. We find that for many of the children who need significant counseling/therapy, the child already knows *what to do*, and may have been taught many times what to do, but deeper factors inhibit the child's *application* of the skills. In the early parts of this chapter, we illustrate progress-inhibiting factors in children's development that suggest an experiential rather than a teaching approach to helping troubled children.

In this chapter, we address aspects of human nature and child development that give power to therapeutic possibilities—especially in the child-centered approach—and make it possible to help children overcome seemingly impossible difficulties. These power-giving aspects of child development include the drive to self-actualize, learn, and master one's environment; the drive to form relationships, to be known, to share experience; the drive to autonomy and self-responsibility; and, when given the opportunity, the drive, and willingness in each individual child to find his own "voice" or own best modes to self-express for self-learning.

A second hurdle for understanding how CCPT can work comes from the common belief, "you can't change the child without changing the parents/family/system." In the latter parts of this chapter, we describe how the child's change can become the system's change or how child change can withstand system pressure against change. One of the most fascinating and hopeful aspects of CCPT is that it provides an opportunity for a child to change her internal world in ways leading to greater happiness, positive behavior, and life success, even without change in key aspects—changes in family/system—of her external world.

## What Gets in the Way of Simply Teaching New Ways of Being, but Also Empowers CCPT for Children's Change?

### The Myth of the Blank Slate

Children develop beliefs about themselves in relation to environment from a very early age. Consider key aspects of the history of thought regarding children. Among the first Western thinkers of the modern era (from the age of enlightenment) to deeply consider the nature of childhood, both John Locke (1632–1704) and Jean Jacques Rousseau (1712–1778) emphasized the importance of caring for children. Perhaps reacting to a premodern lack of emphasis on child development and assumptions of inborn information common in his time, Locke (1693/1964) described infants as something of a blank slate, *meaning that a parent should take great care in child rearing.* He emphasized that from early ages children begin to make associations and should be taught to reason. Rousseau (1762/1895) emphasized that significant developments for children must come from experience and that adults should strive to accommodate the child's natural curiosity and drive to learn and develop. Summarizing implications of these early thinkers for the purpose of considering child psychotherapy, it could be said that children may be taught new ways of acting, but they will need to reason for themselves to implement new ways of being, and they will need to have significant new personal experiences in order to make significant advances in development.

James Mark Baldwin is considered the first in a line of thinkers to recognize that no child is the passive recipient of the behaviors and beliefs of his world, but that he develops a *self* with which to interact with his world (Cairns & Ornstein, 1979). Freud is recognized as emphasizing the importance of very early experiences in shaping one's approach to life (Bukatko & Daehler, 2004). Object relations theory, which grew out of psychoanalytic thought, asserts that unconscious mental images of our earliest relationships shape our emotional life and later relationships (Fairbairn, 1954; Kernberg, 1975). Piaget (1929, 1954, 1971) noted that from as early as infancy, children develop schemas and progress to conceptualize their worlds, meaning that children construct realities based on conception.

## Early Maps of the World

Summarizing from the theories of Alfred Adler (1870–1937), Mosak and Maniacci (2008) explain that each child develops convictions about herself and a "picture of the world" (p. 64) and what it demands of the self at a very early age. For example, second-, third-, and fourth-born children are thought of as finding a different approach to establishing significance in the family constellation in contrast to older siblings who have mastery over their preexisting approaches. The child then develops a very early map into which new experiences are incorporated. If the map is fundamentally flawed, perhaps based on a powerfully

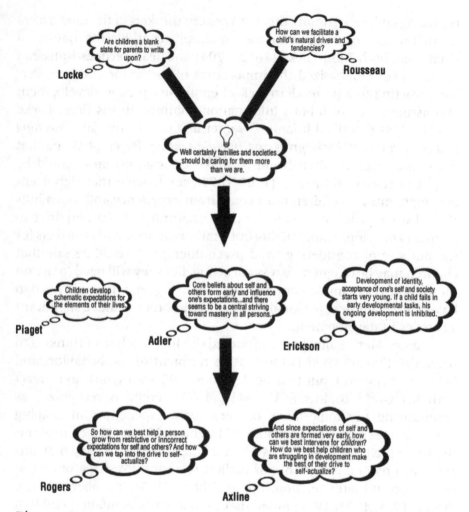

*Figure 2.1*  **A Progression of Thinkers Leading to CCPT**

confusing early experience, a core mistaken belief is formed regarding self in relation to others. It can then be very difficult to teach a child that the map is wrong, much as it was difficult for many in the time of early Western long-distance sailors to believe that the world was not flat and to risk sailing to new worlds.

J. L. Cochran and N. H. Cochran (1999) illustrated from research an example of core mistaken beliefs. Putting adult thoughts on child thinking, they describe children with conduct disorder (APA, 1994) as, for example, holding a core belief that says something like, "I can't be liked or loved and I will be rejected. And I won't be able to stand that rejection." Such a worldview likely formed from real or perceived abandonment in formative years. J. L. Cochran and N. H. Cochran assert that many children with such a map of the world employ the behaviors of conduct disorder in order to drive others away before the "intolerable" rejection occurs. Other children may react to similar mind-sets with withdrawal, lack of effort, or self-destructive behaviors. Whatever the behavioral outcome, the map of self and others is hard to change. It may often be impossible to teach such a child that the "world is not flat," so to speak—that she can and should act differently in the world that she sees, and that she can "sail on" to new relational possibilities with much less fear than that which drives her current pattern misbehaviors.

CCPT provides a new experience through self-expression in a therapeutic relationship—a new experience that need not be long or encompass multiple hours per week because it is rich and deeply felt and because deriving meaning from experience is facilitated within the therapy. To return to the previous metaphor, in CCPT, children take opportunities to experiment and test their "map" in the safer confines of play and within the context of a therapeutic relationship. Then, in the moments and days between sessions, children take further actions, try new behaviors, to test out if the world is really flat, or if, instead, it really does have room to explore, grow, and travel or "sail onward!"

## What About Shaping Behavior in Sessions by Responding Positively to Desirable Behaviors?

Operant conditioning does not apply *within* child psychotherapy. While the notions of behavior management are well accepted, that is, behavior can be shaped by rewards to train a new skill (Bukatko & Daehler, 2004) to accomplish this consistent rewarding across time is critical. Therefore, while you may be able to help a well-functioning teacher or parent employ new ways of interacting that shape behaviors in new directions (this can be a wrap-around service provided in conjunction with CCPT), there are a number of difficulties to overcome: This work takes diligence that requires time and effort of parents and teachers, it takes significant dedication, and it requires a level of unaffected responding that may be unrealistic in the face of significant misbehaviors. So, to attempt to shape behavior through your responses in a single-hour psychotherapy session per week, especially if much of the child's environment is shaping his behavior in different directions, is akin to trying to hold back a flooding river with your hands. It won't work. You will need to provide the child with an opportunity to have a

*Table 2.1* **Elements of Child and Human Development That Empower CCPT**

- The Drive to Self-Actualize
- The Strength of the Drive to Mastery in Children
- Make-Believe Play and Its Role in Developing Social Competencies
- The Inevitability of Choice
- Making Meaning from Experiences
- The Drive to Relationships, to Be Known, to Share Experience
- The Drive to Find One's Voice

profound and deep experience in order to produce lasting internal change. Providing the child this opportunity is the purpose and role of CCPT.

# Elements of Child and Human Development That Empower CCPT

You may be thinking, "Okay, so in many child predicaments requiring therapy or significant counseling intervention, skill teaching will not suffice, but how can CCPT work when lesser interventions do not work?" You may be asking yourself, "How can I provide therapy for a child that goes beyond the limits of help through skill teaching, when skill teaching is not possible or not enough?" In the following pages, we review aspects of child and human development that empower children's change through CCPT.

## Self-Actualization

Numerous developmental and counseling theorists acknowledge a drive to self-actualize—to reach one's full potential. Goldstein (1934/1959) was among the first to assert that people strive to actualize. Erikson (1964), Piaget (1971), Havighurst (1972), and others described stages of development that children seem to almost always go through as they grow, learn, and mature. Adler described a central striving toward completion (1931/1958), perfection (1964), and mastery (1926/1972). Deci's cognitive evaluation theory (Deci, 1975; Deci & Ryan, 1980) holds that people are born with a need for competence and self-determinism. Ellis (2008) acknowledges, "As Abraham Maslow and Carl Rogers have pointed out, that humans have impressive self-actualizing capacities," but that people also develop in "self-sabotaging ways" (p. 195). "Gestalt therapists believe that people are inclined toward growth and will develop as fully as conditions allow" (Yontef & Jacobs, 2008). Rogers (1977) described his wonder at the apparent drive of all species to become the ideal of the species in seeing potatoes stored for winter begin to develop into new plants despite all attempts to retard growth, which makes potatoes inedible. We have often observed that a dandelion can grow out of mere crevices in barren, dry rock and strive to survive on lawns with such resilience that they actually seem to "duck" as the mower passes over them! J. L. Cochran and N. H. Cochran (2006) observed that while every tomato is unique, still we all know when a tomato is ripe or mature. And so it is with persons—while each individual's ideal maturity is unique, there still seems to be an ideal maturity, at least when something is not blocking the way to a person's self-actualization.

CCPT works in conjunction with self-actualization. Given the right conditions for growth, every individual will prosper and grow in ever maturing directions. When the right conditions are present, no therapy is needed. But in the course of life, blocks may come to inhibit or impede this drive toward maturation and normal development. For example, abuse, neglect, and trauma, whether real or perceived (i.e., it may not be enough to be loved, but to see oneself as loved in order to see oneself as lovable) occur all too often from infancy through childhood. CCPT works because it provides the ideal conditions for regrowth in a microcosm.

The same principle is often applied with nonhuman species. If a wild animal is injured or traumatized, it can be given temporary care by veterinarians and then released as a newly strong animal to survive in its wild habitat (Grigsby, 2007). Similarly, a botanist or gardener can tend to a damaged plant by providing its optimal medium for new growth (Ash, Askew, & Kopp, 1996). In an ideal microcosm for new growth, even a single cell can be facilitated in a way to allow it develop into a full and healthy, mature plant of its species (Murch & Saxena, 2005).

For children whose normal path to self-actualization has been diverted, CCPT provides an ideal microcosm for new growth. Elements of this ideal microcosm include the therapists' relational conditions of genuine, deep empathy, and unconditional positive regard (Rogers, 1957), which are addressed further in Chapter 3. The microcosm is described by Virginia Axline's eight principles (1947), which are addressed in Chapter 4. The microcosm is embodied by the communication medium of children's play, because play is the child's natural mode and medium of communication (Axline, 1947). And the microcosm is defined by the skill sets of CCPT that give it structure, make it solid, and put it to work (Part II: Chapters 5–12). The microcosm of CCPT features an ideal environment for child self-expression; for new awareness and new choices; for reevaluating errant schemas, core mistaken beliefs, and flawed maps of a child's inner and outer landscape. In the ideal, the child's new growth in CCPT would be accompanied by changes in his environment (family, classroom, peer relationships), but, fortunately, this is not a requirement for the success of the child. We address how this can be in later sections of this chapter. While the mechanisms of change within CCPT may be infinite and unique to each child, in the following sections we describe the most commonly occurring factors within self-actualization that empower the new growth of children in CCPT.

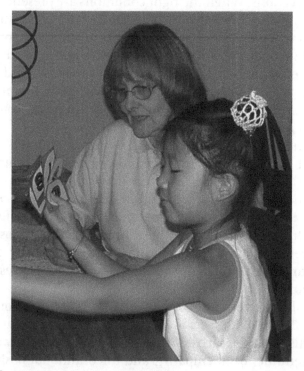

Figure 2.2

## The Opportunity to Revisit Unresolved Tasks and Unmastered Stages

CCPT facilitates children revisiting unmet needs from earlier stages of development. Numerous theorists have described stages in children's development (e.g., Erikson, 1964; Piaget, 1971; Havighurst, 1972). Perhaps most prominent among such stage theories is Erikson's psychosocial theory of development. Erikson theorized that within each stage of development, there are conflicts, such as trust vs. mistrust, autonomy vs. shame and doubt, initiative vs. guilt, that must be mastered for a healthy personality and productive lifestyle to develop. Perhaps you have observed adults that remind you of a child in a certain age or stage of development when stressed. Some almost seem to *tantrum* under certain types of real or perceived crises. Perhaps you can identify pangs of shame or embarrassment in situations that push your buttons of feeling inferior, even when you know there is no rational reason. Perhaps certain behaviors by others with whom you are emotionally invested can push your buttons of mistrust, even when there is no reason to mistrust the person you are involved with in that moment. Such experiences are normal and can be seen as linked to unresolved conflicts from early developmental phases.

But when such unresolved conflicts are extreme or present in the context of ongoing life context difficulties, it can be very important to go back to the unresolved conflicts or unmastered developmental tasks to "rethink" conclusions drawn. In adult counseling, this work can be done in a number of ways. The person-centered relationship (Bozarth, 1998; Rogers, 1951, 1961) is probably most efficient for engaging individuals' processes of self-discovery. In gestalt therapy (Hycner & Jacobs, 1995; Perls, Hefferline & Goodman, 1951/1994), there is the assumption that old relationship patterns are played out and revisited in counseling relationships. Cognitive therapies (Beck, 1995; Ellis & Dryden, 1997) emphasize the discovery of mistaken belief systems, their origins, and their more rational replacements.

The older persons get, the more difficult it can be to revisit and reconsider unmastered stages of development and their negative effects on development. Yet, if you tried to implement a cognitive approach, a child client could not think about thinking, which would be necessary to reevaluate mistaken meanings gleaned from early stages until at least early adolescence, when the necessary intellectual skills begin to be available.

CCPT provides a mode for this process in childhood. If a child has not learned to trust emotional closeness with others, he may act in ways that seek to drive his counselor away, perhaps pushing the limits of acceptable behavior in the playroom. The skillfully applied CCPT relationship and structure can help him master his issues of trust when confronted with emotional closeness. Then, once mastered in the safety of his play therapy sessions, he will be willing, able, and naturally ready to reach out to other appropriate relationships of emotional closeness—because this would have been a normal part of his self-actualization process if unmet needs and unmastered aspects of development had not interfered.

In CCPT, a child may begin play therapy by shunning the toys, perhaps being pseudo-mature, as the expression goes, "8 going on 40." One of the things this child may need most is to feel and enjoy being 8 again—or younger, depending on what he may need to revisit. Without this, he may look "all grown up" without being healthy or mature. When this is the case, in CCPT such a child will grow to play in younger seeming ways, to seem to experiment with unmet needs around giving and receiving nurturing in middle stages of play therapy, before achieving the healthy, balanced, age-appropriate play for his age in the final stage of CCPT. Additionally, a child who is 8, but tantrums and opposes adults like a 2-year–old, may need to work on mastery of feelings vs. being overwhelmed, afraid, and ashamed of feelings. He may need to reexperience some of what it would have been like for him to be a healthy 2-year-old in sessions in order to soon be and act like a healthy, mature 8-year-old out of sessions.

## The Strength of the Drive to Mastery in Children

Sometimes, as adults, we can forget the strength of the drive to self-actualize in children. The drive continues in adults. Unless our normal path is blocked, we continue to acquire new skills and new awareness. But our paths in self-actualization as adults seem to slow down dramatically, as our new physical growth slows.

Rogers (1951) provided an anecdote of the strength of the drive in children.

> Often it is true that the immediate reward involved in taking a few steps is in no way commensurate with the pain of falls and bumps. The child may, because of the pain, revert to crawling for a time. Yet the forward direction of growth

is more powerful than the satisfactions of remaining infantile. Children will actualize themselves, in spite of the painful experiences of doing so. In the same way, they will become independent, responsible, self-governing, and socialized, in spite of the pain which is often involved in these steps. Even where they do not, because of a variety of circumstances, exhibit the growth, the tendency is still present. Given the opportunity for clear-cut choice between forward-moving and regressive behavior, the tendency will operate (pp. 490–491).

In children, unless the drive is strongly and unnaturally inhibited, the drive to learn, explore, and master one's environment is an undeniable force. A child who loves sports play will play and play and play, acquiring new skills all the way. With her, a coach's path need only be to refine the path of her development in small ways and funnel her growth in easily self-rewarding directions, and she can learn many skills and life lessons through her love of sports. A child who is inclined to academic development will make his own games of learning, and learning can seem effortless. A teacher's task with this child is merely to lay out a clear path to learning before him and funnel his growth in ever self-rewarding directions. Children in many stages insist on doing for themselves what they have newly become able to do for themselves, much to the chagrin of many a parent who is just trying to get out the door to work, school, or the next appointment.

As Rousseau (1762/1895) emphasized, children are born with natural propensities to act on impulses, but not for wrongdoing. The ideal adult's role in child care is to capitalize on the natural curiosity and energy of children, to facilitate natural tendencies to the social order. While CCPT does not guide children to particular choices or directions in development, the structure of the therapy does focus each child on awareness of self and her relationship to her world, her choices, and her life direction. The early way of referring to the approach as nondirective is really a misnomer. While the child is not directed what to choose, the child is directed, by the structured process and conditions of new growth, to self-reflect and to make more well informed choices. Because the drive to self-actualize moves each person to our individual ideal and the ideal of the species, choices that are well informed by awareness of ourselves and our world are always more mature choices.

## Make-Believe Play and Social Competence

Perhaps as a part of a drive to master one's own environment, Erikson (1950) saw make-believe play as a way for children to learn about their social world and try out social skills. Vygotsky (1978) would concur, adding that make-believe play requires children to initiate and participate in an imaginary situation and to follow a set of rules to logical conclusions, helping children learn to choose between courses of action. Children who are not easily succeeding, maybe all children, seem to need to also work out social skills in role-play, whether solitary or engaged with a play therapist. The make-believe play facilitated by CCPT provides the ideal opportunity for trying out social skills, choosing and trying out courses of action. Especially for children who are not engaging in this play alone, but need the companionship of the play therapist in order to engage in the needed level of make-believe play, it is the only opportunity.

## Choices

The notion of operant conditioning (i.e., that children can be thoughtfully "operated on" through reinforcement systems) is well established (Skinner, 1974). It can be extrapolated that children's environments are inadvertent operant conditioners (i.e., systems that reinforce certain behaviors without clear thought and planning). But children must choose between reinforcers and rewards, especially in inadvertent reward systems. For example, it can be reinforcing to argue with a parent or teacher—the behavior usually gets attended to and sometimes achieves a tangible goal (more TV time, extra dessert, not having to finish an anxiety-producing assignment). But it also can be rewarding to cooperate. The child could gain a feeling of being loved, a hug, a privilege given in appreciation for cooperation, or self-satisfaction with having worked through a difficult task. The notion of such choices is supported by social learning theory (Bandura, 1986), which provides the notion that *at some level children think about rewards*—how to get them and which to choose. For example, social learning theorists have established that children learn from modeling, that they observe rewards being obtained and *decide* to attempt obtainment in similar ways. Further, from social learning theory, we can know that rewards can be intrinsic—pride, self-satisfaction, a sense of accomplishment.

   An adult could bring his choices (and thoughts about choices of rewards) into awareness by talking about just *what it is* that he really wants in life, just *what it is* that he has been doing lately, and whether or not that will get him the things that *he really wants*. CCPT provides the opportunity for the child to play about this same type of questioning and resolutions, for example, to play out certain choices in characters and see what he thinks about the outcomes, or to play out ways of being in role-play and think about how they feel. Children do think and choose, but not in the same ways as adults. Most children do not have the level of cognitive-affective integration required for "talk therapy" until well into their teen years. In "talk therapy," adults bring choices and thoughts about choices into the light of day from the murky semiconscious. The child's way of contemplating his world, of bringing choices into the light of day from the murky semiconscious, is through "play therapy."

## Making Meaning From Experience

While children don't think in words or silent talk, as most adults do, children do make meaning of experiences. We can know from Piaget's work that children develop schemas to interpret what they see and experience of the world, and that new experiences are input (assimi- lated) into existing schemas (1971). In order to alter a long-existing schema, a new experience needs to be quite significant, as there is anxiety connected to significant schema changes, and it is scary for the child to realize that the world is not as previously thought.

CCPT provides and facilitates the significant new experience—in this case, an experience of oneself, one's feelings, thoughts, and choices—in the context of a warm and caring relationship and in the child's natural medium of play that allows him to deeply consider the meanings he has made of previous experience and work through the anxiety related to questioning long-held beliefs that no longer stand up to the evidence of current experience. For example, if a child with conduct-disordered behavior, as illustrated by J. L. Cochran and N. H. Cochran (1999), thinks that he is unlovable, unlikable, and will be rejected if known; that he can't be loved or liked (what Adler might describe as a *core mistaken belief*), but in his work in play therapy, he shows his counselor the worst of himself—all the annoying, ugly, scary parts—and the two of them find those parts to be not that bad in the light of day, he begins to have to accommodate the old schema to a new experience; the core mistaken belief begins to change. If through CCPT he has built a significant relationship with his therapist, knows deep down that she really knows him (deep empathy) and that she seems to deeply care for and like him, that she loves him in a nonpossessive, agape (brotherly love) way (i.e., unconditional positive regard), then there is a significant exception to the core mistaken belief. We can know from Beck's work in cognitive therapy (Beck, Rush, Shaw, & Emery, 1979; Beck & Weishaar, 2008) that once a significant exception to the automatic thought exists, the automatic thought cannot be maintained as is. The child is then ready for change.

## The Drive to Form Relationships, to Be Known, to Share Experience

We can know from Bowlby's work regarding attachment (1969) and others following in that line of research (e.g., Ainsworth, Blehar, Waters, & Wall, 1978; Arend, Gove & Sroufe, 1979; Cooper, Shaver, & Collins, 1998; DeMulder, Denham, Schmidt, & Mitchell, 2000; Kochanska, 2001; Laible & Thompson, 2000; Warren, Huston, Egeland, & Sroufe, 1997) that attachment patterns form with primary caregivers in infancy and that insecure attachments lead to great anxiety and developmental difficulties, especially in future relationships. Bowlby (1973) theorized that from ongoing interactions with parents, children develop mental frameworks or internal working models of relationships, which can then affect their expectations and actions in other close relationships throughout life.

The resulting anxiety of insecure attachment and errant mental frameworks regarding relationships are a significant detriment to self-actualization (i.e., "looking for love in all the wrong places" and seeking it in all the wrong ways). At the same time, the anxiety from a pattern of insecure attachment is also a force that provides power to CCPT. Humans want to be known. This seems especially true for children with a history of insecure attachments. While such a child may begin by attempting to drive his counselor away, he is also drawn to be known by and close to his counselor. In many ways, CCPT is *all about the relationship*, or at least all about child self-expression and learning through and in the context of the therapeutic relationship. It provides a safe, ideal, and absolutely healthy way for a troubled child to explore just what might be possible for him in a caring relationship, what it might be like if he lets himself really be known. Facing parts of oneself that one might not like to see, expressing openly the parts that one believes will bring rejection, considering changes to long-held schemas is scary business. If we humans, especially children, didn't so much want to be known, and weren't so driven to connect with others, we might never do the work needed to redirect or reignite our paths to self-actualization.

## The Drive to Find One's Own "Voice" or Own Best Modes to Self-Express

It seems that, as a part of the drive to self-actualize, each child *wants* to find her own "voice" or his own way to self-expression. CCPT provides the fullest array of opportunities for this within an environment made ideal for self-expression. One child began with the simple instruments of the playroom and composed early songs and break-dancing scenes along the theme of "I'm killin' myself . . . I'm killin' myself!" His later songs evolved to songs of "My Family," which consisted of singing long ballad-type stories of his family—including all the good and bad times. He expressed himself in many ways in play therapy, but always returned to song and dance, about one per session, ending his play therapy with a joyous song and dance expression of, "I wanta be, I wanta live, I wanta dream!" Other children express themselves with movement and energy release, using that as a medium for self- and therapist-appreciation (i.e., "look what I can do!"). Some, mainly older or pseudo-mature children begin saying or implying that the toys are "stupid," "for babies," "not for school," and prefer to talk or draw. Some may never use the toys but may invent their own competitive games or creative projects in the sand tray. Many make great use of dramas in which they are the star, director, producer, villain, and hero. Quite a few children check in, at least periodically, with art. One client who was known by his therapist to have an intense abuse history at age 5 worked through much rich symbolic play and then in one day completed a book in the playroom called "It Happened to Me" (Alexander, 1992). The important thing is that each child who is struggling finds the means and creates just the perfect mode to express herself. That is a primary goal and function of CCPT.

## Why Play?

The answer to this question is obvious to play therapists and to others who have a great deal of experience with children. As Virginia Axline (1969, p. 9) explained in introducing play therapy:

> Play therapy is based upon the fact that play is the child's natural medium of self-expression. It is an opportunity which is given to the child to "play out" his feelings and problems just as, in certain types of adult therapy, an individual "talks out his difficulties.

So, play is a child's "natural medium of self-expression" and by adolescence and adulthood, talk becomes the natural medium. Since in CCPT we want to facilitate children's self-expression, to reignite their self-discovery by facilitating their finding their own voice, it only makes sense to provide ample opportunities in play. A child can choose to talk in CCPT, and at least part of the adult's responses are given through talk. Although we've met some children in therapy who began with talk—possibly it was what they assumed we expected—we've not met a child yet who didn't find her voice in play. As Garry Landreth has wisely and poetically summarized, "Birds fly, fish swim, children play."

## Underlying Concepts from Existential Thought: The Family of Counseling Theories

The following well-accepted principles from the field of psychotherapy are frequent change mechanisms in CCPT. We address the application of each in CCPT below.

### The "I-Thou" Encounter

We can take from great thinkers related to existential therapy that as individuals develop existential awareness (awareness of being and experience), individuality and responsibility develops, but so does a sense of aloneness and anxiety (Bugental, 1978; May, 1967; 1978; Yolum, 1980). Clinically speaking, individuals can be seen as "suffering beings" (Rank, 1936). Out of this human condition we are driven to relate to others and relationships are key healing factors. As Buber (1955) wrote:

> A great relationship . . . breaches the barriers of a lofty isolation, subdues its strict law, and throws a bridge from self-being to self-being across the abyss of dread of the universe. (p. 175)

CCPT is the ultimate "I-thou" relationship. The therapist strives to come to the relationship with absolute nonpossessive warmth, a simple desire to know the child. The child comes with a desire to be known, no matter how defended with mistaken behavior he may be. Many children in CCPT test limits in at least mild attempts to see what would prompt rejection from the counselor. And we have seen some to work hard to test the possibility of rejection, act in ways that should and would drive most adults and peers away, and in the face of continued warmth and empathy, with necessary limits on actions, come to be authentic. Many a child shows his counselor his big, mean, ugly self, as well as his small, needy, regressed self—and comes to be his authentic, calm, and balanced self in the ideal, through the child-to-adult "I-thou" relationship.

There can be loneliness to pretending alone. A child may have work that he needs to accomplish in pretend play—something big that he needs to *think* through. But many will avoid facing the thoughts and feelings they need to face if the only option is facing them alone. Rogers (1980) noted that our internal worlds can be bizarre. So, many people, children and adults, won't go to the scary places of self-discovery that are often needed in order to make well-self-informed new choices. But as Rogers explained, through deep connection in counseling, the therapist is the clients' "confident companion" (p. 142) to the internal world of the bizarre. Through the deep empathy of the child-centered approach, the child is safe with his play therapist to boldly go places that were previously frightening, to go places that he would avoid without the companionship of his therapist. (For more on why empathy is important, powerful in counseling in general, see J. L. Cochran & N. H. Cochran, 2006.)

## Development of Internal Locus of Evaluation and Control

In many or perhaps all forms of effective counseling or psychotherapy, individuals shift to an internal locus of evaluation and control. Rogers (1987) wrote that through psychotherapeutic experiences persons tend to "become more realistic and objective" (p. 43) and "tend to move away from 'oughts'" (Rogers, 1967, p. 25). Such self-direction is also a value of gestalt (Yontef & Jacobs, 2008) and existential approaches (Mendelowitz & Schneider, 2008), which value making fully aware choices from a personal place of authenticity. And moving away from *"shoulds, oughts, and musts"* is a major tenet of Rational Emotive Behavior Therapy (Ellis, 2008, p. 201).

In CCPT, children come to see themselves, their thoughts, feelings, and actions, in the light of conscious awareness. Thus, in CCPT each child makes ever-maturing choices, with each new choice based on who the individual child wants to be, based on the rational meaning she makes of her experience, rather than the shoulds, musts, and oughts internalized from external sources ranging from well-intentioned caregivers to the salacious, undulating, ever-insinuating and insistent, but uncaring world of media influences upon self-perception.

## Every Choice Is a Choice of Life Direction

There is a moment of video illustrating limit setting in CCPT that is often shown in skill-training workshops by the National Institute for Relationship Enhancement (Nordling, 2009). The video is of a boy with a toy dart gun. He points the gun at his therapist, perhaps hoping to find out just how far he can go, just what the limits are in CCPT. But with acceptance and empathy for his urge to shoot her, his therapist informs him that this is one of the things that he may not do. As he shoots near her once and aims again, she lets him know with continued warmth and empathy for his desire to shoot her that if he shoots her again, his special playtime will end for that day. There is a moment where he seems to vacillate between an idea to shoot her or to shoot the light overhead. His therapist waits, attentive and calm, with occasional unobtrusive reflection. Her way of being with him focuses his attention on his choice. Having viewed the moment a number of times, it becomes clear to us that he is not just choosing "shoot her or shoot the light," but is choosing something bigger, like, "Who am I and who do I want to be? I want to be with her. I want her to know me. Do I want to be the one who drives away this caring other, or do I want to be the one who finds another way to test and express what I need?" In CCPT, there is no need to state the existential choice in words for the child—if that were possible, play therapy would not be needed. In CCPT, his moments of attended reflection bring his choice into his conscious awareness. And there is both no need and interfering harm to be found in succumbing to the temptation of making the choice for him. In that moment he is choosing a direction to affect all his moments to come, just as we are when we choose to take care of ourselves or not, choose to get up and go to work, choose to take time to care for others in large or small ways, just as we are in every action or inaction. The difference in CCPT is that the choice is made in full awareness vs. routine.

## Experience/Emotions Are Useful

If a child has a hurtful way toward others, outside of CCPT, he will avoid feeling how yucky it feels. But in the structure and therapeutic relationship of CCPT, he cannot avoid feeling how yucky that way of being feels. With this realization in his awareness, he will choose what feels right to him inside. (For more on the emotions as useful and other such concepts underlying counseling in general, see J. L. Cochran & N. H. Cochran, 2006.)

## The Push-Pull of Self-Responsibility

Self-responsibility is both intriguing for children and anxiety provoking. In the course of normal development, all children strive to grow and do more and more for themselves. Greater power and self-direction is desired. But greater self-direction brings awareness of responsibility. As a person begins to sense his responsibility for his life directions and his very safety, it is natural to be tempted to recoil. When the self-actualization process is significantly inhibited, the temptation to avoid responsibility can take over. When this has happened, CCPT provides the safe, nurturing environment that facilitates the desire for self-responsibility over the temptation to recoil from responsibility.

## Developing Awareness—Making the Unconscious Conscious

From Freud (1915–1917) through almost all modern approaches to psychotherapy and counseling, a key goal and theme is to make the unconscious conscious. This is a central process in CCPT because CCPT is focused in client self-expression within a warm, reflective, empathic therapeutic relationship. Because the child-centered therapist holds no other agenda above client self-expression within the therapeutic relationship, there is nothing in CCPT to interfere with the process of ever-increasing self-awareness.

## *"You Can Change the Child Even When You Can't Change the System"*

Sometimes it is not possible to change key adults in a troubled child's life—personal change tends to come much easier for children than adults. Fortunately, personal change for the adults is not necessary in order to help the child. CCPT provides the ideal microcosm for a child's progress, a therapy hour specially designed for self-reflection and internal growth to strengthen the child to grow up in the world that is his to grow up in. When done well, CCPT is powerful enough to initiate irreversible progress regardless of context and can be the bright spark that ignites the chain of progress that changes the systems in which the child lives.

## Pandora's Box in Reverse

A metaphor for irreversible progress is the story of Pandora's box in reverse. In the ancient myth, Pandora was said to have opened a box that released evil into the world. Once open, evil could not be returned to the box. Once open, evil was within and a part of the world forever. An opposite thing happens with children's self-awareness in CCPT. Once self-awareness is initiated, it is ever growing, with each new awareness leading to another. Once one has obtained a new under-standing, one cannot become unaware of it. So once the child's awareness is "out of the box," it cannot be put back in and the process of self-awareness will always be alive and growing within him. Once a child realizes the yucky feeling of being mean to others, it does not mean that he will make no more mistakes toward others, but it does mean that he will make fewer mistakes toward others because he can no longer deny the yucky feeling that it brings. Once a child corrects a mistaken self-perception to see herself as lovable, as she came to see that her therapist knew and cared deeply for her, even when she shared her darker inclinations, and as she came to accept herself in the therapeutic relationship, she may have doubts and self-criticisms, as we all do, but she can no longer believe the flawed absolute that she is unlovable. When a friend or a caregiver reaches out to her in love, she will sense the sincerity of the affection and will be empowered to receive it. We have seen many children experiment with old misbe-havior following CCPT, only to reject it and maintain the better path they had chosen in CCPT. Likewise, we have seen many children who were closed to positive friendships or outreach from potential care-givers, such as mentors, principals, and teachers, become open to and flourish in those relationships following progress in therapeutic relationships.

# Children Learn to Tell One Coke Machine From Another

Another concept that allows a child to change behavior even if signifi-cant parts of his behavior do not change is the fact that children can learn to tell one Coke machine from another. Let us explain. Have you ever had the experience of frequently using one Coke machine at work that always works—you put in your money and get your drink? Yet, there is another Coke machine that looks just like it on the pier that you frequent on family beach trips. It is so tempting to look at it thinking of the nice cold drink, but you know that about half the time it won't accept dollar bills and sometimes keeps them without giving the drinks. You may notice the behavior of some would-be patrons when frus-trated by this machine that seems to promise consistent rewards (drinks) for behaviors (putting in money), but sometimes fails to meet its promise. The first thing some people will do is to put in more money (try the behavior again). Then some will try to get the drink others ways (reach up in the machine, shake it), and some will get mad and bang the machine a bit.

Some children live in chaotic homes, where attempts to manipu-late with lies or anger are quite effective. When this is the case, such a child can come to choose new ways of being through his work in CCPT. And that child may not change his behavior much at home even after his work in CCPT. It may be that a new behavior from him isn't asked for (by "asked for" we mean that the desire for the new behavior is not clearly communicated, and in fact the new behavior may make no sense in that environment). But such a child can recognize that school is a different environment, just as you can remember the Coke machine that works consistently and the one that does not. If he has made progress in CCPT and the new behavior is "asked for" at school, he can enact the new way of being at school, whether it makes sense at home or not.

# The Very Large Boat in a Small Pond

Another possibility beyond changing the child if you don't change the system is that the child may change the system. Consider that if you drop a rock in a puddle, the rock causes a ripple, but the water fills the gap the rock made on its way through, the ripples subside, and the puddle is pretty much back to its same balance or homeostasis.

However, if you could drop a large boat into a small pond, the weight and size of the boat could forever change the size and shape of the pond. The incredibly strong drive to self-actualize in children, combined with the power of CCPT to reignite the forces within that drive, can be the mechanism to build the large boat in the small pond. Stepping out of the metaphor: We would much prefer to change the whole family or system for the child, to be a strong advocate in his context—in later chapters we delve into opportunities for this work combined with CCPT—but when that is not an option, it is important to us for you to know that your and your clients' work in CCPT can be enough.

## "It Takes Two to Fight"

One explanation of how the child's behavior can change the system comes from the old adage, "It takes two to fight." We find this adage quite true. We have worked with numerous clients in which parent and child seemed constantly at each other, picking and fighting like troubled siblings. This is no good way for a child to grow up. But in some of the families we served, we found the parent highly reluctant to consider new ways of relating with her child. Yet, as the child was open to change through CCPT, we noticed that they stopped fighting. It seems that before the child's change, both got some sort of psychological benefit out of the ongoing fuss. But after her work in CCPT, the child no longer enjoyed it. She found only misery in the fussing. And so, as she withdrew, the fussing ended. Mom then came to see daughter in a different light, and their relationship grew in positive directions. We do not mean to illustrate that this is always possible. But we do want you to see that there are many possibilities for helping the child change and affecting the system, even when adults in the system are reluctant to change.

## Activities for Further Study

- *Activity A:* Reread the application focus issues. Consider and discuss or journal how much you might have accepted the opening statement of each as true before reading and studying this chapter and how much you still do (note that we would not expect your views to have completely changed short of having your own conformational experiences with effective CCPT).

- *Activity B:* Describe three to four concepts that resonate with you in contradicting the opening statement in each application focus issue.

- *Activity C:* Search original sources from the references and investigate child development theorists whose work helps explain how CCPT works and why it can be particularly powerful.

- *Activity D:* Review sources referenced related to self-actualization and the power of its force in childhood. Relate what you learn back to what you are learning about CCPT.

- *Activity E:* Observe children in your life and compare notes/ impressions with peers regarding the incredible drives among children to develop new skills, knowledge, self-direction, self-responsibility, and voice. Also, observe and note or discuss children you have known of where these drives seemed inhibited. How do you understand the differences between children in which the drives seemed normally strong and those in which the drives seemed weak or off-track?

- *Activity F:* Explore the meaning of close relationships, especially counseling or therapeutic relationships in your life. Discuss what you have found most helpful about those relationships and what you have found difficult. Consider how this may or may not relate to your potential work with children in CCPT.

- *Activity G:* Expand your knowledge of child development. Suggested resources include:

  - The Gesell Institute Child Development Series, which begins with *Your One Year Old* (Ames & Ilg, 1991) and continues by year to *Your Ten to Fourteen Year Old* (Ames & Haber, 1991). We have found the series very helpful and also find them to be a valuable waiting room item for parents to review when dropping in or when their child is in session.
  - *Play and Child Development,* by Frost, Wortham, and Reifel (2005).
  - *The Excellence of Play,* by Janet Moyles (2005).
  - *Parenting: A Skills Training Manual,* by Louise Guerney (1995), which, besides being an excellent resource for counselors and therapists helping parents, contains excellent sections on child development.

- *Activity H:* Describe and discuss the personal difficulties that you have or expect to experience in helping children change in situations in which you do not expect the adults in their family or other key systems to change.

- *Activity I:* Revisit the Primary Skill Objectives for this chapter and see if you have mastered them to your satisfaction at this time. If not, seek additional readings, practices, and discussions for clarification and in order to master them to your satisfaction. In order to become an excellent play therapist, you should become a scholar of counseling and therapy, children and child development, human development, and play.

# The Ideal Therapist Qualities: Deep Empathy, Unconditional Positive Regard, and Genuineness

## 3
### Chapter

*The therapist's role, though non-directive, is not a passive one, but one which requires alertness, sensitivity, and an ever-present appreciation of what the child is doing and saying. It calls for understanding and a genuine interest in the child.*

—*Virginia Axline*

*The therapist may be taller or shorter than others, or she may have a memorable face, but no physical differences exist that can signal to the child that this person will be special. The differences between an effective play therapist and other adults, therefore, must come from within as the self of the therapist is made fully present and available to the child.*

—*Garry Landreth*

*Perhaps what is most essential is the "being" of the play therapist. This registers in openness and receptiveness to child life. The therapist must love children, enjoy playing with children, and be able to enter the child's world and learn directly from his or her unfolding processes and directions in play.*

—*Clark Moustakas*

## Application Focus Issue and Overview

Deidre, Scott, and Yi-ying are graduate students in a mental health counseling program who are all interested in specializing in counseling work with children and adolescents. They have completed three courses in play therapy, and have most recently finished a course focused on learning and intensive practicing of child-centered play therapy (CCPT) skills in mock role-play scenarios. All requested internships where they could use CCPT under supervision to help the children they will see. Deidre was placed in a mental health agency, Scott was placed at an elementary school, and Yi-ying, partly because of her background in nursing, was placed in a hospital pediatric ward. All sites have potential for CCPT to be used to help the children served in these locations.

Deidre has just spent her first child-centered play session with a highly anxious and unhappy 5-year-old boy named Garth. Garth began by announcing, "I'll mess this place up," and then swiped all the toys off the shelves, and dumped out all the bins of blocks, cars, and action figures. He continued this "messing up" until, seemingly all tired out, he crawled under the art table with a bin of action figures and played alone until the session ended. Afterwards, as suggested by her supervisor, Deidre reviews the taped session and takes notes on her initial reactions and feelings about the session. She feels exasperated and distressed just watching the tape. She feels so sad for this little boy, but also guiltily, she thinks to herself, "Perhaps he isn't right for CCPT . . . maybe he won't return for his second session."

Scott has been working with 8-year-old Penny for 6 weeks now. He is videotaping sessions to show to his university professor, who is supervising his CCPT work. Penny is painfully shy. She talks at home, but rarely, if ever, talks in school. She is very smart and finishes her schoolwork, but never answers the teacher or takes part in class conversations. During recess and lunch she finds her cousin, Brittany, who will speak for her. This is something Penny's parents always thought she'd outgrow, and they are at their "wit's end" and are considering having her evaluated by a psychiatrist if she doesn't soon begin to talk at school. Scott hopes he can help Penny, but he admits he feels compelled to want to help by "getting Penny to talk" eventually. He is beginning to feel frustrated because he knows that in CCPT, the child leads the way, and having an agenda for the child is not helpful. Penny comes willingly to sessions, and seems to enjoy her time, but she has never spoken to him, and she remains completely silent throughout her play sessions.

Yi-ying's first client, 7-year-old Greta, has been hospitalized repeatedly since she was diagnosed with childhood leukemia at age 4. In the past three years she has been hospitalized 35 times, for a total of 125 days. Her current prognosis is very good; however, she is now hospitalized for tests while awaiting an upcoming bone marrow transplant. Yi-ying has seen Greta for six sessions and is concerned that Greta keeps "playing the same thing over and over" where Yi-ying is asked to play the role of a little girl or boy who gets many tests and shots and has to "cry out." Yi-ying is mainly worried that she does not talk to Greta enough. Because Yi-ying has a strong accent, she is also worried that Greta doesn't always understand her when she speaks to her. She tells her supervisor that from the beginning of the play session to the end she is always immediately ordered into a character for a role-play, or asked to watch and "make loud crying" while Greta gives shots to the dolls. During the last play session, one doll "dies and goes to heaven." Yi-ying knows that Greta has known other children in the hospital who have died. She wonders if Greta needs to "talk more" about this.

All of these beginning child therapists are in the process of developing skills in CCPT, and as a result are becoming rapidly aware of some of their own inner struggles to accept and have faith in the theoretical underpinnings of the child-centered approach. All are wondering what it takes to become a "good play therapist" and if there are ideal therapist qualities that facilitate a child's work—can these be developed over time with supervision and experience, or must a therapist "have it all together" from the very beginning? Deidre, Scott, and Yi-ying have studied and feel at ease with the person-centered approach to counseling, and believe strongly in deep empathy, unconditional positive regard, and genuineness as the necessary and sufficient conditions for therapeutic growth. But now, as they begin work with children, they wonder just how these conditions manifest in their child-centered play therapy. Are the ideal therapist qualities—these core conditions—coming through in their work, attitudes, actions, and personalities?

This chapter is provided to highlight the ideal therapist's qualities of deep empathy, unconditional positive regard, and genuineness—known to be the "core conditions" of therapy when working with adults and children. The vignettes of beginning therapists, Deidre, Scott, and Yi-ying are provided to help you identify with therapists and counselors who are under supervision, and are discovering their own personal strengths through experiences with their young clients. As you read along, some of your own questions concerning your development as a play therapist may arise. We encourage you to reflect on these questions not only now at the beginning, but throughout the study of this book.

## Chapter Overview and Summary

The qualities of contact and connection through empathy, un-conditional positive regard, and genuineness (congruence) are widely accepted as the core conditions of counseling, introduced by Carl Rogers as needed to foster new growth and recovery or as Rogers termed, "the necessary and sufficient conditions [for] constructive personality change" (1957, p. 95). In the early decades of Rogers's work, Virginia Axline adapted this therapeutic relationship work to help children with play as the medium of connection (see *Play Therapy*, 1969). In this chapter, we demonstrate how each core condition is therapeutic for children and, therefore, how each core condition is *an ideal therapist quality* to be developed through experience and supervision by those wanting to successfully provide CCPT.

## Primary Skill Objectives

The following Primary Skill Objectives for this chapter are provided to guide the reader through the chapter and for reflection and review after completing the chapter reading and exercises. By reading and working through the chapter exercises, readers will:

1. Define the ideal therapist qualities of empathy, unconditional positive regard, and genuineness regarding their roles in CCPT and their relationships to each other.

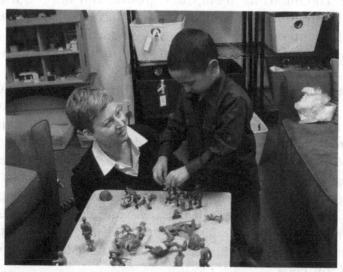

Figure 3.1

2. Explain the particular meanings of "deep empathy" in consideration of what we mean to clarify about empathy, especially in CCPT.

3. Describe and/or provide examples of the challenges to ways of being known to be effective, and the challenges in development of ideal qualities that new play therapists may face.

4. Anticipate and describe the challenges to most effective ways of being that you can anticipate facing with the clients that you will serve, and the lessons that you anticipate needing to learn through experience working with children.

# The Core Conditions and the "Being" of the Child-Centered Play Therapist

## Deep Empathy

It is important to realize that empathy is not a thought process. Empathy is never a matter of "figuring out" what the child is feeling. Rather, you should feel the emotion in the moment between you. As you connect with your child client, emotional experience should be evoked in much the same way that listening to a great classical music performance evokes emotion in you without saying a word. Animals and babies can sense what others are feeling without the need for "figuring out" or assessing the signs of various emotional experiences. So, you can, too, when you strive to connect with openness.

J. L. Cochran and N. H. Cochran (2006) illustrated some of the powerful change mechanisms from empathy as: "joining on a scary journey" (p. 50), "self-experience" (p. 51) and "a profoundly different relationship" (p. 52). The notion of "joining on a scary journey" can remind you that many people, even children, won't go alone to some of the scary psychological places that are sometimes needed for significant new growth and recovery. This principle seems to be true whether the thoughts, feelings, or new self-awarenesses are scary for good reason or are only imaginary "monsters under the bed." The accompaniment of your stable (congruent), loving/caring (unconditional positive regard) connection through deep empathy helps your clients complete the psychological journeys of self-discovery that they need in order to become their constructive best.

The notion of "self-experience" should serve to remind you of the reflective nature of empathy. Empathy assists and promotes self-reflection—awareness of one's experience in the present moment—awareness of such things as the connections of one's thoughts, feelings, and actions. Deep empathy should not be "all about emotions." Rather, deep empathy should be about a total shared experience, including all key elements of the child's experience in the moment. Deep empathy may often include thoughts, feelings, and actions. For example, "You don't like that. It's *yucky* to you. You're getting it as far away from you as you can." But note that we don't want you to take this verbalization example to mean that you should say all those words. To do so could take you far into your "heady head" and away from the present moment, and it might make your client have to divert from her experience to interpret *all those words*. In later chapters, we address the skill balances around responding with empathy in CCPT, but for now, think of focusing yourself on striving for empathy more than planning words for responses—as a skilled play therapist, you can be most free to let your vocal expressions of empathy bubble up in you as you strive to connect.

The notion of "a profoundly different relationship" can serve to remind you that *responding with deep empathy usually does feel awkward at first*. If such a way of responding were common in everyday relationships, significant counseling interventions would hardly be needed. But, fortunately, while it can take time to master, success feels good to both client and counselor.

We use the term *deep empathy* to note the striving for deep and full empathic connection. By referring to deep empathy, we mean to clarify that in CCPT empathy is much more than the common misperception of interpreting and naming client feelings. With your child clients, naming the feeling can be a distraction, especially if he doesn't know the word or has to stop to contemplate its meaning. A strength of working with children is that children are much more attuned to what others are feeling than they may be later as rational, "heady" adolescents and adults. So, when you are empathically attuned, much less needs to be said with your child clients.

There is a preponderance of literature underscoring the therapeutic value of empathy. Bohart, Elliot, Greenberg, and Watson (2002) conducted a highly sensitive analysis of empathy's effect in explaining positive outcomes across counseling. Bohart et al. conclude that empathy is a "key change process in psychotherapy" (p. 93), explaining significant portions of positive outcome even with the fact that it cannot be separated from Rogers's other therapeutic conditions in practice, and assuming research difficulties such as client satisfaction being among the outcome measures and a general lack of appropriately sensitive measures for measuring its effects. In the Norcross (2002) review of reviews, empathy is included as one of the few general elements of therapy relationships considered to be "demonstrably effective with extensively replicated research results" (p. vi).

## Unconditional Positive Regard

In various writings, Rogers associated the terms *warmth, acceptance,* and *prizing* with unconditional positive regard (Wilkins, 2000). Warmth can be taken to mean your nonpossessive attitude of caring, meaning that what you communicate with your way of being is "I care," not "I care for you if you [behave] thus and so" (Rogers, 1961, p. 283). Regarding acceptance, Rogers (1980) wrote, "The therapist is willing for the client to be whatever immediate feeling is going on—confusion, resentment, fear, anger, courage, love, or pride." With children in play therapy, the possibility of *being the feeling* is ever present and real, in ways that many therapists serving adults might only aspire to. And the notion of "prizing" suggests to us that you hold an attitude that each child you serve is a treasure to encounter, a prize to be uncovered as the two of you connect.

The benefits of unconditional positive regard in CCPT can seem obvious and also require contemplation. Please consider (and discuss, if possible) the following concepts related to the benefits of unconditional positive regard in CCPT:

- As you accept your clients, your clients come to self-accept. Self-acceptance can be seen as a prerequisite to honest self-discovery, followed by new, clear-sighted decisions for change.
- As you maintain unconditional positive regard, you create a safe space for your child clients to self-express with as few external reasons for inhibition as possible.
- As you remove the qualifications of your acceptance, your child client's locus of evaluation and control grow—in the vacuum of sessions without your criteria for acceptance, your child client will fill the void in learning to honestly and deeply self-evaluate.
- And as a final rationale, connecting with unconditional positive regard is a joyful thing to both counselor and client. In its pure form, it may be rare. When it's there, it feels right and therapy will happen.

There is also a preponderance of literature supporting the value of unconditional positive regard in therapeutic relationships. As Wilkins (2000) concluded, unconditional positive regard is a "major curative factor in any approach to therapy" (p. 23) and is *the* curative factor in the context of congruence and empathy. From their review of process and outcome in psychotherapy, Orlinsky and Howard (1978) concluded that client perceptions of therapists' manner as affirming the value of their person is significantly associated with good therapeutic outcome. And from their meta-analysis and review of reviews, Farber and Lane (2002) concluded that unconditional positive regard "seems to be significantly associated with therapeutic success," that it "sets the stage" for other positive interactions, and "may be sufficient by itself to effect positive change" (p. 191). The Norcross (2002) review of reviews considers the quality one of the most promising general elements of therapy relationships that work.

## Genuineness

Of course, a "pretense" of empathy or unconditional positive regard is not therapeutic. Child clients have an uncanny ability for knowing, at some level, when you are faking it. While even the best therapists may have to fake it for a moment or two, for therapy to happen, your empathy and unconditional positive regard must be real. While it is and should be a pleasure, it is your responsibility (with help from supervisors, scholars, friends, and colleagues) to keep yourself ready for real empathy and unconditional positive regard.

Rogers also referred to this quality as congruence, meaning that at least in the therapy hour, the therapist is an integrated person open and available to the connection. Fortunately, at least for us, this does not mean that therapists must operate all the time at the level of focus and attention balanced with self-awareness that she must bring to her sessions. We doubt that anyone could live up to that, and would add that it may not be practical even if possible. But we have often experienced CCPT sessions as meditative, in the sense of being almost entirely "one focused," with the object of your focus being holistic awareness and involvement in the experience of your client in the present moment, with also significant but peripheral awareness of yourself, your context, and your experience separate from your client's experience. We find CCPT sessions to almost never be "hard work" and almost always to be centering, even calming. Because the sessions require us to "get ourselves together," we do, at least for the hour, and are the better for it.

And there is, of course, significant and strong literature support for the quality of genuineness. As it is the most difficult of the core conditions to separate for study, much of the literature into genuineness or congruence addresses, the quality within the core conditions. Patterson (1984) explained that this is "a body of research that is among the largest for any topic of similar size in the field of psychology" (p. 431). Related to or as a part of genuineness, numerous studies have explored the importance of the match or mismatch between counselors' overtly expressed messages and implied messages (e.g., how things are said, nonverbal communication). For example, Haase and Trepper (1972) found that congruence is an essential underpinning to communicating empathy and that incongruent nonverbal messages undermine spoken messages that otherwise might have stood as highly empathic; Graves and Robinson (1976) found that counselor inconsistency may prompt clients to maintain greater interpersonal distance; Sherer and Rogers (1980) found that counselor nonverbal behavior impacts client perceptions of warmth, empathy, and genuineness. The Norcross (2002) review of reviews considers congruence, along with positive regard, one of the most promising general elements of therapy relationships that work.

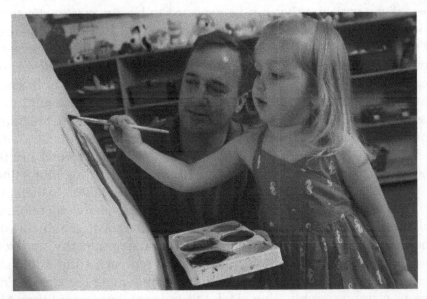

Figure 3.2

## The Core Conditions Overall and the Child-Centered Approach

There is, of course, strong evidence supporting the power of the core conditions as a set (e.g., Bergin & Lambert, 1978; Krumboltz, Becker-Haven, Burnett, 1979; Orlinsky & Howard, 1978; Patterson, 1984; Peschken & Johnson, 1997). As Norcross (2002) pointed out, "quantitative reviews and meta-analyses of psychotherapy outcome literature reveal that specific techniques account for only 5% to 15% of outcome variance (e.g., Beutler, 1989; Lambert, 1992; D. A. Shapiro & D. Shapiro, 1982; Wampold, 2001)" (p. 5). As Glauser and Bozarth (2001) pointed out, there has arisen in the counseling and psychotherapy field a myth of specificity that would hold that specific techniques could be matched to specific problems or groups of people.

Like Glauser and Bozarth, we doubt such prescriptions could be made accurately. Especially because of the tremendous power differential between adult therapists and child clients, we see a danger in well-intentioned, but tremendously inefficient, nontherapy to dominate the work of professional helpers with children. While specific "techniques" may often seem to grow out of CCPT, they are always child-created, child-generated, and child-led. In a sense, the child creates his own "technique" or "metaphor" for healing. We appreciate the nature of CCPT to focus on the therapeutic relationship and thus the set of key therapeutic variables that can be expected to be universally effective. Additionally, our approach to CCPT is to provide CCPT within a context of services (see Chapter 14). In our approach, CCPT and the therapy hour can and should always remain pure. If a specific skill seems to need to be taught, we would be most likely to help a parent or teacher promote this skill, or to help teach the skill in the classroom guidance lessons that are often provided in elementary schools. Thus, the therapy hour remains dedicated to what we know works best in therapy, and the therapist can work separately to facilitate specific mental health and inter- or intrapersonal skills that seem lacking, thus promoting growth in the key relationships of children's lives in addition to therapy.

The primary goal of CCPT is to create an atmosphere wherein the child has an authentic relationship with his therapist (genuineness), one where he is deeply understood and valued (deep empathy) and free to express all feelings without judgment or reproach (unconditional positive regard). This goal is reached not by providing the ideal set of toys or playroom or by using playful techniques, but instead through the "being" of the play therapist. Actions, words, attitudes, and

personality combine and are conveyed in relationship with the child—
these ideal therapist qualities are necessary and sufficient.

## Considering the Ideal Qualities in Action

Now that you have read about the ideal therapist qualities of deep
empathy, unconditional positive regard, and genuineness, consider the
following three excerpted scripts from the previously mentioned sessions of beginning child-centered play therapists Diedre, Scott, and
Yi-ying. After reading each, consider which of the ideal qualities seem
most prevalent to you in the vignette and speculate how the quality
would seem to be therapeutic in that context. If reading alone, note
your thoughts on which qualities stand out to you, and why and how,
after reading the vignette. If you are reading through the vignettes with
classmates, you may want to discuss how you see the ideal therapist
qualities at work in the vignettes, and note how each would seem to be
therapeutic for the child. Supervision comments on developing each
therapist's ideal qualities follow after the third and final vignette of this
chapter. We invite you to consider the ideal qualities we identified as
most prevalent following each vignette, consider the supervision notes
for each vignette, and compare your responses to ours.

## Example 1: "Deidre and Garth"

Deidre knows from background information that her first child client,
5-year-old Garth, is having serious behavioral difficulties at home and
school. He and his mother have seen psychologists and therapists at
the agency since he was 3, but he has not had consistent individual
sessions. He has a diagnosis of attention deficit/hyperactivity disorder
(ADHD), and his mother describes him as a "Jekyll-and-Hyde" personality and "therapist savvy." She tells Deidre that she has doubts that
"any type of play therapy" will help him. When Deidre meets Garth in
the waiting room, she notices at once that he seems terribly unhappy
and disgruntled. To Deidre, it is "as if he is sitting under a dark cloud."
She can really *sense and feel* his fuming and anxiety. She bends down
to his level, warmly introduces herself, and says, "Garth we can go to
the playroom now." He remains sitting on the floor, hunched over,
and doesn't make eye contact. His mother waits a minute, and then
teasingly says, "Garth . . . Garth . . . Earth to Garth . . . come in,
Garth!" Garth ignores this and seems to withdraw further into himself.

His mother changes her strategy and sternly says, "I mean it, Garth . . . get up . . . it's time for your appointment!" With this, he obeys and, though clearly angry, he quickly gets up from the floor and follows Deidre from the waiting room. As they are walking down the hall, Deidre quietly acknowledges Garth's reluctance by saying, "You aren't happy about it, but you'll come anyway." Once in the playroom, Deidre gives Garth the opening message: "This is a special room. In here, you can say anything and do almost anything. If there is something you may not do, I'll let you know." While she is saying this, Garth walks past her to the opposite side of the playroom. He looks straight at her with a blank stare.

> **GARTH:** *Okay then . . . I'll mess this place up . . . [walks over to the shelves and swipes the basket of puppets to the floor].*
>
> **DEIDRE:** *You'll mess this place up . . .*
>
> **GARTH:** *[Dumping out bins of blocks and toy cars]*
>
> **DEIDRE:** *[With a matter-of-fact tone] Out those go . . . right on the floor. . . .*
>
> **GARTH:** *[Dumping another bin of plastic food] Someone will have to pick all this up, too. . . .*
>
> **DEIDRE:** *You are thinking about that . . . someone will have to pick this up.*
>
> **GARTH:** *[Smiling with a snicker]. You will . . . that's who . . .*
>
> **DEIDRE:** *You're telling me I'll have to pick all this up. . . .*
>
> **GARTH:** *[Scooping a big cup sand from the sand tray, and holding it up menacingly]*
>
> **DEIDRE:** *You've got that cup of . . .*
>
> **GARTH:** *[Slings the sand in a swoop across the room]*
>
> **DEIDRE:** *[Getting up quickly from her chair to approach Garth, but then with a calm, but firm tone] . . . You want to throw sand . . . Garth . . . one of the things you may not do in here is throw the sand. . . .*
>
> **GARTH:** *[Dodges around her and runs toward the chalkboard and begins scribbling all over it]*
>
> **DEIDRE:** *[Backs away and sits back down on her chair] You scribbled all over that. . . .*
>
> **GARTH:** *[Grabs a roll of paper towels and unrolls it about the room, then falls over on the beanbag. He rests there for a few minutes, and then rolls over and grabs a bin of action figures and crawls under the art table with it in tow].*
>
> **DEIDRE:** *You're taking those . . . and going under there now. . . .*

## Elements of the Ideal Qualities Seen in Example 1

Evidence and use of all the ideal qualities are indicated in this example, but which one seems most prevalent to you? Take time to contemplate and respond to how you see the ideal qualities that resonate most from the vignette. Which of the therapist's qualities do you think were likely the *most apparent* to Garth through Deidre's mannerisms and actions during her first contact with him? Which do you think Deidre may have been struggling with the most? Which do you think, in a situation like this, you might struggle with most? Why?

Deep empathy

Unconditional positive regard

Genuineness

In terms of congruence, from what you can see or imagine from this vignette, what might be some challenges?

## Example 2: "Scott and Penny"

Eight-year-old Penny begins her seventh session by spending a long time—25 minutes—silently playing at the dollhouse. At times, Scott notices that her lips move as if she is *almost* whispering to herself. He catches himself secretly thinking, "If only she would speak to me." He feels this pressure, as her counselor, to help with her with problems stemming from her selective mutism. He has shared the pressure he feels with his supervisor, who has assured him that "getting Penny to talk" isn't necessary. Still, the pressure is there. During the session, Scott reminds himself to remain patient. After all, this is Penny's special playtime, and it belongs to her. Scott attends with acceptance and empathy, tracking her actions with the doll family. Every now and then, Penny turns around and gives a shy smile, seemingly in reaction to his tracking. After about 20 minutes, she gets up, yawns, and stretches, and takes a look all about the room before going to the art table.

> **PENNY:** *[Begins to intentionally sort out and arrange the different colors of tempera paints. She then very carefully pours some water in a cup, and places three different sized paintbrushes into the cup. She glances back at her therapist, Scott.]*
>
> **SCOTT:** *You are getting all those paints and brushes ready. . . .*

> **PENNY:** *[Puts a large piece of paper on the tabletop easel and paints a black circle for a head and a neck. She rinses the brush, dries it, and dips it in the green paint. She adds a shirt while looking back and forth at her counselor, Scott.]*
>
> **SCOTT:** *You are looking at me . . . while you are painting that. . . .*
>
> **PENNY:** *[Penny paints the green shirt and adds blue pants and brown shoes, matching the clothes that Scott is wearing.]*
>
> **SCOTT:** *You are painting . . . me. . . .*
>
> **PENNY:** *[Keeps painting with her back to Scott, but nods her head in the affirmative to indicate he is correct.]*

[Scott watches and smiles while Penny tries to get every detail just right. She is careful to rinse and dry off the brushes between each color. She finishes his outfit and even adds his striped tie, his black belt and gold wristwatch. She is noticeably pleased with her painting. She turns and squints, looking closely now, directly at his face. She dips a small brush in the red and paints a large smile—from ear to ear. She almost laughs out loud, but quickly catches herself. She then looks at Scott directly in the eyes. She finds a larger brush and dips it first in water, and then in the brown paint. She paints one brown eye, and then, just as she is about to paint the other eye, the watery brown paint runs down the "face" of the painting. Penny makes an audible gasp, and she is clearly upset by this.]

> **SCOTT:** *[With a soft tone, acknowledging her disappointment] Oh, no . . . that's not what you wanted to happen. . . .*
>
> **PENNY:** *[Shakes her head slowly back and forth. She spends a seemingly very long moment there, just standing completely still, staring at the picture. A tear rolls down her cheek.]*
>
> **SCOTT:** *You are sad . . . you don't know what to do now. [Another seemingly very long moment passes. Scott wants so much to do something to help . . . to fix it . . . make it better for Penny somehow.]*
>
> **PENNY:** *[Lets out a long audible sigh. Picks up the largest paintbrush, washes it thoroughly, dries it, and then dips it in the thick white tempera paint. She begins in slow, even strokes to paint back and forth . . . back and forth . . . back and forth . . . back and forth . . . until the entire painting is covered in white.]*
>
> **SCOTT:** *You painted it all white.*
>
> **PENNY:** *[Dips the brush again in the thick white paint—and again in slow, even strokes begins re-covering it . . . painting back and*

*forth . . . back and forth . . . back and forth . . . back and
forth. . . . ]*

**SCOTT:** *You covered it again . . . all in white.*

**PENNY:** *[Continues with her brush, painting back and forth . . . back
and forth . . . back and forth . . . back and forth. . . . ]*

**SCOTT:** *[Notices Penny has visibly become more relaxed now, and it
seems she is breathing in almost complete synchronicity with the
motion of the paintbrush.] You keep brushing it . . . back and
forth . . . back and forth. . . .*

**PENNY:** *[Continues with her brush, painting back and forth . . . back
and forth . . . back and forth . . . back and forth . . . ]*

**SCOTT:** *[Leans in and watches in complete silence for moments that
seem long at first, until he finds himself relaxed, and simply watching
as Penny in her silence paints back and forth with the brush.]*

**PENNY:** *[Clears her throat and in a hoarse, soft voice] . . . I'm painting
air . . . clouds and air. . . .*

## Elements of the Ideal Qualities Seen in Example 2

Evidence of the ideal qualities is indicated throughout this example,
but which seem most prevalent? Take time to contemplate and respond
to how you see the ideal qualities that resonate most to you from the
vignette.

Deep empathy

Unconditional positive regard

Genuineness

From the background of this example, what does Scott's foremost
struggle seem to be? How do his "reminders" to himself (not to have an
agenda for Penny) come through in his actions to convey unconditional
positive regard for her? With a little girl like Penny who struggles with
shyness and selective mutism, and who remains completely silent for
many play sessions in a row, what do you think some of your own
challenges might be?

## Example 3: "Yi-ying and Greta"

Seven-year-old Greta is a wiry and very imaginative girl. Despite a long
battle with leukemia, she is always feisty and full of energy. Her
rapid-fire demanding style in her first six play sessions is something
that—if nothing else—caught her play therapist, Yi-ying, completely

off-guard. During her seventh session, Yi-ying notices that Greta is much more subdued. She paints a picture for Yi-ying and one for her mother. She spends a long time at the water tray. She adds blue paint and then black paint to the water and swirls it around until the water is a deep dark blue. She drops some marbles in and searches for them with her hands. Finding them all, she drops them back in. At some point she turns and asks Yi-ying to get a flashlight out of the doctor kit.

> **GRETA:** *Let's turn off the lights . . . okay? I got a idea. . . .*
>
> **YI-YING:** *[Pulls the flashlight out of the doctor's kit] You want the lights off. It will be okay to turn off lights, Greta.*
>
> **GRETA:** *Good, 'cuz for this we need dark . . . turn on the flashlight now 'cuz I'm turning out the lights.*
>
> **YI-YING:** *[Turns on flashlight] Okay, Greta, flashlight is on now. . . .*
>
> **GRETA:** *[Picks up a baby doll and brings it over to Yi-ying.] This will be your baby. She is very sick and you are the mommy. It is dark because she is very, very sick and needs to sleep . . . now give me the flashlight.*
>
> **YI-YING:** *[Holds the baby doll, rocking it, and hands the flashlight to Greta.]*
>
> **GRETA:** *[Walks slowly around the room with the flashlight, shining it on the walls . . . on the ceiling. When she shines it on the table she finds the doctor's kit and picks it up. She walks over to Yi-ying.] Shhhh . . . we have to be very quiet. I'm the doctor. I'm going to look at the baby now. [She shines the flashlight on the baby doll's face.]*
>
> **YI-YING:** *[Whispers] Doctor, you are here to look at my baby . . . doctor?*
>
> **GRETA:** *[Flips one of the doll's plastic eyelids open and shines the light on the baby doll's open eye] Yes, I'm here to check . . . is she all right or not? . . .*
>
> **YI-YING:** *[Whispers, as an aside] What you want me to say, Greta?*
>
> **GRETA:** *Ummm . . . you say . . . doctor . . . is the baby still sleeping, doctor?*
>
> **YI-YING:** *Doctor . . . is the baby sleeping, doctor?*
>
> **GRETA:** *No . . . something is wrong. She won't wake up. [Greta pauses for a minute and looks directly at Yi-ying.] I'm going to try to wake her up with this flashlight . . . I hope it works.*
>
> **YI-YING:** *Okay, doctor. I hope it works.*
>
> **GRETA:** *[Turns the flashlight on and off and on and off in the baby doll's face for some time, then shakes her head back and forth sadly.] Nope . . . it's not working.*

YI-YING: *[Whispering as an aside] Greta, what you want me to say now?*

GRETA: *Ummm . . . you say . . . doctor . . . is she dead, doctor? [Yi-ying is taken aback by how this feels when Greta says this, and she is glad it is dark because, even in her pretend role, she tears up. She maintains her composure, though, as she follows instructions.]*

YI-YING: *Doctor . . . is she dead, doctor?*

GRETA: *[Officially . . . nodding her head slowly up and down in the affirmative] Yes, I'm afraid so, Mrs. Ying-Ying.*

YI-YING: *[Sits, thinking maybe she ought to say something . . . maybe she should talk to Greta about how she feels about the role-play . . . but then she remembers her skills . . . to follow Greta's lead . . . and Greta seems to have moved quickly on to something else altogether.]*

GRETA: *[Turns quickly and walks away. She stands in the middle of the room and turns in a circle shining the flashlight on the walls and ceiling as she turns]. You know what, Ying-Ying?*

YI-YING: *What is that, Greta?*

GRETA: *I'm not afraid of the dark anymore. I used to be . . . like when I was 3 or 4 . . . but not anymore.*

YI-YING: *So you want me to know . . . you are not afraid of the dark . . . not anymore.*

GRETA: *[Happily] Nope. I guess I'm getting older!*

## Elements of the Ideal Qualities Seen in Example 3

Evidence of the ideal qualities is indicated throughout this vignette, but which seem most prevalent? Take time to contemplate and respond to how you see the ideal qualities that resonate most to you from the vignette.

Deep empathy

Unconditional positive regard

Genuineness

From the background and script of this example, what does Yi-ying's foremost struggle seem to be? How do her strengths as a therapist come through in her actions (following directions from Greta and "playing a role") to convey deep empathy and unconditional positive regard for Greta? With a little girl like Greta, what do you think some of your own challenges might be?

## From Ideal Qualities to Virginia Axline's Eight Principles of Play Therapy

While the beginning experiences of Deidre, Scott, and Yi-ying may seem challenging, we find that it is not unusual for beginning play therapists to successfully meet such challenges in CCPT early on, and to be able to use their previous learning and skills "to fully be" in play sessions while conveying the ideal qualities of deep empathy, unconditional positive regard, and genuineness. In the following discussion, we provide examples of how we see the ideal qualities—deep empathy, unconditional positive regard, and genuineness—illustrated in the actions, attitudes, and personalities of therapists Diedre, Scott, and Yi-ying. Compare to your own responses, and begin to contemplate how Carl Rogers's teachings on the core conditions became the therapist ideal qualities, which then became the perfect guide for his student and colleague, Virginia Axline, as she began her work with children and the development of the Eight Principles for Play Therapy (introduced in the following chapter).

### Ideal Qualities in Example 1: "Diedre and Garth"

The ideal qualities that particularly strike us in Deidre's work are her *ability to connect* from the very first moments with this little boy who is trying so hard to remain disconnected. Deidre initially has doubts about the success of her first session with Garth, yet admitting this in supervision and talking about it helps her see that *from the very first moment of contact,* something "shifts" for this young boy. This "shift" is necessary for Garth, who is described as out of control and defiant both at home and at school. Deidre's first internal emotional reaction to Garth is her "sensing that he is sitting under a dark cloud." She feels his sadness, and this puts her into an empathic mode—as opposed to a reactive mode. Deidre meets Garth's reluctance to connect (or look at her) with steady and warm attentiveness. As he follows her to the playroom, she takes time to acknowledge his reluctance to come. In the playroom, she begins and *then holds true* to her beginning message to Garth—that this is his time for him to decide what to do, and she will let him know when it comes to something he may not do. She does not try to talk him out of his disgruntlement or immediately limit him when Garth begins to test the limits through the dumping of bins of toys. Such mess making is dangerous neither to Garth nor to her. In his more aggressive testing of limits, Deidre sets a limit, as she knows that her genuineness in responding (and congruence) would be at risk if she were to allow sand to be thrown. Deidre reacts quickly, but without too much alarm, when she successfully sets the limit by getting Garth's attention by saying his name: "Garth, one of the things you may not do is throw sand." Her next action of sitting back down *opens the experience* to Garth to decide what to do next, and this indicates to him that his therapist, Deidre, is once again giving him the right to decide. She acknowledges his next action of scribbling on the board by saying without judgment, but with acceptance, "You scribbled on that."

Meeting Garth's limit testing with warmth and with *recognition of his feelings of not wanting to immediately warm-up to her or the setting* additionally works very well to convey *unconditional positive regard* for Garth, who likely is not experiencing this very often (or at all) in other settings.

## Ideal Qualities in Example 2: "Scott and Penny"

The ideal qualities that particularly strike us in Scott's work are his ability to strive for and convey *unconditional positive regard* for Penny. Even with his internal pressure to "help Penny talk," he maintains an attitude of respect for her right to be silent. He is self-aware and admits to his inner pressures, but does not let this affect his actions and attitudes toward Penny in her special play therapy time. We can see how it might be tempting for many beginning play therapists to feel pressure "to fix" things for a child, and to show quick evidence of the effectiveness of their work through helping the child overcome difficulties, symptoms, and presenting problems. From the child-centered perspective, to do so would be to focus on work that the child may not be ready for, and which would likely foster more withdrawal and defensiveness. At the very least, such direct interventions show disrespect for the child's therapeutic process in the "here and now" by which she is symbolically working through important issues. Penny's actions in play therapy are about her experience in that moment, and that present moment experience is what she can (and does) learn from her therapy experience with her counselor, Scott.

## Ideal qualities in Example 3: "Yi-ying and Greta"

The ideal qualities that particularly stand out for us in Yi-ying's work with Greta are her acceptance of direction while taking part in role-plays without interfering, thus conveying *deep empathy* and "here-and-now" connectedness to Greta's processing in therapy. When Yi-ying is unsure how to react within her role, she asks for direction, which allows Greta to be in control and to experience personal empowerment. Whatever level of symbolic directness or indirectness is utilized by Greta is viewed as equally beneficial and effective for Greta's therapy. This faith in Greta and allowance for Greta to decide how to spend her special play therapy time also conveys *unconditional positive regard*. Though Yi-ying questions her ability to communicate empathy and understanding without "talking to" Greta about the feelings surfaced in themes surrounding hospitalization, doctors, and death, she does not waver in her child-centered approach of letting Greta take the lead in the therapy hour. It is through offering the opportunity for Greta to have control (without questioning or interrupting to "talk about" the meaning behind symbolic play) that Greta is able to process, heal, strengthen, and grow.

## Concluding Comments

In our work as supervisors of CCPT, we often find that beginning play therapists have a propensity to meet the very children that they need to "teach" them, the children that will give them the experiences they need to hone skills and strengthen their faith in the child-centered approach.

We hope this chapter introducing deep empathy, unconditional positive regard, and genuineness as the ideal therapist qualities sets up a "strong base to build upon" as you read on and begin to add on to your learning, first with Virgina Axline's Eight Principles, and then with each of the Essential Skill Sets chapters that work together to make CCPT a powerful and effective child therapy.

## Activities for Further Learning

- *Activity A:* We highly recommend reading Carl Rogers's original works, especially his classic book, *Client-Centered Therapy: Its Current*

*Practice, Implications, and Theory* (1951) and *A Way of Being* (1980). While many may have read these works before, a return to the original source is always refreshing and enriching.

- *Activity B:* Observe how the ideal therapist qualities are and are not common in our day-to-day reactions and communications with one another as adults and in our reactions and day-to-day communications with children. Journal or discuss your observations, including your speculations on the likely impacts. Remember that therapy or significant counseling intervention is, by definition, very different from an adult's and a child's usual set of experiences in life. It may not be practical or possible to provide the ideal qualities in many nontherapeutic contexts, but what happens when we do and do not?

- *Activity C:* Consider reviewing key chapters regarding the core conditions in *The Heart of Counseling* (J. L. Cochran & N. H. Cochran, 2006). This text addresses the core conditions in greater detail in the broader topic of general counseling skills or "talk therapy."

- *Activity D:* Review the seminal and clarifying work of Wilkins (2000), especially for Wilkins's explanations of what unconditional positive regard is and is not through exploration of the meaning and reversals of meanings of each of its elements.

- *Activity E:* While the benefit and necessity of genuineness to empathy and unconditional positive regard may be obvious, consider the relationships of empathy and unconditional positive regard to each other and to genuineness. How might each empower or at times simply enable the others in your work and that of other play therapists. Consider their applicability with particularly difficult client situations that you know of or can imagine.

- *Activity F:* Revisit the Primary Skill Objectives for this chapter and see if you have mastered them to your satisfaction at this time. If not, seek additional readings, practices, and discussions for clarification and in order to master them to your satisfaction.

# The Eight Principles in Child-Centered Play Therapy

4

Chapter

*The basic principles which guide the therapist in all non-directive therapeutic contacts are very simple, but they are great in their possibilities when followed sincerely, consistently, and intelligently by the therapist.*

*—Virginia Axline*

## Application Focus Issue and Overview

Now that you have a beginning understanding of how key aspects of child development are employed in child-centered play therapy (CCPT), and of the ideal therapist qualities that facilitate a child's work, you may want to know: What are the foundational principles that underlie the CCPT methodology? You may also wonder: How do these essential foundational principles guide the play therapist's actions, and translate into specific skill sets? From the beginning of modern play therapy, the essential, foundational keys have been Virginia Axline's Eight Principles of Play Therapy.

If you as reader are new to play therapy, it may be encouraging and helpful for you to know that Virginia Axline, the "mother" of the non-directive or client-centered approach to play therapy, started out in much the same way as you are now. She began with a strong understanding of child development, and she understood that play was a child's primary mode of communication—a way of expressing, contemplating, and making meaning of his experiences. She brought to her counseling the ideal therapist qualities of deep empathy, unconditional positive regard, and genuineness that she had learned from her teacher,

Carl Rogers. So, she began by letting the "language of play" be her child clients' primary mode of expression in therapy sessions. She experienced considerable success and periodically stopped to contemplate what seemed to be working and why. She searched her work for the core principles that would guide others to success. From this important work with children, she developed the "Eight Principles of Play Therapy" and wrote her classic books, *Play Therapy,* and *Dibs: In Search of Self.* In this chapter we help you gain initial understanding of each principle by "seeing it in action" and contemplating its possible implications. We state each of Axline's eight original principles with minor modifications made for additional clarity. Following each principle we add our own comments in order to provide additional understanding of the therapeutic importance of the principle and to note how these principles are translated into therapist skills. We then offer vignette examples from CCPT sessions to exemplify sets of principles.

## Primary Skill Objectives

The following Primary Skill Objectives are provided to guide you through the chapter and for reflection and review after completing the chapter reading and exercises. By reading and working through the chapter exercises, you will:

1. Be able to identify the principles in action.
2. Gain an *initial* understanding of the eight principles of play therapy (Axline, 1947) (note that it takes experience and supervision to deeply understand the eight principles, their interactions and implications).
3. Begin to understand the therapeutic values and interactions of the eight principles in CCPT.
4. Begin to see how the eight principles translate into concrete skills in CCPT.

## The Eight Principles of Play Therapy

1. **Establish Rapport.** Rapport means a warm friendly relationship with the child. The child will need to trust the therapist to feel free to self-express and play freely. Rapport helps establish this trust.

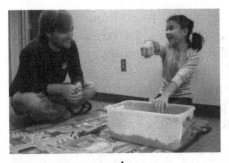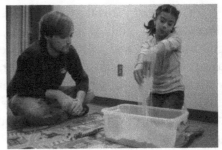

## Figures 4.1 and 4.2

*Comment:* The therapist establishes rapport primarily through the therapist skills of "tracking" and "empathic responding," which demonstrate acceptance of the child's behaviors/choices and emotional expressions, respectively. Although the therapist establishes the conditions for rapport to develop, the therapist does not attempt to force a relationship with the child, but instead allows the child to feel comfortable in choosing to develop such relationship.

2. **Accept the Child Completely.** Refrain from judgments or diagnosis. Put personal feelings of like and dislike out of your mind.

*Comment:* Although the counselor ultimately wants the child to experience a reduction of symptoms that are causing distress, and more positively to experience development and growth, the counselor also realizes that it is the valuing of the child in the present moment that establishes the therapeutic relationship and context for healing. Paradoxically, by not having an agenda or targeting the symptoms the child is experiencing, the counselor creates the conditions for the child to choose the optimal therapeutic path for such changes to occur.

3. **Establish a Feeling of Permissiveness.** This is "so that the child feels free to express his feelings completely" (Axline, 1947, p. 25).

*Comment:* The therapist creates an atmosphere that facilitates the child's confidence that he will still be valued and accepted even when he brings out his "bad side" or engages in actions or behaviors in play that others may object to or attempt to restrict. This permissive environment also assists the child in developing confidence in making choices and decisions and in taking risks at developing a relationship of trust with the therapist.

4. **Recognize and Reflect Feelings.** Be "alert to recognize the feelings the child is expressing and reflect those feelings back to him in such a manner that he gains insight into his behavior" (Axline, 1947, p. 75).

*Comment:* Through the use of empathic responding to feelings, likes/dislikes, beliefs, motivations, and desires for relationship, the child's actions and feelings expressed in play are brought to the child's awareness in an accepting manner, which allows them to be worked with therapeutically rather than being seen as threatening and bringing about defensiveness. The counselor provides this empathic responding and acceptance as a constant mode, and the experience allows for insight on the part of the child.

5. **Maintain Respect for the Child.** Parts of this respect are of the child's ability and responsibility to solve his or her own problems when given an opportunity to do so. Thus, the therapist does not offer solutions.

*Comment:* The therapist's role is to create an atmosphere where the child feels accepted, valued, and free to express herself. In such a therapeutic climate, the therapist trusts that the CCPT methodology will support the child in surfacing the essential therapeutic issues via their play and interactions with the therapist.

6. **Let the Child Lead the Way.** Don't try to direct the child's actions or conversations. This will limit self-expression, damage rapport, and lengthen therapy.

*Comment:* The therapist trusts that children, when in an emotionally safe environment, can and will choose the most effective way to work on therapeutic issues. In doing so, children will often choose play activities that symbolically represent their therapeutic issues rather than to talk about their problems. Even children's choice of symbolic play may vary in terms of how easily the content of the play can readily be linked to the actual therapeutic issues of the child. The therapist respects the healing path chosen by the child and does not try to force the child to either address therapeutic issues verbally or more directly.

7. **Remember That Therapy Cannot Be Hurried.** Personal growth can be a gradual process. Be patient. Often, well-meaning therapists stray from the eight principles by trying to hurry the process. Unfortunately, this often has the effect of lengthening the process.

*Comment:* Three of Axline's principles stress the need for patience, resistance for urges to become directive, and ultimately the cultivating of a deep respect for the child's ability to engage in a therapeutic process if the right conditions are established by the therapist. If the therapist is inconsistent in the implementation of the method, and attempts to blend CCPT with other approaches, this may result in uncertainty, defensiveness, and confusion for the child, and will slow or in some cases inhibit therapy altogether.

8. **Use Limitations Wisely.** So as not to limit the child's self-expression, use as few limits as possible. However, you will need enough limits to anchor the therapy to the world of reality and to make the children aware of their responsibility to the relationship. For example, it is usually off limits in therapy and in society to harm yourself or others.

*Comment:* The power of the CCPT model lies in the balance between establishing an atmosphere of acceptance and positive regard, which promotes self-expression and emotional growth, while also having reasonable limits which preserve safety in the playroom, the development of a relationship between child and therapist, and that foster the capacity for self-control.

## Considering the Eight Principles in Action

Now that you have read about the eight principles, consider the following session examples. After reading each, consider which of the eight principles seem most prevalent to you in the vignette and

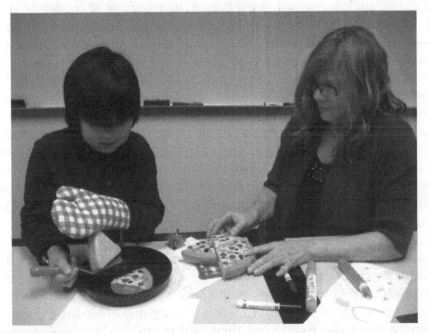

Figure 4.3

speculate how the principle would seem to be therapeutic in that context. If reading alone, note your thoughts on which principles stand out to you, and why and how, after reading the vignette. If reading with classmates, you may want to discuss how you see the eight principles at work in the vignettes and note how the principles would seem to be therapeutic for the child. We invite you to consider the principles we saw as most prevalent following each vignette. Our comments on those principles follow the third and final vignette of this chapter.

## Example 1: "Brianna and the Mad Spider"

Eight-year-old Brianna was recently removed from her family and placed in foster care. She has been coming to her school counselor for CCPT sessions for 5 weeks. She was told by her foster mother that she must "talk" about "what happened to her" in order to feel better. This message has served to make Brianna very suspicious. Brianna was removed from her home after "talking" to a lady using puppets and dolls—and she now feels very wary about this new counselor and her toys. The counselor has given Brianna the opening message: "This is a special room. In here, you can say anything, and do almost anything. If there is something you may not do I'll let you know." In addition, the counselor has explained the meaning of confidentiality to Brianna. As Brianna begins to explore the playroom, the counselor consistently responds to requests for guidance and direction by emphasizing that Brianna can make choices in the playroom, and can decide how to play and what to say. Nonetheless, Brianna is slow to trust and warm up to the idea of being free to self-express. She wants to turn the responsibility over to the therapist to decide "what to do or not to do." She timidly approaches all play activities— even those that she feels confident in—like drawing or painting. She sits at the table and fidgets with the toys and then begins to stare off in silence, or simply watch the clock. The counselor remains accepting, patient, and empathic. She *feels* how difficult this is for Brianna. During the third CCPT session, Brianna begins sorting through a basket of hand puppets, and puts on a large spider puppet. The counselor notices that Brianna becomes rather emboldened as she begins waving it in the air. She makes it jump in the direction of her counselor, and laughs with delight when her counselor backs away and pretends to be scared of it. She begins a game of having the spider jump around the room, and then "sneak up" on the counselor to "scare" her again and again. At one point during this game, Brianna raises the puppet high and sweeps it along the table, accidentally knocking off a few blocks and small toys. She stops and looks at the toys on the floor. She looks a little unsure, but shrugs her shoulders and smiles before saying to her counselor:

> **BRIANNA:** *Ooopsie!*
>
> **COUNSELOR:** *Ooopsie . . . some fell off.*
>
> **BRIANNA:** *Uh-huh, the spider did it—'cuz he hates toys!*
>
> **COUNSELOR:** *That spider hates toys!*
>
> **BRIANNA:** *ARGHHHHHHHH! [Brianna shouts as she waves the spider in front of the counselor's face, and then swoops down to "accidentally" sweep more toys off the table.]*
>
> **COUNSELOR:** *ARGHHHHHHHH! That spider is getting those!*
>
> **BRIANNA:** *Yeh . . . and killin' them!*
>
> **COUNSELOR:** *And killing them!*
>
> **BRIANNA:** *He's mad!*
>
> **COUNSELOR:** *He's mad!*
>
> **BRIANNA:** *And he's not a very nice one, either.*
>
> **COUNSELOR:** *And not very nice either . . .*
>
> **BRIANNA:** *Uh-huh . . . now watch this . . . [Brianna, using the spider hand puppet, starts to pick up various toys off the table and throw them about the room]. Get away! [She yells as she picks up the baby doll and tosses it into a corner]. I said . . . get awaaaaay! [She yells as she throws hand puppets one by one all about the room. Finally, out of breath but looking happily energized, she extends her arm across the table and, with one broad sweep of her arm, clears the table of all the remaining toys.]*
>
> **BRIANNA:** *ARGHHHHHHHH! [She dances and waves the spider hand puppet high in the air, as if in triumph] I got 'em all!*
>
> **COUNSELOR:** *You got 'em . . . every one of 'em!*

## Elements of the Eight Principles Seen in Example 1

Evidence and use of all the eight principles are indicated throughout this example, but which seem most prevalent? We list the ones that come to mind most for us from the session. Take time to contemplate and respond to how you see the principles that resonate most with us from the vignette.

1. Establish Rapport
3. Permissiveness

5. Maintain Respect
6. Let the Child Lead
7. Remember That Therapy Cannot Be Hurried

## Example 2: "Raymond and the Safe House"

Seven-year-old Raymond has been living at a domestic violence shelter with his mother for the past two months. He has been seeing the agency therapist for CCPT during that time, and has made a lot of progress. He is usually very energetic and animated and immediately engages his therapist to watch or take part in one of many prolonged battles between the dinosaurs. During his eighth session, however, he begins by spending a long time with his back to the therapist, quietly building a structure out of wooden blocks in a far corner of the playroom. Though this is a different way of beginning than in previous sessions, the therapist attends quietly—tracking and making empathic reflections now and then—especially about how important it seems to Raymond to get this structure "just right." When he finishes and seems satisfied with his structure, Raymond leaves the area where he has been building with blocks, and walks over to a table to sit across from the therapist. He dumps out the small plastic toy dinosaurs.

> **RAYMOND:** *Okay, now let's get started here!*
>
> **THERAPIST:** *You are ready to get started!*
>
> **RAYMOND:** *[Sorts through the bins until he finds the small ''baby'' pterodactyl, and then goes through the larger plastic animals to find the large ''mama'' pterodactyl, a large T-rex, and a large saber-toothed tiger.]*
>
> **RAYMOND:** *They is gonna fly off today. [Raymond places the little pterodactyl on the big pterodactyl's back.] See how the baby fits right on the mama's back?*
>
> **THERAPIST:** *It fits just right.*
>
> **RAYMOND:** *They practice flying . . . [Raymond flies the big pterodactyl over to pick up the little one.] Hop on my back, baby! [Spends some time making sure that the little pterodactyl can balance on the big pterodactyl as it flies. It is hard to get it to balance and it keeps falling off, but he tries it again and again.]*
>
> **THERAPIST:** *You keep trying . . . you really want that little one to stay on mama's back while she flies.*
>
> **RAYMOND:** *Uh-huh. But it don't work so easy.*

THERAPIST: *It's hard, but you keep trying.*

RAYMOND: *It's okay though. [Raymond puts the two pterodactyls aside and picks up the tiger.] Tigers like these ones and T-rexes live in volcanoes.*

THERAPIST: *Hmmmm . . . that's something you know . . . where tigers and T-rexes live.*

RAYMOND: *Yup [Lifts the tiger high, and "leaps" it across the room to bring it down hard on the wooden table]. BOOM! BOOM! BOOM!*

THERAPIST: *I hear some big BOOMS!*

RAYMOND: *BOOM! BOOM! BOOM! BOOOOM!! [Raymond becomes louder and louder, emphasizing each landing as he makes the tiger jump up and down on the wooden table.]*

THERAPIST: *That tiger makes big loud booms wherever he jumps!*

RAYMOND: *Yep . . . and the mama . . . she hears it and flies off to get the baby. . . . [Raymond picks up the large and small pterodactyls.]*

THERAPIST: *The mama hears and goes to get the baby. . . .*

RAYMOND: *She's gonna teach him how to fly . . . 'cuz he don't know how.*

THERAPIST: *He doesn't know so she'll teach him.*

RAYMOND: *[Softly] They practice flyin' together. [Raymond puts the little pterodactyl on the big pterodactyl's back.] Hop on my back, baby!*

For a few minutes, Raymond flies the two pterodactyls, holding them tightly together, about the room until they reach the corner where he has built the wooden block structure. Just as they are about to land, Raymond stops and begins to swirl and twirl the little pterodactyl as it falls, slow-motion style, off the big pterodactyl's back.

RAYMOND: *[Spoken with broken, agonized pauses] I . . . can't . . . make it . . . maaaa-maaaaaaa. . . .*

THERAPIST: *[Spoken with concern] The baby is falling . . . and crying out for mama.*

RAYMOND: *Uh-huh . . . but . . . then . . . the mama comes back . . . [Raymond flies the big pterodactyl over and lets it hover over the little one.] Hurry up baby! [Raymond then flies the mama ptero-dactyl back and places it carefully inside the wooden structure.]*

THERAPIST: *The mama goes and calls for the baby to hurry, then flies off to the house.*

RAYMOND: *[Picks up the little pterodactyl. He spins slowly in a circle, making the little pterodactyl fly around in a circle as he does.]*

THERAPIST: *The baby is up now, flying on his own.*

RAYMOND: *Uh-huh . . . he . . . the baby . . . he learnt how to fly. "Swishh . . . whirrrrrrr . . . swish . . . whirrrr!" [Raymond flies the little pterodactyl, doing loop-the-loops all around the room, and then lands near the wooden house of blocks. He carefully places the baby pterodactyl beside the mama pterodactyl. He lies down and peers inside at the two together side by side. For some time he is silent, just peering in like this.]*

THERAPIST: *[Softly] You're looking in at them, right there together.*

RAYMOND: *Uh-huh . . . there they is . . . back at the safe house.*

THERAPIST: *They're back at the safe house.*

## Elements of the Eight Principles Seen in Example 2

Evidence and use of all the eight principles are indicated throughout this example, but which seem most prevalent? We list the ones that come to mind most for us from the session. Take time to contemplate and respond to how you see the principles that resonate most with us from the vignette.

2. Accept the Child Completely
4. Recognize and Reflect Feelings
5. Maintain Respect for the Child

## Example 3: "Jamal and the Handcuffs"

Five-year-old Jamal is very small for his age, and because of his September birth date, he started school earlier than many in his kindergarten class. He is very smart—a real charmer—and he often wins the attention and "help" of girls in his class who love to carry him around like a baby. Teachers (and other adults in his life as well) find themselves doing things for Jamal and assisting him with tasks that he is developmentally able, but not always willing, to do. His teacher wants him to spend an extra year in kindergarten and is very concerned—especially about problems with fine motor skills, his tendency to "give up" and not persist on tasks, and his physical immaturity. But at a child-study team meeting, the members of the meeting are in disagreement. Jamal's mother emphasizes that Jamal is very bright and already reads. She is adamant that retention will hurt and not help Jamal. There are three months left in the school year. The school counselor offers CCPT as an intervention, to see if this will help Jamal with self-efficacy and readiness for first grade.

It is Jamal's fourth CCPT session. He enters the playroom, sits down, and immediately puts his foot up on the chair beside his counselor.

> **JAMAL:** *Can you get my sock up? It's all scrunched up inside there . . . [Jamal is already looking through a bin of toys, not at his counselor, as he says this. He finds his favorite toy gun.] I wish I could take this gun home with me.*
>
> **COUNSELOR:** *You're looking through the toys, and you've found your favorite gun. You also have something wrong with your sock that bothers you.*
>
> **JAMAL:** *[Looking somewhat incredulous] It's all scrunched up . . . please fix it!*
>
> **COUNSELOR:** *I see that it is all scrunched up, Jamal. You want me to pull it up for you. [She moves forward to assist him, but hesitates while keeping her focus more on his experience than on his sock.]*
>
> **JAMAL:** *Well . . . watch me. When I try, it gets . . . stuck . . . [Jamal pulls hard on his sock, and to his surprise it pulls out of its ''scrunched up'' position in his shoe.] Oh! There it goes . . . that feels better.*
>
> **COUNSELOR:** *You pulled hard and got it out, and it feels better now!*
>
> **JAMAL:** *AHHHH! Much, much better! [He stretches his leg out and wags his foot back and forth and laughs.]*
>
> **COUNSELOR:** *[Sharing his laugh] It* really *feels much better now!*
>
> **JAMAL:** *[Changing the subject and holding up the toy gun with a pleading, flirtatious look] I really would bring it back . . . please let me.*
>
> **COUNSELOR:** *You really do like that toy gun . . . so much you want to take it home, but one of the things you cannot . . .*
>
> **JAMAL:** *I knowwww. One thing you can't do is take the toys!*
>
> **COUNSELOR:** *You know . . . but you still don't like that!*
>
> **JAMAL:** *No, I don't like it one little bit! [Jamal laughs and pauses for a minute. He still holds the gun, and now picks up the handcuffs.] I'm going to have to lock you!*
>
> **COUNSELOR:** *You're gonna lock me up!*

Jamal struggles for some time, figuring out how to open the handcuffs. He almost asks for help, mutters to himself that it is "too hard," but then works and works at it until he gets them open.

> **COUNSELOR:** *You worked and worked on it until you got them open . . . now you're gonna lock me up!*

> JAMAL: *[Excitedly and obviously pleased with himself]* Yep. Now put out your hands!

The counselor puts her hands out. Jamal slowly and carefully puts the handcuffs on his counselor, making sure they aren't too tight, but that they click together. He smiles a big, satisfied smile as he picks up his favorite toy gun.

> JAMAL: *Now I've got the gun . . . and you're all locked!*
>
> COUNSELOR: *You've got the gun, and I'm locked up.*
>
> JAMAL: *[Picks up keys, and twirls them in the air] You're locked . . . and I got the keys!!*
>
> COUNSELOR: *You've got the keys!*
>
> JAMAL: *[Walks around the room for awhile . . . twirling the keys and shooting the gun in the air.] Now I'm going to let you out! [Jamal comes over and tries one key in the handcuffs. He turns it, but not quite far enough, and the handcuffs don't open. He tries the other key—still no luck.] This is hard. . . .*
>
> COUNSELOR: *You tried both keys, but neither seems to work. It's frustrating.*
>
> JAMAL: *Wait . . . just . . . one . . . minute . . . here. I have an idea. [Jamal takes the keys and, in a very "official" manner, gives one a little "lick" with his tongue.] This might just work. . . . [Jamal puts the key in one of the handcuffs, turns until he hears a click, and this time it slips right open. He then uses the key to open the other handcuff]. See . . . that worked! [Smiling broadly and with obvious pride]*
>
> COUNSELOR: *It worked . . . you thought of something and made it work. That feels good to figure it out!*
>
> JAMAL: *Uh-huh. I had an idea, and it worked. Watch . . . I'll do it again.*
>
> COUNSELOR: *Now you want to do it again.*
>
> JAMAL: *[Putting the handcuffs back on the counselor] It's gonna be rough, but don't worry . . . I know how to do it. If it gets stuck . . . just give it a little lick!*
>
> COUNSELOR: *You know what you're doing!*

## Elements of the Eight Principles Seen in Example 3

Evidence and use of all the eight principles are indicated throughout this example, but which seem most prevalent? We list the ones that come to mind most for us from the session. Take time to contemplate and respond to how you see the principles that resonate most with us from the vignette.

4. Recognize and Reflect Feelings
5. Maintain Respect for the Child
7. Therapy Cannot Be Hurried

## From Principles to Skills

In the following discussion, we provide examples of how we see Axline's eight principles—and the concrete CCPT skills soon to be introduced—illustrated in this chapter's examples. Compare to your own responses, and begin to contemplate how *each principle becomes a concrete skill* in CCPT.

## Eight Principles in Example 1: "Brianna and the Mad Spider"

**Principle 1: Establish Rapport.** In these moments, the therapist is meeting Brianna's reluctance to engage and her initial aggressive testing of just what is possible here with a warm attentiveness. This is helping Brianna believe that she really can trust that the therapist wants her to self-express and play freely, that it isn't a test or a trick.

**Principle 4: Recognize and Reflect Feelings and Principle 2: Accept the Child Completely.** The trust Brianna is beginning to develop in her therapist is supported by the fact that her therapist recognizes and accepts Brianna's feelings. The therapist does not try to talk her out of reluctance or discourage her when Brianna begins to test the limits of what is possible with her therapist through the spider's aggression and mess making. Meeting her reluctance and initial limit testing with warmth and with recognition of her feelings (empathy) also works to convey that the therapist accepts her completely and establishes a feeling of permissiveness, which Brianna begins to relish and use with growing abandon in these early moments. Recognizing and reflecting feelings, or empathy, can be seen as the golden road to  the core of the person (Cochran & Cochran, 2006). Accepting and meeting her expression of feelings, both her initial reluctance and her more aggressive (seeming) testing of limits, equals accepting Brianna as she really is in that moment in time.

**Principle 6: Let the Child Lead the Way** and **Principle 8: Use Limitations Wisely.** It is critical to her growing sense of free expressiveness that the therapist does not try to talk Brianna out of her reluctance to "jump right in" in the beginning sessions. Doing so would have likely created more reluctance and suspicion. Plus, Brianna has a right to her reluctance. Even if we didn't know the background reasons for it, we know that **Therapy Cannot Be Hurried (Principle 7)** and that trying to make a child be emotionally in a place that they are not or have an emotional experience that she does not naturally have in a given moment is certainly possible and often necessary in life (e.g., for parents and teachers), but this is more of the same constriction that the child must live with on a regular basis and does not provide for a therapeutic experience.

## Eight Principles in Example 2: "Raymond and the Safe House"

Two of the principles at work in this vignette that particularly strike us are **Principle 5: Maintain Respect for the Child** and **Principle 7: Remember That Therapy Cannot Be Hurried.** We can see how it might be tempting for many beginning play therapists to fall into analytic mode—to try to figure out what his play says about his relationship with his mother, and to interpret in order to try to speed up therapy. From the child-centered perspective, to do so would be to try to focus on insights and realizations that the child is not ready for and which are likely to foster defensiveness. At the very least, such interpretations would interrupt, and thus show disrespect for the child's therapeutic process in the "here and now" by which he is symbolically working through important issues. His actions in play therapy are about his experience in that moment (thus **Principle 4: Recognize and Reflect Feelings**). That present moment experience is what he can learn from. As the therapist uses empathic responding to  actions during the child's symbolic role-play, over time the child will become more aware of and work on his need for nurturing. The child becomes more open to reaching out to the persons in his life who would be willing to offer appropriate nurturing, if he were not hardened against it. He can also practice/is practicing this openness to nurturing in his sessions in other role-plays or more directly with the therapist. Importantly, he is practicing it with a person who stands ready to provide what is asked, but not to force it (again, **Principle 7: Therapy Cannot Be Hurried**).

It should be noted that in CCPT children may use direct or indirect symbolic ways of working therapeutically with important life issues. A child whose parent has died may use very symbolic play such as conducting a funeral scene, or may be much more indirect by doing a role-play where animals go for a walk and one of the big animals gets lost. In CCPT, the therapist trusts that insights into the connection between the meaning of the child's play and real life do not need to be made for therapeutic change to occur. Therefore, whatever level of symbolic directness or indirectness is utilized by the child is viewed as equally valuable and effective in bringing about change. The therapist therefore uses empathy with whatever the child chooses to do in the "here and now" and avoids making analytic interpretation about the relationship of the "here and now" to the problems experienced by the child outside the playroom.

## Eight Principles in Example 3: "Jamal and the Handcuffs"

The "scrunched-up sock" incident suggests to us the attitude of **Principle 5: Maintain Respect for the Child.** His counselor respects him enough to attend to him warmly **(Principle 1)** while letting him do what he can do for himself (fix his sock himself).

We might also point out that this is an example of **Principle 6: Let the Child Lead the Way.** His counselor *lets* him lead the way in fixing his sock. This is different from her *making* him lead the way (i.e., "Now Jamal [scolding tone], you know you can do that. Why would you ask me to do what you can do for yourself?"). By the way, we are not saying that letting him lead the way in that moment means he will pick up and start doing all things that he should for himself from that moment on. If the needed change were that simple, the change would already have been made. Rather, that moment of interchange helps to establish the kind of therapeutic relationship that will facilitate his making the deeper internal change.

You can also see a clear example in this vignette of the counselor applying **Principle 8: Use Limitations Wisely,** with **Principles 1: Establish Rapport, 2: Accept the Child Completely, 3: Establish a Feeling of Permissiveness,** and **4: Recognize and Reflect Feelings.** The limit is needed to keep consistent toys in the playroom. But notice that the counselor reflects Jamal's feeling, his *wanting* the gun, his *really* liking it, before the limit, and she reflects his feeling in response to the limit. Her warmth and empathy in establishing the limit conveys that "even when your actions must be limited, I accept you," that "even though there are some things you may not do, I still welcome and recognize your right to express yourself in this permissive atmosphere (e.g., not liking not being able to have the gun "one little bit," as Jamal put it!).

## Concluding Comments

As you can see, Axline's eight principles are a set that works together to create a sense of emotional safety, acceptance, nondefensiveness, and willingness to explore and work on therapeutic issues. While each is important in and of itself, none alone suffices for successful implementation of the CCPT model without working in synchronization with the whole set. For example, "Letting the Child Lead the Way" could be an especially curative principle, or potentially harmful principle without the safety and structure that the principle, "Using Limits Wisely" provides. Remembering that "Therapy Cannot Be Hurried" is wise only if the therapist structures client self-expression through "Establishing a Feeling of Permissiveness" and "Recognizing and Reflecting Feelings." And while "Establishing Rapport" is critically important to the other seven principles, it has no value or meaning without the other seven principles, which work together to ensure that the child in therapy feels valued, free to emote, open to relationship, and safe. We hope that this chapter introducing Axline's eight principles sets up a good "springboard" as you now delve into the core of this book and study each of the following skills chapters: chapters that work together to make CCPT a powerful and effective child therapy.

## Activities and Resources for Further Study

- *Activity A:* There is no substitute for returning to the source of the approach. We encourage you to read Virginia Axline's original works, especially her classic books, *Play Therapy* (1947/1969) and *Dibs: In Search of Self* (1964). If you are interested in this sort of work, it is the kind of book you might read in an evening. While her approach has been refined by therapists and contexts over the decades, it continues to define play therapy for all who follow.

- *Activity B:* Observe how the eight principles are and are not common in children's lives. Journal or discuss your observations, including your speculations on the likely impacts. Remember that therapy or significant counseling intervention is, by definition, very different from a child's usual set of experiences in life. It may not be practical or possible to provide the eight principles in many nontherapeutic contexts, but what happens when we do and do not? Which principles seem better able to be applied on their own outside of therapy with children in our daily lives? For instance, what is the value of "not hurrying" children when the time allows? Or "reflecting feelings" before asking questions when they are expressing themselves?

- *Activity C:* Revisit the Primary Skill Objectives for this chapter and see if you have mastered them to your satisfaction at this time. If not, seek additional readings, practices, and discussions for clarification, and in order to master them to your satisfaction.

# Preparing Your Setting for Providing Child-Centered Play Therapy

## 5
## Chapter

*The play therapy room is good growing ground for the child.*
—*Virginia Axline*

*To different children, objects have different meanings. In children's imaginations sand, clay, water, and the like may symbolize almost anything—a parent, a sibling, a painful experience, fears, food, love and hate, hostility. . . . Objects with more definite structure, such as cars, knives, soldiers, guns, boats, also may symbolize many things to children. The therapist accepts the child's symbolism exactly as it is and does not in any way try to enforce society's labels on children's play.*
—*Clark Moustakas*

*The feeling in the playroom should be like putting on a well-worn, warm sweater.*
—*Garry Landreth*

## Application Focus Issue

Corrine is a child-centered play and filial therapist in private practice. She shares an office space with Rochelle, who counsels adolescents and adults. Corrine uses a large corner of the room to set up a "play area" for her younger child clients, and in addition uses Rochelle's more structured "office area" and arts/crafts table with older child clients, and for parent consultations. Corrine finds that this "blending" of office space has advantages when an older child is uncomfortable with "baby toys." Corrine's main challenges in this shared office have been in limit setting with her more rambunctious youngsters.

Javier works at a mental health agency as the child and adolescent therapist. He has a wonderful, spacious, well-stocked playroom, and a separate office space that is connected to the playroom. Main difficulties for Javier have arisen in explaining the effectiveness of play therapy to his coworkers, and in structuring the waiting room experience for his child clients, whose siblings are often in tow, and whose parents, at times, want to give full, detailed reports of the child's problem behaviors in the waiting room before each session.

Maura is a school counselor who has limited mobility and, many times, must be in a wheelchair. She has a large playroom with a separate office area. For CCPT she structures her sessions so that all toys and art supplies for play are on a large table in the middle of the room, and she has adequate space to move about in her wheelchair. Maura's challenge was in knowing how to structure her space for sessions, and trusting in her ability to provide play therapy—despite her physical limitations—with some adjustments to setting and style.

Aliah is a graduate student in mental health counseling on internship. She works in two small inner-city elementary schools, where space is limited. Sometimes, after arriving at the school, she finds that her space is being used, and without notice, she is moved to another area such as the art room or auditorium for the day. This continual need to be flexible in changing spaces, and dealing with the resulting effects on her child clients, has been Aliah's main challenge.

In our work as play therapists, we have had the opportunity to provide services to children in many different settings. As supervisors, we have also been fortunate to help play therapists in a wide variety of situations find the way to provide child-centered play therapy (CCPT). This chapter will share what we've learned from these experiences, and help you in preparing your space and collecting materials and toys for providing CCPT. Learning how to bring to the sessions a feeling of openness, freedom, and warmth and safety—even when you must structure for personal reasons, or your work setting isn't ideal—will be covered. Demonstrating how "you are the best toy in the playroom" is a goal of this chapter.

## Chapter Overview and Summary

Preparing your space and collecting materials and toys for providing CCPT will depend in many ways on the setting and work situation that you find yourself in. Play therapy is provided in schools, mental health clinics, hospitals, private practices, and "on the road," with the therapist traveling from place to place with a rolling duffle bag of toys. Play therapists are found in a variety of diverse settings: in emergency shelters and refugee camps, hospital pediatric wards, and elementary schools.

This chapter will address the preparations that a therapist needs to consider in developing the space and appropriate toys to provide play therapy. The range of children that CCPT is appropriate for, and the basics of gaining coworker, parental, and teacher support will be introduced; however, the main purpose for this chapter is to consider the physical preparation of your space and environment including selection of toys, playroom setup, ideal settings and reasonable compromises in setting needs, and the fit of CCPT within agency, school, and private practice settings.

## Primary Skill Objectives

The following Primary Skill Objectives for this chapter are provided to guide your study, and for reflection and review after completing the chapter reading and exercises. By reading and working through the chapter exercises, you will be better able to:

1. Select appropriate toys and supplies to set up a playroom (or modify your playroom) in a school, agency, or private practice setting.
2. Select appropriate toys and supplies for a traveling play kit.
3. Understand what to do (and what not to do) to accommodate for older children (10–12 years) in CCPT.
4. Explain the meaning and significance of the saying, "You're the best toy in the playroom," and how development and experience in CCPT helps all play therapists better accommodate and be adaptable in providing CCPT in a wide variety of settings.

## Play Materials Commonly Used in Child-Centered Play Therapy

The following list should help those who are interested in setting up a play therapy room in a private practice, mental health agency, or school counselor office setting. In general, the toys should be chosen to promote expressive and imaginative play. Toys should be durable (not easily broken or with too many small parts) and easy to use by small hands. The quantity of small toys (Legos, toy soldiers, plastic animals) should be limited to help with clean-up time; for example, no more than 20 toy soldiers—10 green and 10 tan—for each "side" of the battle, and an adequate selection and variety of Legos, but not the full set of 5,000 pieces.

There should be an assortment of appealing toys; however, the toys chosen for CCPT should not be associated with pop culture or current trends, and should be more generic in nature. Toys should be chosen that allow for energy release (foam balls, Hula-hoop, and punching bag), artistic and musical expression (crayons, paints, clay or Play-Doh, and a small set of musical instruments such as a small keyboard and drums), and sociodramatic expression or role-play (sunglasses, two or three large scarves, costume jewelry, play money, play food and utensils, handcuffs, and gun).

The toys and structure of the room should remain consistent from week to week. The child in play therapy will feel safer within this consistency, and, in addition, this structuring of the toys/space helps make the "therapy hour" more time efficient. Once engaged in CCPT, a

Table 5.1   **A Suggested List of Play Therapy Materials**

Sturdy doll house with family dolls (multiethnic)
Baby (nursing) bottle, 2–3 small baby dolls (multiethnic), and blanket
Hand puppets (various animals, family)
Art supplies (paints, crayons/markers, paper, gluestick, tape, scissors, Play-doh or clay)
Music supplies (small drum, small electronic keyboard, pretend microphone)
Mix of transportation vehicles (trucks, airplanes, cars, boats)
Mix of small plastic animals (forest animals, farm animals, dinosaurs)
Toy soldiers and "wrestling" action figures
Legos, wooden blocks, peg-pounding set
Dishes, play cookware and utensils, play food
Small broom
Small spray bottle (with water)
Diecast (metal) play handcuffs, soft foam dart gun, toy (rubber) knife
Play doctor's kit
Play money, small handbag or suitcase
Sunglasses, large scarves, play telephones and/or walkie-talkies
Small set of toy construction tools
Bop bag or "Bobo"
Soft foam swords (or bats)
Soft (foam) basketball and hoop set
Jump rope, Hula-hoop
Ring toss game

child will often return to the same themes and patterns of play, and will tend to gravitate toward what is easiest and most *individually natural for his self-expression.* For this reason, toys should be readily available, easily accessible, and organized in bins, so that the child can find them quickly and without undue frustration.

## Other Play Materials Recommended When Space and Money Allow

Water tray

Sand tray

Painting easel, paint smock, and washable paints

Puppet theater

## Criteria for Toy Selection in CCPT—What to Include or Exclude, and Why

In summary, selection of toys from the list of commonly used play materials above helps to ensure that:

1. Toys are included that may be logistically related to a given stage (warm-up, aggressive, regressive, mastery) in CCPT (see Chapter 10 for understanding stages of CCPT).
2. Toys are included that support role-play and sociodramatic play.
3. Toys are available and can be used for creativity: artistic/musical/ dramatic expression.

To ensure that toys may be logistically related to a given stage in CCPT, "aggressive release"–type toys as well as more "nurturing release"–type toys should be available. Toys that can have multiple purposes are helpful (i.e., toy gun could be used to symbolize aggression, protection, or rescue; absent a toy gun, a drill can serve as one pretend gun, and a toy carpenter's square as another). Overly structured puzzles (including jigsaws with over 25 pieces), board games with rules, and video games should not be used. While a child may need, especially in warm-up stage, to have available toys that she is used to seeing in everyday life, a deck of playing cards, papers and paints, and soft balls for playing catch will suffice for this purpose.

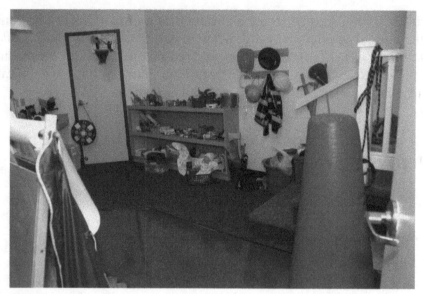

Figure 5.1

## Ideal Criteria for the Space and Environment of the Playroom

Ideally, the space should be not too big and not too small (approximately 200 square feet), should have adequate light and ventilation, and when possible have easy access to a child-size sink and bathroom. Privacy is assured through outward facing (to the outdoors) or curtained windows, soundproofing panels in the walls, and/or a "white noise" soundproofing machine placed outside the door. If a two-way, mirrored window is part of the room, it should be curtained during play sessions. Organization of the room might include one wall space with an arts/crafts table and another with a bin/shelf area that arranges assorted toys by category (plastic animals, trucks and cars, etc.) for easy access. One corner of the room might have a "dress-up" trunk and another corner a large bin of foam bats and balls. Foam basketball and hoop sets are designed to be hung over the doorjamb, so if using these, leave some open space around the door area. If possible, and available, the art easel, sand table, and/or water table should be in an area of linoleum flooring (for easy cleaning of the flooring underneath). The opposite section of the room could include a small rug area with a beanbag chair. One wall space could be used to hang a wipe-off board with low-odor markers and an eraser. In general, it is best to leave ample open space for movement (energy release such as dancing, jumping, punching the Bobo [bop bag]) in the middle of the room.

The arts/crafts table area can be standard (adult) height, but should have appropriately sized chairs for seating older children (10–12), as well as a higher chair for younger children. A sturdy stepstool is also helpful and will tend to be used by all different-sized children for "reaching higher" or "being taller." Along with the art supplies suggested on the list, an abundance of nonstructured "disposable" scrap art supplies such as pipe cleaners, cotton balls, Popsicle sticks, scraps of paper, paper towel tubes, small cardboard (shoe) boxes, Styrofoam "popcorn," and multicolored plastic bottle tops should be available for the child to use for a variety of play activities and projects.

The room should be one where you will not worry about things getting messy or broken; however, if CCPT must take place in an office that serves dual purposes, limit setting may include structural limitations (i.e., play can be limited to the table top or one area of the room) when necessary.

## The Traveling Play Therapist

If you are a traveling play therapist and have the ability to request a room to use solely for CCPT, some of the aforementioned suggestions can be shared with the school or agency when communicating your needs in finding a space for providing CCPT. However, if a room is not consistently available, many traveling play therapists find a quiet, out-of-the way section of the hallway far from "hustle and bustle" or an area of a room regularly used for art or music to work well as long as it is consistently available, and *confidentiality is not compromised*. A folding screen and soundproofing "white noise" machine can be used for an extra sense of privacy and structure. Consultation rooms in agencies or schools can be arranged for play therapy and are often open or can be signed up for scheduled times. Other excellent options include coordinating alternating times with the school psychologists' testing schedule or those who provide speech/language and physical therapy services. Many traveling play therapists have found that the key is in *building strong relationships with others who must travel from school to school*, and in coordinating schedules with these other child helpers, who also must share space in schools and agencies.

There are many possibilities for carry-along (traveling) play kits— and because a special playroom for CCPT is not always available, spaces can be modified to provide CCPT within your budget and space limitations. A private area set aside with a rug and toys can suffice for a play area. A folding dollhouse with a mix of multiethnic family dolls; animal hand puppets; wooden blocks; nursing bottle and two or three small multiethnic baby dolls; crayons; Play-Doh; colored pencils; drawing paper; watercolors; a spray bottle with water; scarves; sunglasses; play telephones; a toy gun and handcuffs; a selection of small plastic animals and transportation toys such as cars, trucks, and airplanes; soft balls; and a cotton jump rope all fit well into a large rolling duffle bag or small toy bin. As a substitute for a punching bag, it is easy and affordable to purchase several punching balloons for "punching" and energy release. A small, mobile sand tray can be devised using a plastic container (medium size, 30-quart) with a snap-on top. While this is a heavy item, it is also a great one to include. Some of our traveling play therapists have one stored at each school/agency they visit, to avoid having to haul one in and out each week. A folding tabletop easel, paper, and paints might also be included. An extra-large T-shirt (for keeping clothes clean while painting), a box of tissues and hand sanitizer to reduce spread of germs, and disinfectant wipes should be included in the traveling kit for quick cleanups and sanitizing toys between play sessions.

## Children in the 10- to 12-Year-Old Range: What to Do (and Not to Do) to Accommodate Older Children in the Playroom

Child-centered play therapy is an appropriate counseling intervention for children 3–12 years old, and has been adapted for use with adolescents as well (J. L. Cochran, Fauth, N. H. Cochran, Spurgeon, & Pierce, in press). Some 10- to 12-year-old children in CCPT and pseudo-mature children may feel disgruntled (early on in warm-up stage) and may report not liking "baby toys" and being "bored." They may repeat wanting to bring in their DS or video games because in that case, at least, they "would have something to do." The skilled play therapist is sensitive to this awkward phase for an older child, or a younger child who feels intimidated by the toys, and is careful during this time to acknowledge that "this is different, and it is difficult to find something you want to do." However, complying with the requests for "something more to do" is not recommended. Often, with empathy and the acknowledgment of feelings the child is having during this rapport-building time, the child will move in the directions he needs to, and begin taking the lead through talking, playing cards, drawing, or exploring the room and making different comments about the toys. Older children, and those pseudo-mature children who may fear "being seen playing," particularly need to be reassured of *consistency and confidentiality* of sessions.

Remember that some initial awkwardness and disgruntlement is to be expected, and for many older children this initial time of rapport building is a crucial time in the therapeutic process. Older children who have been "play deprived" due to chaotic, traumatic, or even merely overly structured lives, can be given an opportunity to self-express and heal through CCPT if given the chance in a safe, consistent, confidential setting. Patience, therapeutic listening, and responding with empathy will allow these children due time to build trust, take the lead, and fully utilize the therapy hour "to say anything and/or do almost anything"— to play, paint, act, create, and self-express—on a self-directed path toward healing and growth. In our experience, most of these children

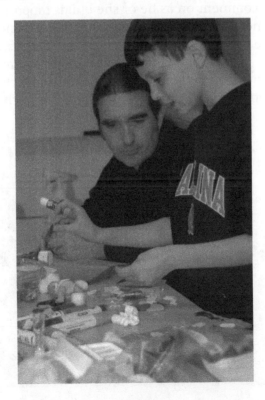

Figure 5.2

embrace the chance to become self-directed, free to be, free to self-express *all* thoughts and feelings, and play. Most, though initially awkward, do take the lead and move through the stages of CCPT. If necessary for the therapy process, most also utilize this chance to revisit periods of childhood development that *words alone would have not been adequate to express,* and otherwise may have been left behind, and not attended to in therapy.

That being said, providing some additional supplies (that an older child might find more engaging both during warm-up stage and throughout therapy) is an accommodation some play therapists find helpful. An "older child box" of supplies on the art table might include origami paper and instructions, paper airplane folding kits, snap-together car models, colorful beads to string for making necklaces and bracelets, air-dry clay, and a variety of higher quality multicolored markers/colored pencils and art pad. A high-quality yoyo, a deck of cards, "squishy" stress balls, magnetic "paper dolls" with multiple outfits, and small toy skateboards—the miniature type with tools—provide the older child something familiar to create with, play with, fidget with, or comment on as he or she builds rapport. A sand tray is highly recommended for play therapists that commonly see older children in the 10- to 12-year-old range, as well as adolescents in their playroom. While some of these items might add more expense to your play supplies tab, this box can be added for those children who are older and removed or put away when you are seeing very young

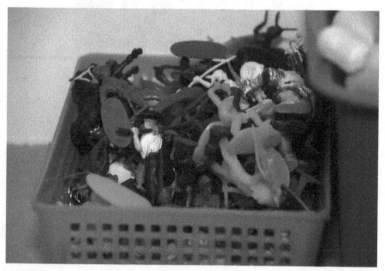

Figure 5.3

children (3–6 years) for which small beads for jewelry making and small parts for snap-together models are not age/developmentally appropriate.

## Suggestions for Setting Up Your Playroom on a Shoestring Budget

As mentioned earlier, for the best selection of generic toys and a large selection of multiethnic dolls/puppets and play foods, we have found discount school supplies for preschool and school-age children to be the most durable and affordable. Stores and catalogs that sell these usually have toys arranged by category (sociodramatic play, arts/crafts supplies, etc.), and they are meant to be purchased for use with young children, so are more hard-wearing than toys from the variety of stores that sell everything for "just a dollar."

Yard sales and "flea markets" can be wonderful places to find a variety of children's used toys that are still in good condition. Many papers advertise these sales and include in the advertisement if children's toys are the main product or included. For finding materials for a "dress-up trunk," the catalogs and stores that sell costumes for Halloween often have sales after that event, and it is possible to find an abundance of suitable props for dress-up.

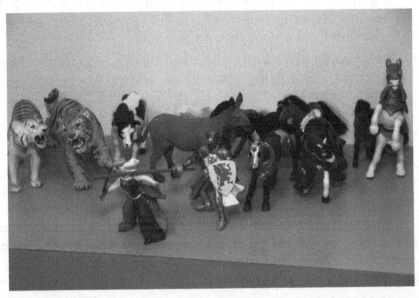

Figure 5.4

Additionally, our interns have often set up "new" playrooms in schools and have found the faculty and staff to be more than generous in donating from their attics to fill a list of toys for the playroom.

## Common Problems in Preparing Play Space and Choosing Materials

Depending on the work setting that you are in, some of the following common problems will be unavoidable. For instance, if you share a space with another therapist, you may need to use structuring and limits around certain items and areas of the room (coworker's desktop). The list is provided to help therapists and counselors in a variety of settings avoid some difficulties by structuring/organizing their space and materials ahead of time, and preparing through awareness of some common challenges other play therapists have reported.

- Avoid toys that cause frustration on the part of the child or worry on the part of the counselor. Toys that raise safety issues due to spread of germs (face masks, musical toys such as harmonicas, horns) and mechanical toys that make obnoxious, repetitive sounds can be a source of worry and frustration for the therapist. Broken toys (a partial train track without all the pieces, Bobo punching bags that pop easily or lose air) can be a source of frustration for the therapist and the child.

- Avoid having items in the playroom that the therapist is overly concerned about being damaged or broken (laptop computer; framed artwork or diplomas; personal items; family pictures; fragile, expensive toys).

- Avoid food or snacks in the playroom or surrounding area. No food in the playroom is a basic structural limit; for safety reasons (choking hazard) it is best that children do not have hard candy, gum, or snacks in CCPT sessions. However, in some shared spaces, candy dishes in waiting rooms or in office spaces are common. Talking with coworkers about removal of these, or simply removing these during play therapy, can prevent your having to deal with this during your sessions.

- Try to be aware of board games, personal items, and artwork in shared spaces with other counselors and therapists. Some therapists use a large screen to divide off the section of the office not being used. Large, locking cabinets where certain items can be put away and safely stored during play sessions works also.

- Avoid problems caused by too many toys (or not enough toys). Both can be a problem. Toys and space should be balanced. The child should have plenty of room to play and not have to sort through mounds of toys.

- Avoid problems due to an imbalance of toys (those appealing more to a certain age range, gender, culture/ethnicity). Always try to have a variety of toys for multicultural populations, differing ages, and stage levels of play.

- Avoid toys that are too sensational and are representative of pop culture, such as characters from popular children's television programs and movies, and therefore have a preset or established symbolic value or meaning.

- Try not to have too many bins of blocks, plastic figures/animals/toy soldiers or small pieces that make for longer cleanup time for the therapist (hundreds of soldiers, thousands of Legos, 50 small plastic dinosaurs).

- Avoid the "do not play here" atmosphere created by an overly organized, overly clean room full of all brand new toys. Children need to feel that the toys are "ready to use," so when you are first preparing a playroom, mix in toys that have some previous use.

- Avoid replacing toys too often or adding new toys unnecessarily. Children (especially in the warm-up stage) may request or suggest certain toys that they would like to have in the playroom. While this request is acknowledged with empathy, it is a common mistake to comply with such toy requests. Adding toys at the request of a child sends the wrong message and lengthens the therapeutic process.

- Avoid "clutter" and the disorganized playroom. This common problem is easily solved by using shelves in the playroom or plastic bins with tops in small travel kits to organize toys.

- Avoid filling up small spaces or not having enough space in general so that the child feels crowded. In cases where this can't be helped, try to make the area seem more open and spacious to the child by removing unnecessary furniture, large objects, and toys. In rooms that are too large, use a room divider or screen to section it off.

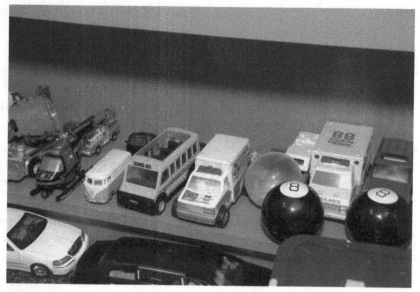

Figure 5.5

- Avoid including toys that are not hard-wearing and break too easily. One counselor found that she had to replace her Bobo (punching bag toy) so often that within four months she had spent more on cheaper varieties than if she had initially invested in a more durable punching bag.

- Avoid not having enough supplies and disposable, easily replaced art materials (paper towel tubes, cotton balls, pipe cleaners, small cardboard boxes, colorful bottle caps). Children like to use "lots and lots" of materials—at times with abandon—as they create and play. It helps if these materials are easily replaced and not so expensive.

## Further Suggestions as You Begin to Collect Playroom Toys and Supplies

- If you find a toy that is sturdy, works well, and is used a lot in the playroom or in your play kit, purchase more than one so that you have an extra in case you misplace it or it gets broken. For toys that are used and need more frequent sanitizing (nursing bottle), it is especially helpful to have some extras on hand to quickly replace when needed.

- Files should be kept for each child to keep artwork in. Children will often leave artwork behind in the room. This should be kept in a secure, confidential place regardless of whether the child asks you to keep it. Artwork should not be displayed on the wall or discarded.

- Wet wipes and hand sanitizer should be in the playroom for quick clean-ups between sessions. Just as in a day-care setting, toys, especially those that have been "mouthed," should be quickly wiped and sanitized between sessions.

- As mentioned previously, try to include some sort of "punching bag" or large stuffed animal, but avoid the cheaper (dollar store) variety punching bags.

- Multicultural doll families do not have to take up space. Toy companies sell small, bendable families and allow for a mix of dolls representing Asian, African-American, Caucasian, and Hispanic backgrounds.

- When setting up your playroom in a school setting, check with the school principal about tolerance for items such as toy swords, guns, and knives. While most schools will allow such toys for purposes of therapeutic play, it is always best to consult with the principal ahead of time and to explain the rationale for inclusion of these toys.

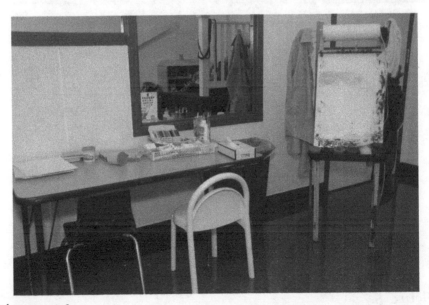

Figure 5.6

# Remember That "You're the Best Toy in the Playroom!"

While preparing your setting to provide CCPT—selecting toys and creating a comfortable space—is important, nothing is more important than *how you are:* your "way of being," in the words of Carl Rogers. The ideal therapist qualities of deep empathy, genuineness, and unconditional positive regard that you convey each time you meet with the child, and skills that you develop in practice and supervision, prepare you to provide CCPT well and consistently. To return to our opening quote by Garry Landreth, when you are working at your very best, the therapeutic opportunity you provide will feel to the child like "putting on a well-worn, warm sweater"—familiar and "comfy" with room to stretch and grow. The child will find safety—a haven—within the warm relationship you provide consistently from week to week. This is what allows for therapy to happen, and this will surpass any toy or setting.

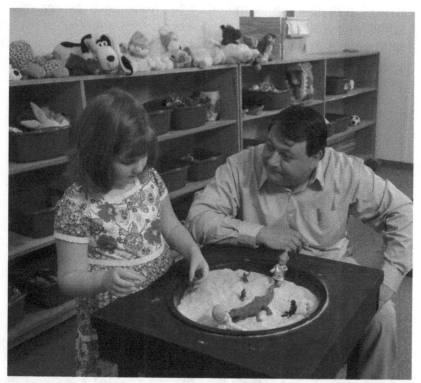

Figure 5.7

## Concluding Thoughts

After reading through this chapter, we hope you will feel confident in being able to put together a selection of toys appropriate for CCPT, and being able to provide CCPT in a variety of work settings. Over your career, if you decide to work with children and provide CCPT, you may move from setting to setting. We hope this chapter has helped to make this adaptability possible, and will help you avoid some of the common problems made when first starting out.

## Activities for Further Study: Questions for Discussion and Review

### Contemplation and Practice of Key Concepts

Contemplation and academic practice can help you develop confidence, depth of understanding, and comfort with newly acquired learning. The following activities and questions are provided for this purpose. They can be completed on your own, but most are designed to be completed with a partner or in a small group or classroom.

- *Activity A:* Return now to our opening counselor and therapist scenarios. Read through each scenario again. What types of other difficulties do you think you might encounter in a situation like Corrine's? What might you do to remedy these problems? What advice might you give to Javier about his difficulties in the waiting room? How might he educate his colleagues about CCPT? What might you do to advise Maura about her concerns due to her disability? What other modifications in structuring come to mind for a counselor who has limited mobility? If you were Aliah, what do you think you might try to do to improve your circumstances?

  If you are working in a class or group, compare your answers with others. You'll be surprised at the different (and creative) responses you and others may come up with. For comparison, our sample "solutions" are included at the end of the book in Skills Support Resource A.

- *Activity B:* If you are currently providing or have in the past provided play therapy, do you have any trouble spots, "sticky situations," or funny stories that come to mind—situations that could have been handled better or improved by changes in the structure of your setting or toys/supplies? Do you have helpful suggestions to add? If so, share with your peers.

- *Activity C:* If you are setting up a play area or gathering toys and supplies for a traveling play bag, has this chapter helped you to determine supplies to add or subtract in the future? Have you or are you currently working as a "traveling play therapist?" If so, do you have some funny stories or difficult situations to tell others about? Do you have any helpful suggestions for others? If so, share with your peers.

- *Activity D:* If you have a playroom that you currently use for play therapy, after reading this chapter, are you able to determine some changes that may make providing CCPT more efficient and enjoyable? If so, share these changes with the group, and give your reasoning for these changes.

- *Activity E:* Revisit the Primary Skill Objectives for this chapter and see if you have mastered them to your satisfaction at this time. If not, seek additional readings, practices, and discussions for clarification and in order to master them to your satisfaction.

# The Two Core Therapist Skills: Tracking and Empathic Responding

**6**

**Chapter**

*When a child is in the midst of strong emotions, he cannot listen to anyone. He cannot accept advice or consolation or constructive criticism. He wants us to understand him. He wants us to understand what is going on inside himself at that particular moment. Furthermore, he wants to be understood without having to disclose fully what he is experiencing.*

*—Haim G. Ginott*

## Application Focus Issue

It has happened—one of your greatest dreads. It is the first session with 8-year-old Billy, who has very reluctantly entered the playroom. He sits quietly with a furrowed brow, and after you give him the opening message, he glares at you briefly and then looks away. He is clearly angry and not at all happy to be there. What are you to do? How can you communicate acceptance and unconditional positive regard to Billy in the face of such obvious defensiveness and resentment so that a therapeutic relationship can develop?

In an accepting tone that captures some of Billy's clear displeasure, a skilled play therapist could say, "You don't want to be here right now." Billy, clearly a bit surprised at having his experience acknowledged in such an accepting way, shouts, "No! My mom forced me to come." The therapist replies, "You are pretty angry at her for bringing you up here." Billy, clearly less defensive now says, "She thinks I am bad because I hit my little brother." The therapist replies, "You believe she thinks you are bad, but you don't think so." Billy replies, "No, he deserves it!" In an accepting tone, the therapist captures some of Billy's tone of righteous indignation, "You have your reasons for hitting him that your mom doesn't understand."

Billy is clearly engaging her at this point. She is not seen as someone who views him as bad and who is here to fix him. Billy goes over to the table and picks up the toy knife and a baby doll. He says, "This is what this baby deserves!" and stabs the baby doll with the knife. He then looks defiantly at the therapist, wondering what the therapist's response will be and clearly expecting the therapist to confront him. The therapist maintains her accepting tone and captures a bit of Billy's anger, "You are mad at the baby and giving it what you think it deserves." Billy, a bit shocked by such acceptance, smiles and stabs the baby doll again in the stomach. The therapist responds, "You are sticking the baby again, right in the stomach." Billy, again shocked at his ability to express his anger so directly, asks, "You mean I can do that in here?" The therapist replies, "You are surprised that you can do things like that in here. In here, you can do almost anything you want."

Billy smiles and moves on to explore what other toys are in the playroom. In a very short time, Billy has moved from viewing her as the "enemy" to understanding that the playroom is a nonthreatening place where he feels accepted and is able to express his feelings, and where he is not judged. His initial defensiveness and resentment have diminished, and the therapeutic relationship is developing. By the time he leaves the first session, he is actually looking forward to coming back next week.

## Chapter Overview and Summary

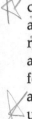

A major goal of the child-centered play therapy (CCPT) model is to create a therapeutic atmosphere in which children feel nondefensive and comfortable in expressing themselves and developing a therapeutic relationship with the counselor. The counselor's attitude of acceptance and unconditional positive regard for the child serve as the foundation for creating this atmosphere. The two core therapist skills of tracking and empathic responding embody the attitudes of acceptance and unconditional positive regard. Through the use of the tracking skill, the counselor demonstrates acceptance of the child's behaviors and sends a clear message of the expanded opportunities for self-expression in the playroom. Through empathic responding, the counselor provides the child with the experience of being understood and promotes the child's further expression and working through of therapeutic issues.

Tracking and empathic responding skills are among the most frequent responses made by the counselor. They are often used in tandem with each other, with the counselor first making a tracking response to note the child's behavior and following it up with an empathic response that identifies the feeling, preference, motivation, belief, or relationship issue underlying the behavior. Making skillful tracking and empathic responses entails active identification with the experience of the child, proper pacing, correct level of directness, avoidance of repetition, and willingness to accept any corrections made by the child. This chapter provides the counselor with insight into the importance of these two core skills, as well as providing models of skilled statements and an opportunity to practice these skills.

## Primary Skill Objectives

The following Primary Skill Objectives for this chapter are provided to guide your study, and for reflection and review after completing the chapter reading and exercises. By reading and working through the chapter exercises, you will be better able to:

1. Explain the therapeutic purposes of the two core therapist skills of tracking and empathic responding and how they are often used in tandem in response to children's play.

2. Demonstrate how to skillfully use the tracking skill.

3. Identify five dimensions of empathic responses: feeling, like/ dislike/preference, intention/motivation, belief, and desire for relationship.

4. Explain and demonstrate how to effectively make an empathic response:
   a. Identify the relevant dimensions of the child's experience.
   b. Decide what level of directness to utilize in the empathic response.
   c. Make corrections when an empathic response is inaccurate.

5. Handle special situations requiring the use of the tracking and empathic responding skills, including:
   a. What to do when children react negatively to use of the tracking skill or empathy skill.
   b. How to use empathic responding when children want to talk for extended periods rather than play.

    c. How to use tracking and empathy skills during times when children choose to play games with the therapist, including handling it when children "cheat" during games.

## The Therapeutic Purpose of the Tracking and Empathic Responding Skills

In responding to children's play, the therapist is actively attempting to create a therapeutic climate in which the child feels accepted, valued, and free to make decisions and choices. The two therapist skills of tracking and empathy are foundational to creating such an environment in the playroom. A tracking response is one in which the therapist acknowledges the child's behavior (or one or more characters in the child's role-play) in an accepting tone of voice. Tracking responses serve two therapeutic purposes. First, the child realizes that the therapist is attending to and valuing the child's activity. Second, because the tracking response is delivered with an accepting voice tone, the child recognizes that the behavior in which he is engaging is acceptable in the playroom. In short, in using tracking responses, the therapist communicates indirectly to the child: "I am present, I am valuing and accepting of what you are choosing to do, and your choices are ones that do not violate the limits of the playroom." As the recipient of the tracking response, the child experiences: "You are interested in me, you are aware of the things I am doing and are accepting of them. It is okay for me to express myself like this in here."

    An empathic response is one in which the therapist acknowledges the underlying feeling, preference, intention/motivation, belief, or relationship desire expressed in the actions of the child (or characters in the child's role-play). Empathic responses serve to make the child more aware of the emotional meaning of his play. In addition, empathic responses leave children feeling understood and often facilitate their willingness to broaden and deepen their emotional expression in play, and to be more aware of and work through the therapeutic issues present in their play. By the use of empathic responses, the therapist communicates indirectly, "I understand the meaningfulness of this play to you, and you are fully valued and accepted—even when you express sides of yourself that others might reject." As the recipient of the empathic response, the child experiences: "You deeply understand me, you help me understand myself more, you accept me—even the sides of me that others reject—and I feel safe in expressing myself in here."

In the playroom, tracking responses and empathic responses are the most frequent responses made by the therapist. Given that nearly all human behavior is motivated and emotionally meaningful, the therapist frequently will use tracking responses and empathic responses in tandem. Following are some examples in which tracking and empathic responses are used together in a single response by the therapist:

1. You are smiling (tracking) because you are happy about hitting the target (empathy).
2. You are erasing that part of your drawing (tracking) because it didn't turn out the way you wanted (empathy).

However, since it is not always possible for the therapist to be aware of the emotional meaning of the child's play, when there is significant uncertainty about the meaning of the child's play, the therapist may simply need to make a tracking response alone.

## Making Skillful Tracking Responses

Skillful use of tracking requires that the therapist consider such issues as using the proper voice tone, the pacing/frequency of responding, and avoidance of too much repetition. As mentioned previously, tracking responses involve the therapist's verbally noting the child's behaviors. In order for such responses to accomplish their therapeutic purpose, tracking responses should be made in a voice tone that reflects the energy level and emotional tone of the child. In the case of a child whose play is slow paced, subdued, and lacking much energy, the therapist's tracking responses are less frequent, softer in volume, and match the low energy and subdued emotional level of the child. However, in the case of a child who is energetically participating in a very active role-play, the therapist's responses will be more frequent and louder in volume, and will reflect some of the enthusiasm of the child.

One common mistake made by the therapist new to the CCPT model is to try to infuse more energy and enthusiasm into tracking responses than is being experienced by the child. Sometimes this may be done as an attempt by the therapist to communicate acceptance of the child, but more often is experienced as jarring and intrusive by the child. Another common mistake is for the therapist to decrease the frequency of responding and/or to fail to match the emotional tone when children are engaging in play that expresses negative emotion or has maladaptive content. For example, in a role-play, if a child decides to angrily slap a baby doll because it won't stop crying, the therapist may fail to make a tracking response or, if she does respond, may not reflect the child's anger when making the response. In short, it is important for the therapist not to respond differentially in either the quantity or quality of tracking responses made based on either the content or affect expressed in the child's play.

Another factor in the making of skillful tracking responses involves frequency/pacing. Generally, for most types of play, a frequency of four to eight tracking and/or empathic responses per minute allows for adequate communication of connection and acceptance of the child without being perceived as intrusive. However, this frequency of responding may need to be decreased for children whose play is very quiet and reserved, or in the case of children who are engaging in repetitive play for long periods of time. In making tracking responses, the therapist is not noting every behavior of the child, but simply periodically noting the child's behavior so that the child experiences the therapist as present and attentive, and so that the child perceives acceptance of his emotional expression and activities.

Finally, in using tracking responses, the therapist should be careful not to become too repetitive. Repetition can take the form of making the same response over and over: "You are hitting the bop bag . . . You are hitting the bop bag again." Alternatively, the therapist may find himself using a similar sentence structure over and over. For example, as a child is drawing a picture of a house, the therapist may respond: "You are putting a roof on the house . . . you are putting a door on the house . . . you are putting a window on the house." Too much repetition can leave the child feeling intruded upon and result in expressions of annoyance. Even slight variation of tracking responses, especially when utilized in tandem with empathy, can help transform them into vehicles for communicating welcomed attention and acceptance. For the last example, note the difference when only slight variation and empathy is used in the tracking response: "You are putting a roof on the house . . . you want to make sure there's a way to get in so you are adding a door . . . . you think it needs a window, too."

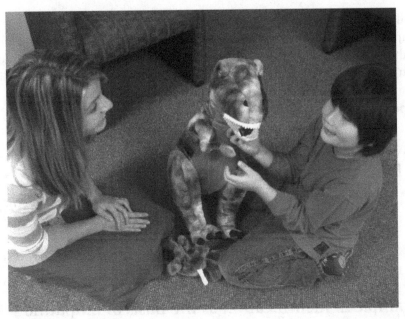

Figure 6.1

## Empathy: Foundational Skill, Foundational Attitude

As mentioned previously, the empathic skill serves to help the child feel deeply understood, which in turn supports the child's further expression and working through of therapeutic issues. In many ways, empathic responding is the most foundational of all the therapist skills in that empathic responding is an essential component of other play therapy skills, such as limits setting, responding to questions, and responding to requests/commands, and is also utilized by the therapist as children engage in role-play either alone or interactively with the therapist. These therapist skills will be discussed in later chapters.

However, empathy is much more than simply a technique or skill employed by the therapist. Empathy requires the therapist to engage in an active process of identification with the inner life of the child, and this is not truly possible without the core therapist attitudes and values of acceptance and unconditional positive regard. In its purest form, empathy embodies these values, and the therapist puts his own emotional life in service of the child through a process of identification in which the therapist actually experiences much of what the child is experiencing in her play. Although it is possible for the therapist to utilize a more passive approach to making empathic responses whereby empathic responding is approached primarily as a cognitive task of deduction, where the therapist states what he believes underlies a behavior, this will generally result in lower quality responses than would have been possible if the therapist had identified with the experience of the child.

## Example 1: Cognitive Deduction as the Basis of Empathic Response

> **CHILD:** *[Child has said that she wants to paint a picture and reaches for a jar of paint. She begins twisting the cap on the jar but is stuck; she grimaces and struggles on unsuccessfully.]*
>
> **THERAPIST:** *[Sees that the child wants the top off]* You are trying to get that paint top off so you can paint.

## Example 2: Identification as the Basis of Empathic Response

> **CHILD:** *[Same situation as above]*
>
> **COUNSELOR:** *[Through identification, the counselor's hand tightens and a slight grimace ensues as he experiences the tension experienced by the child.]* Oh . . . it's on so tight! You really are trying to get it off but it just won't budge. But you are determined to keep on trying because you really want to paint.

It should be noted that this active process of identification is not easy for the counselor to maintain all the time, and a lapse into empathy as a cognitive task or technique is inevitable. However, it is helpful for the counselor to be aware of this distinction.

## Five Possible Dimensions of Empathic Responses

Five different dimensions of the child's experience serve as the focus of the therapist's empathic responses: feelings, likes/dislikes/preferences, intentions/motivation, beliefs, and desires for relationships.

### Example 1: Feelings as Focus of an Empathic Response

> **CHILD:** *[Runs into the playroom; sees her favorite toy, a doll; and cheers.]* It's still here!

THERAPIST: *You are so happy to see it is still here so you can play with it again.*

*Example 2: Likes/Dislikes/Preferences as Focus of an Empathic Response*

CHILD: *[Begins to draw a picture of a house. Starts to draw the door, frowns, erases it, and starts over again.]*

COUNSELOR: *That didn't turn out quite like you liked, so you are going to try it again.*

*Example 3: Intentions/Motivations as Focus of an Empathic Response*

CHILD: *[Child is coloring a picture and does so slowly and deliberately, using her other hand to make sure that she does not stray outside the boundaries of the drawing.]*

THERAPIST: *You are trying really hard to stay within the lines as you color.*

*Example 4: Beliefs as Focus of an Empathic Response*

CHILD: *[While doing a solitary role-play involving two squirrels, one squirrel is asked to divide a pile of nuts but is clearly putting more nuts into his pile than in the pile of the other squirrel. Child is adopting the role of the squirrel with fewer nuts in his pile.] Hey! You are taking more nuts!*

COUNSELOR: *He doesn't think it's fair for the other squirrel to get more. He's pretty upset about that.*

*Example 5: Desire for Relationship as the Focus of an Empathic Response*
Although children's desire for relationship are sometimes expressed directly, as in the case of a child who suddenly hugs the therapist, in many cases desire for relationship is expressed more subtly and is mixed with other dimensions of the child's experience.

CHILD: *[Finishes her drawing, jumps up, and runs toward the therapist with a big grin on her face.]*

THERAPIST: *You are coming over here because you want me to see what you drew. [Desire for relationship dimension] You are proud of it! [Feeling dimension]*

After careful review of the preceding examples, you will see that in most cases the child's experience actually contains a combination of expressions of feelings, likes/dislikes/preferences, intentions/motivations, beliefs, and desires for relationships and that empathic responses often focus on more than one dimension of the child's experience. In cases where such complexity is clearly present, the therapist need not worry that they have to identify all such dimensions of the child's experience in their empathic response. Making an empathic response that captures one or two dimensions of the child's experience is preferred to becoming excessively wordy. If a given empathic response does not quite capture the child's experience, the child will generally clarify this either verbally or through additional play.

*Example: Child's Clarification in Response to Empathic Response*

> **CHILD:** *[In the child's role-play, a mommy leaves its baby behind, and the baby begins to cry; a male stranger passing by picks the baby up and begins to feed it.] Here baby, you must be hungry. Here's a bottle. [The baby stops crying.]*
>
> **THERAPIST:** *The stranger stopped to help the baby. He's feeding the baby so it won't be hungry.*
>
> **CHILD:** *Yeah, the baby feels a little better, but he still wants his mom.*
>
> **THERAPIST:** *The baby misses his mom and is hoping she comes back.*

## Table 6.1   Five Types of Empathic Statements

1. Identifying feelings:
   "You are happy you won the game."
   "The squirrel is mad at the chipmunk for taking his nuts."

2. Identifying preferences and desires:
   "You want me to have the red car and you to have the yellow one."
   "You wish there were more blue paint."

3. Identifying intentions, motivations, and effort:
   "You are trying really hard to get those dominoes to stay up."
   "You are aiming carefully so you can hit the target."

4. Identifying knowledge and beliefs:
   "You know the rules of the game 'Go Fish.'"
   "You don't think teachers should yell at kids."

5. Acknowledging relationship:
   "You want to show me your drawing."
   "You are sad that I won't come to your birthday party."
   "The baby misses his mom and wants her to come home."

## Making Skillful Empathic Responses

As mentioned previously, the most skillful empathic responses will generally occur when the counselor engages in a process of identification with the child and her experiences. Indeed, through identification with the child, empathic responses seem almost to come automatically and effortlessly. However, counselors new to the CCPT methodology often have to practice the more deliberative, deductive, and technique-oriented approach to making empathic responses first. It is important to note that even the best play therapists fail to engage in identification with the child's experience all the time. It is even more important to note that even when empathic responding is used as a technique, rather than as a form of identification, it can accomplish the therapeutic goals of the child's feeling deeply understood and facilitating the child's expression and therapeutic work.

Components of making a skillful empathic response include identifying the relevant dimensions of the child's experience, deciding what level of directness should be used in making the empathic response, making the empathic response, and responding to the child's correction of the counselor's empathic response.

## Identifying the Relevant Dimensions of the Child's Experience

The first step in making an effective empathic response is to identify the important feelings, likes/dislikes/preferences, intention/motivations, beliefs, and desire for relationship expressed in the child's play. It is important for the therapist to realize that access to the child's experience can occur through observation of the child's behavior and verbal statements by the child (with the accompanying voice tone communicating important information), as well as by nonverbal communication such as the facial expression of the child. For example, while drawing a picture, a child may frown (nonverbal facial expression) and say, "That's not it" (verbal expression), and then erase a part of the picture and redraw it (behavioral expression). Any of the three forms of expression may result in the therapist's saying, "You don't like how that turned out."

## Deciding What Level of Directness to Use in the Empathic Response

Given that the true test of an empathic response is whether it is instantly accepted by the child as part of his experience and results in a feeling of being understood, it is important for the therapist to capture the expression of the child in a manner that does not leave the child feeling shame, guilt, or defensiveness. For example, the child may say: "I hate my mom!" The therapist has a wide range of possible empathic responses, ranging from direct to indirect ones:

"You hate your mom." (very direct)

"You are really mad at your mom." (moderately direct)

"You are upset with your mom." (less direct)

"You don't like some of the things your mom does." (much less direct)

Given that the criteria for a successful empathy resides in the child in that the empathic response must be accepted by the child and leave the child feeling understood, the goal of the therapist is to choose the level of directness that will not be rejected by the child. In most cases the therapist can make an empathic response that is similar in directness as that made by the child, but the therapist needs to be open to correction by the child. For example:

> CHILD: *I am very, very mad at my mom!*
> THERAPIST: *You are very mad at her.*
> CHILD: *No, I am not super mad.*
> THERAPIST: *You are not very mad, but you don't like some of the things she does.*
> CHILD: *Right.*

From this example it can be seen that although the child may in "reality" be very angry at his mom, it is the task of the therapist to capture the experience of the child in a way that is not threatening. In this case the therapist may have been accurate in his assessment of the child's feelings of anger, but his first response, although seemingly close to the child's level of directness of expression, was not perceived by the child as an empathic response. Fortunately, most of the time, if the therapist stays close to the level of directness expressed by the child, it will be accepted by the child. But it is important for the therapist to remain open to correction.

In addition to the issue of what level of emotional directness the therapist should use in empathic responses, another issue of directness emerges related to whom the therapist should attribute the emotion to when the child is engaging in role play. For example, consider the following scenario. In role-play, a child assigns herself the role of a "sassy child" and gives the therapist the role of a schoolteacher; then the child in role says, "You are a stupid teacher!" Which of the following empathic responses should the therapist make?

**Choice 1:** "You are angry at me and are telling me I am really dumb."

**Choice 2:** "The student is angry at the teacher and telling her she is really dumb."

We believe that when a child chooses to engage in a role-play, she is trying to create some psychological safety by distancing herself from the direct expression of her feelings. Therefore, we would opt for respecting this distance by assigning the emotional expression to the characters in the role-play rather than to the child herself (e.g., Choice 2).

## Making the Empathic Response

In making an empathic response, the counselor should match the general emotional tone of the child's expression in a way that shows acceptance of the child's experience, but not to such an extent that the child believes or experiences the response as being a self-expression of the counselor. For example, if the child expresses feeling sadness about leaving early, the counselor captures this in her voice tone as she says, "You are really sad our time is over for today," but without giving the impression that the counselor is expressing sadness. To do this, the counselor identifies for herself what emotion is being experienced by the child, then in her empathic response decreases the intensity of the emotion and clearly assigns the emotion to the child.

Much as with tracking responses, the therapist should avoid differentially responding to positive experiences of the child compared to those when the child expresses anger, urges to hurt or control others, or to get revenge. For example, a common mistake of beginning play therapists is to acknowledge the child's joy at the completion of a drawing, but not the child's clear joy upon getting revenge on an enemy in role-play.

In making the empathic response itself, we suggest that you make empathic statements, without using qualifiers such as "It seems to me that . . . " or "What I hear you saying. . . . " We also recommend that you avoid putting a questioning tone in your voice when making empathic responses.

**Not:** "It seems to me you are mad about what he did."

**Instead:** "You are mad at what he did."

**Not:** "What I hear you saying is that you don't like it when our playtime is over."

**Instead:** "You don't like it when our playtime is over."

**Not:** "You want me to see what you drew?"

**Instead:** "You want me to see what you drew!"

Some therapists prefer to make more indirect empathic statements because they may be concerned about being perceived as forcefully imposing experiences on the child or concerned about the possibility that they are incorrect. We believe that these dangers are minimized if the therapist is in a mode of identification with the child while making empathic responses, and if the therapist simply refrains from making empathic responses when considerable doubt about the child's experiences exists.

In addition, we believe there are distinct advantages of being more direct in empathic responses. First, we believe that the use of more directness in empathic statements avoids calling attention to the therapist. Phrases like "It seems to me that . . . " or "What I hear you saying is . . . " are actually self-expressions of the therapist. Since self-expression is not really part of the CCPT model or therapist skill sets (with the exception of when limits need to be set), we believe it is more consistent with the basic child-centered principles to avoid such indirect statements. Second, indirect empathic statements, such as, "It seems to me that you are feeling mad," can sometimes be experienced by children as an implied question to which children may feel obliged to respond and which can pull the child away from the intense focus of their play. In summary, we believe there are advantages to using more direct rather than indirect empathic responses, and any dangers that may exist with being more direct can be minimized.

It is important to note again that an empathic response does not merely consist of words. As was mentioned previously, a skillful empathic response matches the emotional tone and energy level of the child. But beyond this, because an empathic response emerges from a process of identification with the child, some aspects of empathic responding are even nonverbal. For example, as the child's face bursts with joy upon hitting a target with a dart, a smile also appears on the therapist's face as the therapist experiences the joy of the child.

# Accepting Children's Corrections to Empathic Responses

The final step in making an empathic response is for the therapist to be nondefensive and instantly open to correction by the child. Although the therapist should generally have a relatively high level of certainty about the child's experience before making either a tracking or empathic response, all therapists will fail at times to either accurately or fully capture the child's experience. Corrections by the child should be viewed positively as opportunities to be more effective in our therapeutic work. When a child corrects an empathic response, the therapist should first acknowledge that the initial response did not match the experience of the child, and make a revised empathic response that better captures the child's experience. The therapist need not apologize, since this would be a self-expression of the therapist and might result in the child's being reluctant to make further corrections in the future since the initial correction to the therapist could be seen as bringing remorse to the therapist. Here are some examples of how the therapist could skillfully handle corrections.

> **CHILD:** *That squirrel took the rabbit's carrots and ate them!*
> **THERAPIST:** *He's a bad squirrel! He took the rabbit's carrots and ate them all up!*
> **CHILD:** *He's not really a bad squirrel; he just wanted some food.*
> **THERAPIST:** *He is not bad, just hungry.*

Earlier, we pointed out that at times empathic responding can have nonverbal elements. We recall an example when our mentor, Louise Guerney, made a correction to an error in empathic responding without saying a single word! In a role-play, a child she was working with was elaborately going through a list of items she could use to make sure that no one separated her and Louise. The little girl stated how a knife could be used to fight bad people and a rope could be used to tie them together so they could not be separated. The child then took a pair of sticks and used a rope to tie the sticks together criss-crossed at a right angle. The child then announced with great confidence and a smile on her face, "If everything else fails, this will keep us together." Louise empathically responded, "Even if nothing else works, those sticks will keep us together." The child's face suddenly displayed a combination of disappointment and outright anger. She said, "STICKS!! That's a cross!" Without a single second of hesitation, and without uttering a single word, Louise turned to the cross and bowed reverently. The little girl's face beamed with joy again. It was as if the mistaken empathic response had never been uttered, and she immediately carried on with her role-play. We recount this story because it so clearly illustrates that an empathic response is not just a technique but a process of identification with the child, and that it is the therapist's whole person and not simply words that convey empathy.

Now that we have covered the elements of making a skilled empathic response, we want to give you an opportunity to practice. Then we will finish up by talking about some situations in which making tracking and empathic responses are especially challenging for therapists.

## Practice Activity for Tracking and Empathic Responding

For the following child experiences, identify which of the five dimensions (feeling, like/dislike/preference, intention/motivation, belief, or desire for relationship) appear to be present. Some statements may have more than one dimension present. Then give a possible empathic response for each.

1. Child spends 20 seconds aiming the gun at a target and fires, missing. "Darn! I missed the stupid target."
2. Child is looking through the crayon box, checking each one out until she spots the green one, smiles, and then starts to use it to color the picture of a frog she drew.
3. Child is playing ring toss with the therapist. "You should stand further back because you are bigger than me."
4. The therapist announces that the play session is over for the day; the child runs and frantically puts her arms around the therapist's legs. In a whining voice, she says, "Our time can't be over yet!"
5. The child sets up a role-play in a dollhouse. He has a mom shout at the baby. "You be quiet and stop your crying right now or you won't get any dinner!"

Answers and suggested responses can be found in **Skills Support Resource B** at the end of the book.

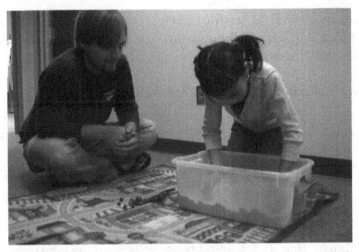

Figure 6.2

## Special Situations Requiring the Use of the Tracking and Empathic Responding

There are a number of special situations regarding tracking and empathic responding that arise during play sessions that require skillful responses by the counselor. These include the child's reacting negatively to the use of tracking and empathy, the need for the extended use of empathy when children want to talk about their lives, and how to use empathy when children want to play interactive games.

### Special Situation 1: The Child Begins to React to the Use of Tracking and Empathy

Even when the counselor observes proper pacing of responses and avoids undue repetition, the child may react to the use of tracking and empathic responses. This reaction may range from curiosity to annoyance. In either case, the best response is for the counselor to respond empathically to the child. In the case where the child is becoming annoyed, the counselor should follow up the use of empathy toward the child's annoyance with a decrease in frequency of tracking and empathic responses for a period of time. For the remainder of the session, the counselor may find it prudent to focus less on making tracking responses (which target behavior) and instead make empathic responses (which target feelings, preferences, intentions, motivations, and relationship), since children who are sensitive to tracking responses tend to be less reactive to empathic responses.

*Example 1: Curiosity in Response to Tracking and Empathy.*

> CHILD: *You are always saying the things that I do. How come?*
> COUNSELOR: *You think I talk a lot different than other people, and you are wondering why.*
> CHILD: *Yeah, like you are trying to repeat what I do. [Child returns to play.]*

*Example 2*

> CHILD: *Quit it! You keep saying the things I am doing.*
> COUNSELOR: *You don't like that.*
> CHILD: *NO! You stop it.*
> COUNSELOR: *[Remains quiet; decreases frequency of tracking and empathic responses with more focus on empathic responses.]*

## Special Situation 2: The Need for Extended Empathy When Children Want to Talk to the Therapist about Their Life

Although certainly allowed, most children will not choose to talk about their problems directly in the playroom, but instead will use play to work through their therapeutic issues. In the CCPT model, when children desire to talk about their life, the therapist moves to a sustained and disciplined use of empathic responding, and avoids getting into a mutual dialogue where the therapist self-discloses or asks questions of the child. Staying true to the CCPT methodology can be very difficult when children begin to talk with us, since it might seem like a "teachable" moment and thus create a temptation to ask questions, self-disclose, give advice, or teach a skill. However, if we do not stay true to the model in such moments, the child may become confused and defensive since our role as therapist has become unpredictable. In some cases, it may be that the only reason the child was comfortable in speaking directly to us about their life was because they felt secure that we would not start to ask probing questions or give advice, which can easily communicate that we are judging or attempting to change the child. In short, we strongly suggest not switching to a more "verbal" therapy simply because the child chooses to talk more directly about his problems. In cases in which the child says something about events in his everyday life that require further exploration or action by the therapist (e.g., disclosure by the child of physical/sexual abuse or suicidal ideation/intent), we recommend that the therapist leave such discussion for after the play session has ended. In some cases, the play session may need to be ended early to allow time for such dialogue to occur, but we recommend careful maintenance of boundaries between the time for therapeutic work and the time for other necessary clinical activities. Following is an example of the extended use of empathy when a child begins to speak about his life:

> CHILD: *[In a role-play in which a mama bird gives more nuts to one baby bird than another. The child's voice becomes slightly sad.] My mom's like that, too; she always gives more things to my sister.*
>
> THERAPIST: *You believe she treats your sister better and you feel sad about that.*
>
> CHILD: *[With some anger in his voice] It's not fair! And when I do something wrong, she screams at me and punishes me . . . punishes me a lot! But when my sister gets caught doing something, almost nothing happens.*
>
> THERAPIST: *You feel pretty mad at your mom because you believe she unfairly treats you harsher.*
>
> CHILD: *[With clear sadness] Yes, sometimes I wonder if she loves me or even wants me around.*
>
> THERAPIST: *You feel really sad because at times you don't feel loved by her. And you feel worried that sometimes she doesn't seem to like being around you.*
>
> CHILD: *[Clearly anxious] She may send me to live with my dad.*
>
> THERAPIST: *You really don't want that to happen. You want to live with your mom.*
>
> CHILD: *Yes, I wish we could just get along.*
>
> THERAPIST: *You would really like things to be better between the two of you.*

In such situations, the purpose of using extended empathy is to assist the child in exploring and expressing himself around the important issues in his life. It is not for the therapist to use questions to get the child to go deeper into the issue than the child himself initiates, to challenge the reality base to the child's feelings/beliefs, or to help the child solve problems more directly through advice giving or social skills training.

## Special Situation 3: Using Empathy When Children Play Games and When They "Cheat" During Games Play

Another common situation that occurs in play therapy is children wanting to interact with the counselor through playing a game. The child may create a tic-tac-toe board on a piece of paper, want to test the counselor's skills through a target-shooting contest with a dart gun, play ring toss, or play a card game. Such situations require the disciplined use of empathy by the counselor because there can be a tendency for the counselor to become so involved in the game that she begins to focus more on the game play and fails to capture the child's experiences through good tracking and empathic responses. To avoid this pitfall, we offer the following suggestions.

First, the counselor should enter the process of games play with neither a desire nor intention to win or lose. So, if the child asks the counselor to play a game of target shooting with a dart gun, the counselor should neither deliberately try to miss the target so the child can win, nor should the counselor give her full attention to applying all her skills. The net result is that the counselor can be more aware of the child and less personally involved with the game. In many cases, such an approach will decrease the intrinsic advantage, if any, that the counselor may have as an adult, but it still is not a deliberate attempt to lose and should not appear so to the child.

Second, when the counselor is involved in games play with the child, she should always be focused on the child's experience or reaction to the game, both the child's reaction to his own performance and his reaction to the counselor's performance. Unlike games play outside the playroom, the counselor should not self-express about her own performance or evaluate the child's performance.

> CHILD: *I hit the bull's-eye the very first time. I can't believe it!*
>
> COUNSELOR: *You are surprised and happy that you hit it after just one shot. [Counselor shoots and hits a lower score area than the child. Counselor observes child's reaction to his shot, but does not evaluate his own shot or express self.]*
>
> CHILD: *Ha! You got a really low score compared to me. I am going to win!*
>
> COUNSELOR: *You want me to know that you were a better shot than me. You are happy because you think you are sure to win.*

Another challenging situation that comes up in games play is when children "cheat" during games. It is important that the counselor not take such behavior personally, but instead recognize it as a way for the child to work through issues of control and the desire to feel competent and effective. When the counselor encounters "cheating" behavior, it is important that the counselor track the behavior of the child and use empathy to make the child aware of the feeling or motivation underlying the "cheating" behavior, rather than confronting or limiting such behavior. Inevitably, children in play therapy become more socialized and able to comply with social norms; however, such learning occurs not through social skills training or confrontation in play sessions, but through personality development in the areas of self-expression, self-understanding, and self-control, which are fostered by the therapeutic relationship.

> **CHILD:** *[Playing ring toss; after missing the first time, she moves the ring peg closer.]*
> **COUNSELOR:** *You have decided to move it closer so it's easier to make.*
> **CHILD:** *[The child tosses the ring and makes it.] Yippee! I made it.*
> **COUNSELOR:** *You are so happy about making it!*
> **CHILD:** *Yes. And if you don't get a point next turn, I win the game! You will never make it!*
> **COUNSELOR:** *You really want to win and you hope I don't get a point.*
> **CHILD:** *[Smiles and moves the ring toss peg all the way across the room.]*
> **COUNSELOR:** *You are moving the peg way over there. You want to make sure that I don't make it because you want to win.*
> **CHILD:** *[The counselor tosses the ring and it is headed toward the ring, but unlikely to go on the peg; nonetheless, the child, standing near the peg, steps in front of the peg and knocks the ring down.]*
> **COUNSELOR:** *You are making sure there is no chance for me to score so you can be sure to win. You just swatted my toss down!*
> **CHILD:** *[The child smiles.] I win! I am the best.*
> **COUNSELOR:** *It feels good to you to be the winner.*

## Concluding Thoughts

Tracking and empathic responding are core skills that are among the most frequent responses made by the child-centered play therapist. Making skillful tracking and empathic responses involves active recognition with the experience of the child, proper pacing and tone of voice, correct level of directness, avoidance of repetition, and willingness to accept any corrections made by the child. Skillful tracking and empathic responding conveys to the child, "I'm right here with you, buddy." By honing these core skills, the therapist is helped to *not go ahead or lag behind* as the child takes the lead in therapy.

## Activities and Resources for Further Study

### Activity A: Practice Activity for Tracking and Empathic Responding

For the following child experiences, identify which of the five dimensions (feeling, like/dislike/preference, intention/motivation, belief, or desire for relationship) appear to be present. Some statements may have more than one dimension present. Then give a possible empathic response for each.

1. Child spends 20 seconds aiming the gun at a target and fires, missing. "Darn! I missed the stupid target."
2. Child is looking through the crayon box, checking each one out until she spots the green one, smiles, and then starts to use it to color the picture of a frog she drew.
3. Child is playing ring toss with the therapist. "You should stand further back because you are bigger than me."
4. The therapist announces that the play session is over for the day; the child runs and frantically puts her arms around the therapist's legs. In a whining voice, she says, "Our time can't be over yet!"
5. The child sets up a role-play in a dollhouse. He has a mom shout at the baby. "You be quiet and stop your crying right now or you won't get any dinner!"

Answers and suggested empathic responses can be found in **Skills Support Resource B** at the end of the book.

### Activity B: Mock Session Practice of Tracking and Empathic Responding

An excellent way to develop your skills for service to children is to practice with a partner in mock sessions. Take turns in the roles of child and therapist. You will find that you'll learn from the role of the child, therapist, or, if you have the extra opportunity, as observer. We find 15 minutes to be a reasonable length for mock sessions. Longer sessions allow more time for practice, but it can get difficult to sustain the role of the child for very long periods. You can limit yourselves to small sets of representative toys at a table or expand to a playroom. If you can establish mock sessions to follow most chapters, try to stay with the same partner to see how your relationship develops. The following practice set instructions can be taken together or separately:

- Engage in a 15-minute mock session in which the person in the role of the child provides you with opportunities to respond within the steady mode of tracking with empathy. Stop and allow the person in the role of the child to give feedback. Ask your partner how it *felt to be in the role of the child* in the mock interaction. Switch roles and repeat this exercise, with you now playing the role of the child and your partner tracking with empathy.

## Activity C: Return to and Review the Primary Skill Objectives

Revisit the Primary Skill Objectives for this chapter and see if you have mastered them to your satisfaction at this time. If not, seek additional readings, practices, and discussions for clarification and in order to master them to your satisfaction.

# Creating an Optimum Environment for Therapy through Structuring and Limit Setting

*Providing a framework doesn't take away children's individuality. In fact, structure generally helps them to be more free because it provides boundaries. It's like a fence that offers security for what can happen inside the enclosure. It can be very frightening for a child not to have limits. Not only can the world outside be frightening, but the world inside, the world of feelings, can also be scary when you're not sure you can manage those feelings by yourself.*

—*Fred Rogers, better known as "Mr. Rogers"*

## Application Focus Issue

Imagine little Gina painting at the easel. After having begun nervously, she is warming up to self-expression, beginning to paint with vigor and excitement. A little paint accidentally splatters beyond the easel and onto the wall. She smiles—a little inward smile—and tilts her head as if she has an idea. Her brush dips lightly into the rich red paint. She lifts her brush and, after taking a quick sideways glance at you, splatters a little paint on the wall! Smiling broadly now, Gina dips her brush deeply into the purple paint, and looks to you expectantly. . . .

Seeing her stance and her facial expression, you have a good idea what's coming next. But what do you do? She's been so restricted, she *needs* to self-express. You have hoped and waited for her to let herself go, to begin to express herself freely and strongly. And you know that she must find her way—that it will never have the same "oomph" and satisfaction, never be as effective if *you* tell her how *she* should express herself. But you can see where this is going. If she can do "almost anything," what she wants to do now is splatter the playroom wall with colorful paints. A bright idea indeed, but it will take *forever* to clean it—if it can be cleaned. What do you do? How do you create an atmosphere where she can self-express with freedom and abandon, but in a manner that is acceptable? How can you find a way to let her freely self-express, to do "almost anything," without her choices being so worrisome as to negatively affect your empathy, genuineness, and unconditional positive regard? Preparing you for such situations and questions is the goal of this chapter.

## Chapter Overview and Summary

In child-centered play therapy (CCPT), limit setting allows the child to feel secure and remain physically safe during sessions. In addition, limit setting may be used for structural purposes and to limit purposeful destruction of materials that cannot be easily replaced. While the therapist acknowledges and shows acceptance of the child's desire to cross a particular limit, the therapist also allows the child the opportunity to control the impulse to cross the limit. In general, this means that the child is given the opportunity to reject the limit imposed and repeat the behavior or find an alternative. The limit-setting process involves a three-step delivery process—the "empathy sandwich" in which the therapist acknowledges and values the child's motivations for engaging in the behavior that requires a limit through empathy. The therapist states the limit in a firm, yet warm and nonthreatening manner, and the child's reaction to the limit being set is acknowledged empathically. In cases where the child does not alter his behavior, and persists in the behavior for which the limit has been set, the therapist informs the child of the consequences, and enforces the consequences when necessary. This informing of consequences and resulting reactions are also delivered with empathy and in a calm, nonthreatening manner.

This chapter explains and demonstrates how, through structuring and limit setting, the therapist creates an optimum environment for the child to self-express and develop self-control as needed. Additionally, this chapter illustrates how structuring and limits set with empathy in CCPT allow for more freedom of expression in play therapy, rather than less. When a therapist is skilled in structuring and limit setting, he is better able to feel secure and maintain consistent acceptance and unconditional positive regard for the child in CCPT. When a child feels this safety, she can then experience self-expression in play to the fullest—with all the feelings and behaviors involved—without fear of criticism or need for repression.

## Primary Skill Objectives

The following Primary Skill Objectives for this chapter are provided to guide you through the chapter and for reflection and review after completing the chapter reading and exercises. By reading and working through the chapter exercises, you will be better able to:

1. Illustrate how limits in CCPT assure safety for the child, therapist, and playroom equipment, and promote the child's development of self-responsibility and emotional regulation.

2. Explain what is implied by the opening statement for CCPT about the structure of CCPT, including what is said and not said, and the meaning of the simplicity of the statement.

3. Demonstrate the correct delivery of the "empathy sandwich" in CCPT, and explain why therapist self-awareness and ability to attend, listen, and convey empathy is vital during this three-step delivery process.

4. Describe the qualities for voice tone, body posture, proximity, and movements, and the demeanor of the child-centered play therapist in limit setting.

5. Explain the role of limit setting for play therapist congruence—for remaining warm and accepting of the child's self-expression while also conveying limits in a clear and absolute manner.

6. Demonstrate limit-setting skills across a range of realistic CCPT scenarios, and general structuring skills across a range of realistic CCPT scenarios.

7. Explain the benefits (flexibility, emotional regulation, and empowerment) that result from allowing the child to come up with alternative behaviors vs. targeting alternative behaviors for the child after a limit is set.

8. Describe common mistakes that play therapists make when attempting to balance permissiveness and freedom to self-express (or freedom to be) with necessary limits.

9. Describe common problems of play therapists in structuring play sessions and setting limits, and avenues for overcoming those problems.

10. Describe the significance of structuring around the ending phase of CCPT (process of termination) for the child, and the importance of assessing for when the child is ready for a "countdown" of CCPT sessions.

## Introductory Notes: The Value of Structuring and Limits to Enhance Autonomy and Self-Regulation

Adults self-limit their behavior based on perceived rules; expectations of normal behavior and social acceptance; assumed societal or other consequences; and desires for mutual kindness, consideration, and fairness from others. Children are in the process of learning about societal rules and developing internal guides for limiting their behaviors. While established "rules" for behaviors and moral teachings provide an external guide for children, our societal norms and early schooling tend to rely heavily on external guides, while forgetting that children have within them *powerful internal resources* that, if nurtured, will help them develop self-regulation (emotional regulation) and autonomy necessary for growth and a strong sense of self-efficacy and esteem. CCPT, including skills for limit setting and structuring, nurtures and grows the child's capacity and motivation to self-regulate. In this chapter, we address the reasons for and methods of limit setting in CCPT, as well as the details of the parameters of the playroom and general structuring skills of CCPT.

## The Established Limits of CCPT

We know from Virginia Axline's historic work, *Play Therapy*, that the eighth principle states that limits are used to "anchor the therapy to the world of reality" and to make the child aware of his or her responsibility to the relationship (1969, p. 128). For instance, in life, it is rarely allowable to physically attack another person or physically hurt oneself, nor is it allowed to purposely destroy property. Additionally, limits are used to make self-expression safe for the child, to create an atmosphere in which he is free to experiment, while a caring, understanding, deeply

Table 7.1  **The Opening Statement to CCPT**

"[Child's name], this is a special room. In here you may say anything you want, and you may do almost anything you want. If there is something you may not do, I will let you know."

accepting adult connects with him and monitors and maintains his safety. For these reasons and others to follow, the standard areas of behavior that are off limits in CCPT include harm to self, harm to others, and damage to the toys and equipment of the playroom. While these established "limits" are provided whenever necessary, it is also important to remember that the eighth principle states that "limits are minimal" and, therefore, it is imperative that the provided space, time, and adult therapist be prepared to offer as free, accepting, and *open* an experience as possible to the child. So, before we delve into the methods and details of limiting behaviors in CCPT, we need to first consider the importance of the *atmosphere* created with the opening statement of CCPT—what is allowed, and how a child first encounters the concept of CCPT. What message is conveyed from the therapist to the child from the very beginning, and why is it imperative to remain true to this message?

## Structuring Begins With the Simple Opening Message to the Child

Based on commonly accepted best practices for classroom teaching and other areas of child care and child guidance, one might expect that the established limits of CCPT or some "basic rules" would be set before therapy begins. However, while limits and structure are necessary for therapy to occur, limits or "rules" should not be mentioned before the need for them arises. In therapy, there is very little advantage to beginning the counseling relationship by telling the child what is prohibited, and this establishment of "rules" may serve to challenge some highly resistant or aggressive children to act out, or inhibit more submissive or perfectionist children from engaging in free play and self-expression. Indeed, the very word *rules*, for most children, only serves to create defensive behavior and distancing from the therapist. Therefore, we maintain that it is best to not use the word *rules*, even when limits are necessary.

The opening statement in CCPT serves to create awareness for the child that the playroom is an optimum environment for *self-generated activity and self-expression*. The statement begins to convey to the child that it is okay to make his or her own decisions in the playroom, and it is used to open the first play therapy session. The statement must also convey to the child that the therapist will establish boundaries when needed. The statement is clear, simple, and may be discontinued after the first few sessions or once it becomes apparent that the child has an understanding of this general structure of the play therapy session. The statement is as follows:

> Shayla, this is a special room. In here, you may say anything you want, and you may do almost anything you want. If there is something you may not do, I will let you know.

Structuring begins with this simple, yet meaningful message to the child; in a sense it is a promise made, and therefore requires that the therapist is prepared to remain true to the message.

## The Meaning of the Simple Opening Statement in Helping the Child to Take the Lead From the Very Beginning in CCPT Sessions

Learning to use and then remain true to this *simple* opening statement is a challenge for many beginning play therapists; however, with experience, therapists learn that children are better able to *take the lead* in therapy when the structuring is simple, understandable, and as nondirective as possible. In order to convey that the experience is *open to the child's first decision*, it is also not recommended that the play therapist try to alleviate the child's or her own anxiety by adding to this statement in any way in attempts to "help" the child get started. It is best, instead, to begin with simple tracking and empathic responding statements that attend to where the child leads—how he or she responds—following this initial opening statement.

Upon hearing the opening statement, most children begin to explore the playroom. Consider the following beginning scenario as an example:

> COUNSELOR: *Shayla, this is a special room. In here, you may say anything you want, and you may do* almost *anything you want. If there is something you may not do, I will let you know.*

good opening

SHAYLA: *[Nine-year-old Shayla moves about the room slowly, looking from toy to toy. She picks some up and holds them close in front of her face to investigate them. Her face conveys that some she likes (finds interesting) and some she doesn't like (finds strange or boring)].*

COUNSELOR: *You are seeing what's here. Some things are interesting to you, and some not so interesting.*

SHAYLA: *My baby sister would like this. [She holds a baby doll up, then quickly puts it back down.]*

COUNSELOR: *The baby doll is something your baby sister would like.*

SHAYLA: *She sure would—she'd like a lot of this stuff. [Shayla approaches the art table.] I like painting mostly . . . or drawing.*

COUNSELOR: *Painting and drawing are things you like to do. . . .*

SHAYLA: *Uh-huh, so . . . can I use these things? [Shayla points to the paints and brushes.]*

COUNSELOR: *You're thinking you'd like to use the paints. In here, you can do almost anything you like.*

SHAYLA: *Okay . . . I'm gonna paint then. [Shayla sits down at the art table and opens a set of watercolors.]*

## Why Not to Use the Word *Play* in the Opening Statement

Perhaps ironically, the introduction to CCPT need not mention the word *play*. To some older children, the notion of play may actually be inhibiting, as that child may worry that if he plays he will look silly. Or for a very serious-minded or pseudo-mature child—a child who, as the expression goes, is "5 going on 40"—the very notion of play may seem threatening, especially in the beginning, to her serious, no-nonsense view of life. In these cases, the use of the word *play* may serve to set up an expectation or perceived directive. Inclusion of a wide variety of therapeutic toys, drama, music, and art supplies—suitable for children from ages 3 to 12—are sufficient to indicate to the child that "play is accepted here." In cases of older children and pseudo-mature children, we have commonly found that initial rejection of toys and play is often the necessary beginning in therapy for such children, and by no means indicates that these children will not eventually choose to engage in spontaneous, self-expressive play as therapy progresses. Also, as an important reminder to the therapist, it helps to understand that what constitutes "play" differs from child to child. It would therefore be helpful to remember a quote from another historic work, *Play in*

*Childhood*, by Margaret Lowenfield. In this book, Lowenfield defines play as all activities "that are spontaneous and self-generating, that are ends in themselves, and that are unrelated to 'lessons' or the normal physiological needs of the child" (Lowenfield, 1935).

In the beginning sessions of CCPT, the therapist must be able to attend with empathy, moment by moment, thereby allowing the child to discover and use his individual "voice" within. From our experience in practice and supervision of CCPT, we have found that because play is a natural mode of self-expression for children, what is most commonly the case is that children move very quickly into spontaneous play and art activity when a child-centered therapist, toys, and supplies are available. However, a child's "play" is *whatever* self-generated activity she finds self-expressive and healing. The quality, intensity, style, and symbolism of the child's activity and self-expression change and develop continually, as we will discuss further in Chapter 10. It is the therapist's role, *from the beginning introductory statement on,* to offer an open and accepting atmosphere or, in the words of Axline, "good growing ground" for the child "to be" (Axline, 1969, p. 16).

## Established Parameters of the Playroom and Structuring Statement Skills

Consistent structuring and established parameters of the playroom help the child to feel secure and make CCPT more efficient. As will be discussed in more detail in Chapter 9, in general, any question asked by the child that concerns structure or boundaries should first include acknowledgment of the child's feeling or motivation behind the question. Some consistent parameters are that the CCPT session has a time limit (usually 50 minutes) and the therapist tells the child when there are 5 minutes left, and then when there is 1 minute left. Toys stay in the room, and the child is not allowed to bring toys of his own into the playroom. Art projects (paintings, drawings, and objects the child makes of clay) may be taken with the child. An exception to taking artwork would be in the case that the child's creation would be provocative to the parent or teacher; for example, if the artwork had violent themes or profane language written on it. Unless the child has toileting problems, or it is apparent that an additional trip to the bathroom is needed, the child may leave once for a bathroom break. If a water fountain is available outside the playroom, the child may leave the session once for a drink of water. These structural limits ensure that the therapy time not become a continual coming and going, which may happen especially in the early stages of rapport building. Common questions that children ask that will require structuring include asking about what is permissible in the playroom, asking about temporal and spatial boundaries, questions about the reason the child is coming to therapy, and questions about boundaries of the relationship. The following section covers some common child questions along with a short structuring statement for each.

> CHILD: *Can I play with this Play-Doh?*
> THERAPIST: *You'd like to play with the Play-Doh. You can choose and play with any of the toys you want to in here.*
> CHILD: *Can I leave early today?*
> THERAPIST: *You're wondering if it's okay to leave early. You may leave early, but if you do, our playtime will be over until next week.*
> CHILD: *Can I say bad words in here?*
> THERAPIST: *You're not sure if it's okay to say bad words while you're in here. In here, you can say anything you want to.*
> CHILD: *Can we go outside to play?*
> THERAPIST: *You'd like to play outside, but we stay in this room for our playtime.*
> CHILD: *Can I go potty?*
> THERAPIST: *You may leave special playtime once to go to the bathroom. [The bathroom trip can generally be avoided by structuring the situation before the session begins by simply asking the child if she needs to go to the bathroom.]*
> CHILD: *Where is my Mommy?*
> THERAPIST: *You're thinking about Mommy . . . your Mommy is waiting right outside in the waiting room.*

These are some common questions asked during the rapport-building stage, and can usually be responded to with empathy (or acknowledgment) and a simple structuring statement. We cover responding to questions in much more depth in Chapter 8.

## Structuring Around Time Limits and Delivering the Departing Message

Because the time the child has in CCPT with a caring, attentive therapist is unique, and a healing time that the child uses fully and commonly enjoys, ending the time can be very difficult for some children.

Structuring with empathy helps with this. In general, the therapist tells the child when there are 5 minutes left, and then when there is 1 minute left. The therapist's message to the child would be, for example: "Sarah, we have 5 minutes more for today."

At the end of the last minute, the therapist firmly, but pleasantly, says: "Our time is up for today, Sarah. We have to leave now." If the child is resistant and reluctant to leave the room, first reflect the feeling (use empathy and acknowledgment) and also use your *body language and voice tone* to emphasize your conviction. It may help to stand up, walk toward the door, and then open it. You may continue to reflect the child's "wanting to stay longer," but then always return to the message, "but our playtime is over for today, and it's time to go." Demonstration of patience by the therapist is important at this time. Although it may take 1–5 minutes longer for the child to exit, this is the child's time to work therapeutically on issues related to attachment and coping with transitions. Most children benefit from having the feelings of "not wanting to go" empathized with, and deal much better with the endings from that point on.

## Maintaining Therapist Congruence While Balancing Necessary Structuring and Limit Setting With Permissiveness or the "Freedom to Be"

Imagine you've given the clear and simple introductory statement, and now you allow the child to take the lead in the session. As you track with empathy, trying to stay *right there with* the child, you notice that he appears both perplexed and intrigued. This seems so different to him. You can almost hear him thinking, "Why isn't the adult telling me what to do?" You notice, at the same time, that he's warming up— at his own pace, in his own way. He explores the toys, tries out activities, and looks expectantly to you for a reaction. It is for the child, to borrow again from Virginia Axline, "a challenge . . . and something deep within the child responds to this clearly felt challenge to *be*—to exercise this power of life within himself, to give it direction, to become more purposeful and decisive and individual" (Axline, 1969). So, now how does the skilled therapist *get out of the way* while still providing the necessary empathic responding, structuring, and minimal limits? How does the skilled therapist provide for the child the optimum freedom to be? How does the skilled therapist maintain an attitude of warmth and acceptance—congruence—as the child tries out expressing himself freely and at times with wild abandon in a purposeful and decisive way?

Perhaps the best way to answer this is to return now to the Application Issue from the beginning of this chapter. Let's say that you are the therapist in session with little Gina, who seems to have quite suddenly "come into her own" and wants to redecorate your office with colorful splatters of paint!

> She smiles—a little inward smile—and tilts her head as if she has an idea. Her brush dips lightly into the rich red paint. She lifts her brush and, after taking a quick sideways glance at you, splatters a little paint on the wall! Smiling broadly now, Gina dips her brush deeply into the purple paint, and looks to you expectantly. . . .

Unless your playroom has a wall for this purpose (provided you have a playroom), Gina's "idea" poses a couple of problems. First, if you are unable to remain accepting and warm as Gina continues to splatter paint on the walls, little that is therapeutic will transpire from that point on. There can be little healing value when the core conditions of empathy, unconditional positive regard, and genuineness are out of balance. In regard to this balance, the therapist must be the one who remains self-aware of his own limitations. Trying to appear "warm and accepting" while feeling "annoyed and anxious" isn't comfortable for the therapist or the child. So, what to do? The following section of this chapter is designed to help therapists enhance skills in this area.

## Established Limits and Limit-Setting Statement Skills: "The Empathy Sandwich"

We have trained and supervised many child-centered play therapists using what we call the "empathy sandwich" model for setting limits in play sessions. This three-step method helps remind the counselor that when it is necessary to limit the child's activity, it is always best to "sandwich" this limit between two "slices" of "wholesome empathy." It is also a reminder that just as a wholesome sandwich can be satisfying, and can nourish a child's physical growth, an "empathy sandwich" can be satisfying and nourish a child's cognitive and emotional growth.

## Table 7.2  "Empathy Sandwich"

When a child approaches something that she may not do in CCPT remember these steps:

• The first slice of bread: Empathy for what the child is experiencing when approaching a behavior that will require a limit. Example: "Gina . . . you like splashing the paint on the wall"*

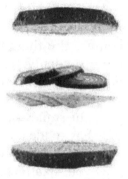

• The middle or "substance" of the sandwich: A clear statement that she has come to something she may not do, with the to-be-limited behavior identified for her. Example: "You would like to use purple next, but Gina . . . painting on the walls is one of the things you may not do."

• The second slice of bread: Empathy for how the child reacts to the limit. Example: "You don't like it . . . you were having fun and that's what you wanted to do."

*The first step may, at times, be skipped for safety reasons; however, empathy and acknowledgment of resulting feelings and next actions should always follow the limit.

These authors have observed that, most times, just by *beginning* with empathy, the child's attention becomes focused on what is being said without defensiveness, and the child is better able and willing to *emote and talk about* feelings surrounding the limit—knowing she will receive an empathic response from her counselor.

So, to return to our aspiring artist, Gina, as an example, you sense that Gina's idea to splatter paint on the walls *feels fun* to her, and it is what *she wants to do*. So, the first "slice" of the "empathy sandwich" shows respect for her feelings and her ability to come up with good ideas, as well as an understanding of her wanting to do it, just for the fun of it. The limit, or middle of the sandwich, is what is needed for you as therapist to maintain warmth and acceptance and need only be stated matter-of-factly and to the point, in accordance with the opening statement. As stated in the opening statement, you have told the child, "If you come to something you may not do, I'll let you know." So, the phrasing need only be a caring, matter-of-fact reminder of this. In Gina's case, the limit might sound something like this:

> **THERAPIST:** *Gina, you like splashing the paints on the wall!*
> **GINA:** *Yes! I'm going to do purple now!! [Gina lifts the brush dripping with purple paint.]*
> **THERAPIST:** *[Slowly leaning in and making eye contact, and in a soft but emphatic tone] You would like to use purple next, but*

*Gina . . . I told you that I'd let you know if there was something you may not do. Painting the walls is one of the things you may not do.*

**GINA:** *Okaaaay! [Sounding disappointed, and a little annoyed, Gina drops the paintbrush back in the paint.]*

**THERAPIST:** *You don't like it . . . you were having fun and that's what you wanted to do.*

**GINA:** *I was going to make it all the colors!*

**THERAPIST:** *You had an idea for all the colors . . . it's disappointing.*

**GINA:** *[Looks around the playroom, shaking her head back and forth] It's too bad . . . it sure would have looked prettier in here.*

**THERAPIST:** *You would have made it a prettier place with your many-colored painting.*

**GINA:** *Uh-huh, I'm a good painter!*

## Self-Awareness and the Genuine Response: Developing Important Therapist Qualities in Structuring and Limit Setting

It is important that the child-centered therapist remember that because limits are not stated before the need for them arises, practice of this skill in mock sessions may help in development of the necessary self-awareness and skill involved. Asking, "How would I normally react to this or that?" as you read through scenarios in this chapter can also be helpful. Voice tone, facial expression, body language, and proximity to the child can all have an effect (positive or negative) on what is conveyed to the child during limit setting. It is therefore also helpful to videotape sessions and watch and listen to yourself as you set a limit or give a structuring statement. During this form of "self-supervision," you might look for answers to the following questions: When there is time, do you use the child's name to gain the child's attention? Does your tone of voice remain neutral and calm and "matter-of-fact"? Do you use proximity control (moving closer to the child) when necessary to gain the child's attention? Are you using empathy—the three-step "empathy sandwich" delivery method of limit setting?

In our teaching and supervision of students, we have found that by practicing in mock role-plays, scenarios that require limit-setting and structuring skills, the child-centered therapist can better develop:

1. An ability to sense the child's feelings or motivation and convey that understanding before setting the limit

2. An ability to use a neutral, caring (yet nonapologetic) tone when stating the limit in clear, to-the-point terms

3. An ability to set the limit with an attitude that conveys the therapist's confidence in the child's ability to self-control, rather than conveying tentativeness or doubt in the child's compliance with limits

4. An ability to use empathic listening to convey acceptance and acknowledgment of the child's emotional reaction or self-expression after the limit is set

While it may take some time, once this process becomes a natural *way of being and responding* in child-centered therapy, both the therapist and child will benefit from the improved therapeutic atmosphere, and the enhanced communication and relatedness it allows.

## Two Limit-Setting Vignettes for Review: Allowing the Child to Come Up With Alternative Behaviors vs. Targeting Alternative Behaviors for the Child

Just as each child brings his own unique style of self-expression to CCPT sessions, each child will differ in the need for limit setting. Some children rarely, if ever, require limit setting, while others seem to engage the therapist from the beginning with a "rapid-fire" form of limit testing. All forms of limit testing are therapeutic opportunities for the child. Many times limits are crossed simply because the child is anxious and wants to know what the parameters are. The child's actions are, in a sense, questions in disguise: "Okay, just *what are* the boundaries here?" "What will happen if I do this?" "Am I safe?" Other times, the child may become so caught up in the spontaneity of exuberant free play that her play may become too rough and tumble or reckless and unsafe.

The following vignettes are provided to illustrate these differences, and to give examples of therapeutic limit setting. As you read through the vignettes, notice how the child-centered play therapist expresses empathy both before and after the limit is set—providing the "empathy sandwich." Notice also how the child-centered play therapist uses a limit-setting method that clearly promotes the child's individual acceptance of responsibility for one's own actions and allows for the child to express a reaction to the limit and have that accepted and empathized with. While some forms of play therapy use a limit-setting message that offers an alternative for the child (you cannot shoot me with the dart gun, but you may shoot the bop bag) or a structuring statement (the walls are not for painting on; paper is for painting on), we recommend allowing the child the opportunity to come up with his or her own alternatives, and maintain that by doing so the child is offered better opportunities for empowerment and developing flexibility and emotional regulation. The following two vignettes are offered as a demonstration of this advantage. As you read through each, try to think of how each child likely benefited in the areas of empowerment, flexibility, and self-regulation. How might the scenario have changed if alternative behaviors were targeted or suggested for the child in each example?

## Vignette 1: Maurice Wants to Slam Dunk the Ball

Ten-year-old Maurice is playing basketball with a Nerf ball and basket that is hooked over the playroom door. He is showing the therapist all his moves, bragging and having great fun! He runs, jumps high, and SLAM! He dunks the ball so hard that the little plastic rimmed net flops down.

> **MAURICE:** [*Rubbing his shoulder, and grinning triumphantly*] *Man . . . did you see that?!! [He clicks the net back into place.] Let's have an instant replay!*

The therapist knows that the net won't stand up to too many more slam dunks like that, and that Maurice will likely want to slam dunk many more! She also notices that in order to get up that high, Maurice has to get a running start that propels him into the hard wooden door with great force. She notices he is rubbing his shoulder and knows a limit is needed to keep Maurice safe from possibly hurting himself, and the basketball basket and hoop from breaking.

> **THERAPIST:** *Wow! You liked that . . . a slam dunk!*
> **MAURICE:** [*Picks up the ball, getting ready to run*] *Watch this one!*
> **THERAPIST:** [*In a firm, but pleasant tone*] *Maurice you're having a lot of fun with your slams, but remember when I said I'd let you know if there were things you may not do in here? One of the things you may not do is slam dunk the ball.*
> **MAURICE:** [*Sighs and drops the ball*] *That's crazy. . . .*

THERAPIST: *It's disappointing and doesn't make sense.*

MAURICE: *Nope, I said . . . it's crazy!*

THERAPIST: *Oh, correction . . . you think it's crazy.*

MAURICE: *[Picks up the Nerf ball and tosses it in the air and catches it] Uh-huh . . . you got any other sports games in here, 'cuz I can't play basketball without playing full out.*

THERAPIST: *You're thinking you'll have to play something else because when you play basketball, you like to play full out.*

MAURICE: *Yep [Tosses the ball over his head backward toward the goal, and then asks with excitement] Hey . . . was that close—did it almost go in?*

THERAPIST: *[Matching the excitement] Yes . . . it hit the rim!*

MAURICE: *Not too bad for a backwards shot, huh?*

THERAPIST: *You think that was a pretty good shot . . . for a backwards shot.*

## Vignette 2: Karina Wants to Wash Her Hair

Five-year-old Karina is having fun filling the big plastic teapot with water from the sink and then pouring it back in. She smiles as she fills it up and then lifts it over her head.

KARINA: *[Excitedly] I'm going to wash my hair!*

THERAPIST: *[Moving in closer, to get Karina's attention] Just a minute, Karina . . . that's your idea to wash your hair and you like it, but remember when I said I'd let you know if there was something you may not do in here?*

KARINA: *[Frowning . . . bringing the teapot down] I can't wash my hair?*

THERAPIST: *That's right. Even though it would be fun, one of the things you may not do is pour the water on your head to wash your hair.*

KARINA: *I'd just pour a little bit. . . .*

THERAPIST: *And you're letting me know you'd just pour a little bit, but one of the things you may not do is pour water on your head . . . even just a little. . . .*

KARINA: *Okay. I'll wash the baby now. [Karina finds a baby doll, undresses it, and puts it in the water table.] I might wash her hair, though!*

THERAPIST: *So, you decided you'll wash the baby now . . . maybe her hair, too.*

KARINA: *Yes! [Putting the doll in the water table and pouring water on its head.] She's getting her hair washed now!*

THERAPIST: *You are washing her hair now!*

## Vignette 1 (Continued): "Maurice Slam Dunks Again"—What to Do on the Occasions That a Child Persists With the Limited Behavior

In most cases, when limits are set with empathy, it is our experience that even the most "limit-testing" children are able to move on and find alternatives for self-expression on their own. In the instance that a child breaks a limit that has just been set (the second time this happens in the session), remind her of the limit and then state with a neutral, and matter-of-fact manner what will happen if the limit is broken again; that is, that the playtime will end for *that day*. For example, to continue from our vignettes above, let's say Maurice decided to continue to play Nerf basketball, and for a while does so without a "slam dunk." Then, quite suddenly, he picks up the pace and slams the ball down hard in the net again. The therapist response would then be something like:

THERAPIST: *You decided to slam dunk again! Maurice, you enjoy playing full out and slam dunking, but I told you that slam dunking is one of the things you may not do in here. If you slam dunk the ball again, we will have to end our playtime for today.*

This warning is given so that Maurice knows that if he slam dunks the ball again, he also knows that the session will end for that day. If Maurice chooses to slam dunk the ball again, the counselor restates the limit, and follows through with the ending of the session for that day. It is important during this "ending" to remain firm, but pleasant. The therapist's response would be something like:

THERAPIST: *Maurice, you really want to be able to slam dunk in here, but remember when I told you that if you slam dunked the ball again, you would have to leave the playroom for today. Since you slam dunked again, our playtime is over for today.*

MAURICE: *[In a pleading, disappointed tone] But . . . you know . . . that's what makes my time fun . . . to play full out. . . .*

THERAPIST: *It's a lot of fun, and you really wish it were something you could do in here.*

A child will begin to learn that he is responsible for what happens to him when he makes a choice to break a limit, after having been told in clear terms previously, and knowing what the result will be. A variation of this limit-setting step would be to remove the toy; however, the ending of the session—while rarely necessary—is generally very effective in helping the child to develop self-control, and it appropriately communicates to the child that although the therapist's positive regard is unconditional, the child must take responsibility in the therapeutic relationship for keeping self, therapist, and property safe.

## Putting It All Together: Limit Setting and Structuring Applied

It is natural for children to strive to be self-directed and independent. It is not, however, natural for children to always behave responsibly, with respect for others, or within safe limits. A basic tenet of the child-centered approach is that if provided the core conditions of empathy, unconditional positive regard, and genuineness by his therapist, the child will strive toward mastery and will ultimately become the "best self" he can be. In order for a child to discover this "best self," he must have the freedom to be—to create, explore, and make choices while relying on an internal locus of control. By allowing this, the child is able to rely on an internal guide or "moral compass" as he makes choices. Some children have rarely experienced any rights to make choices and so, in a sense, have not had an opportunity to "exercise their choice-making muscles." Without this "exercise," a child will come to rely on an external locus of control and will not feel responsible for choices and when making decisions. Without this "exercise," a child's ability to self-regulate does not have a chance to develop and his sense of self-efficacy is impaired. For this reason, it is imperative that the child-centered therapist become skilled in balancing the limits needed for structure and safety with permissiveness or the freedom to be. During CCPT, the child must have a safe and structured time and place to wrestle with what are, many times, confusing and powerful forces—conflicting feelings of good and bad, big and small, powerfulness and powerlessness. Consider the following four vignette examples. Each example is from the first through sixth sessions of play therapy—sessions when children are often still "warming up" and building a sense of trust and rapport. In each scenario, it is apparent that a structuring statement and/or limit setting is needed. After reading through each, write down your personal reactions and feelings. What do *you feel?* What do you assume the *child is feeling?* If structuring is needed, why is this structuring necessary? If a limit is needed, try to come up with ideas of how to best respond to the child using the "empathy sandwich" model provided in this chapter. If it is helpful and you have a play partner, mock role-play these scenarios, taking turns as therapist and child. Try this on your own first, and then check your work, comparing it to some suggested examples of therapists' structuring and limit-setting responses that are provided at the end of this book in Skills Support Resource C.

## Practice Vignette 1: Antonio Doesn't Want to Leave

From his first session, 5-year-old Antonio has always had some diffi-culty with ending his special playtime and leaving the playroom. It is his fifth session, and he has been told he has 5 minutes left in his play therapy session. He immediately comes up with a new idea and starts working quickly, with great gusto and determination, to build a fort. He uses large blocks, chairs, and a blanket to build a wall to hide behind, and then stashes many weapons and supplies behind. He peeks out from behind his "fort" smiling broadly, obviously proud and excited.

> **ANTONIO:** *We're almost ready for the big fight!*
> **THERAPIST:** *Almost ready!*
> **ANTONIO:** *How much time left?*
> **THERAPIST:** *We have 1 minute left today, Antonio.*
> **ANTONIO:** *NOOOOO!!! That's not enough!!! [Antonio becomes tearful] I'm going in my fort now! [Antonio ducks behind his barricade out of sight].*

## Practice Vignette 2: Sam Is Angry and Reluctant to Come to Therapy

It's Sam's first child-centered play therapy session. He has reluctantly left the waiting room but is following the counselor down the hall. He enters the room scowling, making no eye contact with the counselor. As the counselor begins to give the introductory statement, Sam walks right past her and kicks a box of blocks over.

> COUNSELOR: *You're gonna kick that right over!* [*Sam takes a quick sideways glance at the counselor as he walks past her again, and grabs the BoBo (bop bag). He smacks it sideways and laughs loudly.*] *You liked that—smacking that down!*
> [*Sam picks the Bobo up, places it in front of the counselor, and starts to kick it directly toward her.*]

## Practice Vignette 3: Taneesha Warms Up at the "Beach!"

Taneesha's first two play sessions have been difficult. Painfully shy, she has yet to risk spontaneous, self-directed play. She has colored quietly at the art table and explored the playroom, but hasn't been able to stay for more than 20 minutes without asking to leave to "see Mommy now."

To her therapist's surprise, during 3-year-old Taneesha's third session in play therapy, she really seems to open up. At one point, laughing gleefully, she takes off her shoes, and hops right into the sandbox.

> TANEESHA: *Beach!! I'm going beach now!!!* [*Taneesha laughs and digs her hands deep into the sand.*]
> THERAPIST: *You're happy . . . you're at the beach . . . you're digging deep in the sand!*
> TANEESHA: *Yes!! Sandy-sand!! Sandy-sand!! Sandy-sand!!!* [*Taneesha sings out as she lifts large handfuls of sand and begins throwing it over her head in the air.*]

## Practice Vignette 4: Anxious Krista Plays a Game of "Catch"

Ten-year-old Krista enters her third play therapy session with lots of nervous energy. She has difficulty making eye contact and is still obviously warming up to therapy and the relationship with her counselor.

> KRISTA: *Let's play catch—here . . . catch!* [*Krista picks up a Nerf ball and throws it fast and hard toward the ground. It lands at the counselor's feet.*]

COUNSELOR: *You're throwing it hard and low, making it hard for me to catch!*

KRISTA: *That's right . . . [laughing] . . . now throw it back!*

COUNSELOR: *Okay, here it comes! [The counselor picks up the ball and throws it back to Krista, who snatches it from the air and squeezes it. With a mischievous smile, she begins tossing it up in the air and catching it.]*

COUNSELOR: *You're thinking of something while you're tossing the ball. . . .*

KRISTA: *That's right—now . . . CATCH!!! [Krista throws the ball fast and hard directly toward the counselor's head.]*

## Practice Vignette 5: Corey Puts His Favorite Power Figures in His Pocket

Seven-year-old Corey has been playing with the same two power figures consistently every session for 5 weeks. Every battle includes these two guys who can outjump, outfly, outfight, outrun, and outswim any evil force! The therapist sees that Corey has become very attached to these two power figures, as he begins every session by searching through all the power figures and exclaiming, "First, I have to get *my* guys!" Even when Corey temporarily suspends the action in his long battles with evil forces and comes over to the art table to draw or paint, he always has "his guys" close at hand. During his sixth session, Corey has spent most of his session battling evil forces in the sandbox. He stops, and after a long pause tells the therapist that his "guys," now named "Slasher" and "Highjumper," are "all tired out."

THERAPIST: *Whew! Your guys are tired after that!*

COREY: *You would be too . . . after all that fightin' an' stuff!*

THERAPIST: *I'd be tired too, you think.*

COREY: *Yep. I think . . . I think we'd better sleep this one off. [Corey walks over and plops down on the beanbag and cuddles with his two little ''guys,'' holding the small power figures close to his chest.]*

THERAPIST: *You guys are gonna rest now. It's better to sleep this one off.*

COREY: *Yep, nightee-night!*

Corey cuddles close in with his guys. The therapist watches him as he curls into a ball—and unbeknownst to him, she sees him as he "secretly" slips the two little power figures in the pocket of his jeans. He rolls over, closes his eyes, and begins to make soft snoring sounds while pretending to be asleep. After a short time of "pretend sleep" passes, Corey comes over to the art table. He spends the remaining 5 minutes of the play session painting a picture. After the session has ended, just as Corey is about to walk out the door, the counselor gently gets his attention.

## Structuring Around the Ending Phase of CCPT

CCPT, like any therapeutic relationship, is temporary—an intervention that heals and strengthens the child to thrive in her natural and permanent relationships with family and peers. In some settings such as schools, the counselor will continue to have an ongoing relationship and contact (in the hallways, for group therapy, in classroom guidance) with the child, but even then the relationship will change as it shifts to group interaction settings or more casual friendliness.

The ending phase is initiated generally when two criteria are met. First, the child has clearly entered into Mastery Stage play (see Chapter 10) and, second, the parents and teachers are reporting improvement in areas previously established as therapeutic goals. It is best to structure the determination for ending based on external as well as internal measures (see Chapter 12). Use the "Stage Recognition" approach (Chapter 10) to assess each child's internal readiness to end, and external measures and reports from parents and teacher as an external gauge. It is not necessarily the case that a child will be completely symptom free at ending, but he should be functioning in the "normal" or expected range of his peer group.

When the two basic criteria have been met, the therapist begins a "countdown" of CCPT sessions while observing closely the child's reactions to this process both in terms of in-session behaviors and those in outside settings of home and school. Introduce the countdown of sessions with the same even, matter-of-fact tone used for limit setting and other structuring statements. Simply say, at the beginning of the child's scheduled play session, "Carly, I need to let you know before we start, that after today we have six more times in special playtime, and then you will stop coming for playtime here." The number of count-down sessions may vary, but we've found a good number is five to six sessions. You may decide to start with every other week, decreasing the frequency. In which case the structuring statement would be: "Joel, after today, we will be meeting every other week for our special playtime instead of every week."

In general, you do not explain or make any other adjustments to your usual mode of providing deep empathy, unconditional positive regard, and genuineness during each remaining therapy hour, and following the child's lead during this ending phase. In most cases, the "countdown" of sessions is uneventful, and the child reacts matter-of-factly and without negativity or upset. Many times, they use the time to revisit past play themes in a playful "remember this" reminiscent manner. If you have assessed correctly, the child is ready to end. This means he has worked through his therapeutic issues, has new coping skills, and a renewed sense of self and well-being. During the countdown of sessions, he has an opportunity to work through—without stress or overwhelming sadness—the ending of his special play therapy times with you.

For children who have experienced abrupt endings in their lives, abandonments, and broken relationships, this opportunity to have their therapist fully "right there with them" during a time of "good-bye" can be very empowering and healing. The child, because she is in Mastery Stage, at some level—though rarely overtly verbalized—realizes that she is ready. Sometimes this readiness is "seen" by you and "felt" by her in that the "oomph" seems to have gone out of the intensity of her play, and the *need to be there with you* has lessened significantly. Whereas before the child was fully and intensely involved in her play, now you sense some ambiguity, or that the child is "finished." She senses that, too. She also senses her ability to not be overwhelmed by this "good-bye" to someone who has become very special to her. This is quite empowering.

## When a Child Reacts Strongly to the Ending Phase of CCPT

Occasionally, a child may react strongly to the announcement that CCPT sessions will be ending. This may be seen in the child's *clear* return to Regressive Stage themes, or more rarely Aggressive Stage themes. If the child works his way out of this during the countdown, and has returned to primarily Mastery Stage themes by the next-to-last play session, the ending is continued. However, if the play continues to be clearly characterized by themes from earlier stages, and the parents and teachers are reporting a return to struggles outside the sessions, then you may choose to add more CCPT sessions, and you would simply tell the child, "Lamont, I found out that we will have five more times together in special playtime."

## Arbitrary Endings

At times, due to circumstances out of our control, we must help a child who is not in Mastery Stage play through an arbitrary ending. When this happens, if there is an opportunity, you should try to arrange your schedule so that the child may have a 2-day countdown, or even a one-session countdown. If in a school or agency setting, making the extra effort to have a last session can be very helpful, caring, and respectful to a child who has come to know you, and worked hard in special play time. If seeing for one more session, you would inform the child, "Sierra, I have learned that today will be our last meeting for special playtime. I have learned that you and your Mom are moving, and we will no longer be able to meet." We have often seen children briefly return to small themes of their play during this last session, revisiting, and sometimes allowing themselves to "feel the heavy weight of good-bye." We've also seen them seem to figuratively "wrap things up" and "put it all in a back pocket"—as if to wait until another time. Remaining "right there with the child" with deep empathy, unconditional positive regard, and genuineness through the therapy hour respects the reality of the situation. Often, the children we see during one last session due to an arbitrary ending are those who experience this over and over. Having someone offer a time to say "good-bye," even if it's a very brief 30-minute session, is very caring and empowering for the child.

The key to effectively structuring every ending phase, whether it is arbitrary or you have a countdown of sessions, is to use the time to remain true to the original structuring opening statement of "this is *your time* to say anything, and do almost anything. . . . " The ending phase is a time for the child to process, and does not in any way change your promise to him or your "way of being." You facilitate the child's processing in the same way you facilitate all important processes in the different phases, or stages, of CCPT—through deep empathy and unconditional positive regard for the child's felt expressions and actions in his play therapy hour with you.

## Working With Parents and Teachers During the Ending Phase of CCPT

During the ending phase of CCPT, as the child's therapist and advocate, you also work to prepare the parents and teachers of the child to help make this a smooth transition (see Chapter 14). This preparation may include training parents in filial therapy (see Chapter 13) or child-centered parenting skills so that the parents can provide ongoing support and growth opportunities for the child. Teacher consultation may also include sharing of your conceptualization of the child, and enlisting the teacher's help in the transition (finding other school and community activities that would foster success and using new prosocial skills to build relationships with others).

## Common Problems Regarding Structuring and Limit Setting

### Adding Excessively to the Simple Introductory Statement

Sometimes well-meaning therapists forget that children can own their anxiety and, within supportive contexts, *need to* own their anxiety in order to mature and become well functioning and autonomous. As therapists know, it can be quite difficult for some children to enter a new relationship with the therapist—an adult who can be reasoned to be safe but is still a stranger. So a common error is to try to soften the beginning, to ease the awkwardness by changing the wording of the opening statement, particularly for a seemingly anxious child. For  example, a therapist who is caught up in this error might say to a shy or nervous child something like, "Sweetheart, this is our special playroom, and you can play with any of the toys in here, and we can have lots of fun! I just want you to know that anything you do is okay!" From all this, the child's work is already inhibited by an expectation of play and fun, and by the therapist's use of "sweetheart" rather than her name in addressing her. As is mentioned in earlier chapters, children's work in play therapy will not always be "fun"—just like for adults in counseling, sometimes we need to go to scary places with our counselors, sometimes we need to admit parts of ourselves that are "not pretty" or "sweet" or we fear are unlovable. Also, it is not possible that everything a child does in the playroom or in life is "okay." In reality, there are always limits and consequences. Individual choice and personal responsibility are always needed.

While the example above may be exaggerated for clarity, the same error can be present in the tone conveyed (stressed or strained, overly happy and excited, overly sweet and soothing) by inexperienced therapists in the opening statement. We find it helpful to remember that each child can and needs to work through anxiety with the support of adults. In play therapy, the support is the empathy, unconditional positive regard, and safe structure that the therapist provides. Play therapy is a place for a child to work through anxieties in an environment that makes this "working through" possible. For an anxious child, sometimes working through the anxiety of getting started is a huge part of his work. To be overly soothing in *his beginning* would rob him of that opportunity. It's helpful to remember the saying, "I can only get where I'm going by being where I am."

## Omitting Parts of the Opening Statement

Along the same lines as above, it is important not to leave out parts of the opening statement. The most common part left out is the mention of limits, "If there is something you may not do, I will let you know." Probably this error is due to similar therapist anxiety as above. While it is understandable that a therapist would want to offer a child an hour of "fun-filled freedom" without limits, this is unrealistic and anxiety provoking as children need structure and limits from a caring adult in order to feel safe to fully self-express. Therapists sometimes want to avoid setting limits. Some of the best therapists feel a strong pull to be liked by their child clients, which opens the door to misconstrue that avoiding conflict by being overly permissive is the way to ensure this affection from child clients. In fact, just the opposite is true. Setting limits as needed and in appropriate ways makes the therapist genuine. Then, when the therapist is genuine, if there is affection from the child (there almost always is), the affection is real and earned through a solid relationship.

We strongly recommend that therapists not stray from the careful use of empathy and the specific wordings suggested when structuring or setting limits. Such care can prevent many later "pitfalls," and keeps the therapist's work consistent and efficient.

## Letting a Few Too Many Behaviors "Slide By" That Should Have Been Limited

This is an extension from the error in the section above. In this case, the therapist gives the opening statement, but then when limits are needed, he hesitates. He may be trying to avoid conflict, probably fearing a negative child reaction. This is anxiety provoking to the child and inhibiting to the child's work. The therapist who repeatedly makes this error should review his belief systems around what is possible and most facilitative for children in therapy (see the early chapters of this book). The ideal that all play therapists must work toward is to get a solid feel for what should be off limits and then to apply limits with a steady consistency. If this error has occurred, rereading this chapter and working the activities should help. If such errors persist to great length, then additional supervision, consultation, or counseling to discern the reasons for the persistent error would be appropriate.

## Forgetting Empathy Around Limits

A very common beginner error is to skip providing empathy around limits. Sometimes this happens because the novice therapist is trying so hard to get the limit right that her focus on the limit distracts her from empathy. This can usually be worked through with practice, and by working on the skill-enhancing opportunities provided in this book. It can be supervised clinical practice, or it can be through carefully self-supervised work (i.e., record your sessions, with appropriate permission; review your behaviors, voice tone, body language, habits, thoughts, and feelings around necessary limits, periodically stopping the tape to practice saying it just the way you would have in a more "perfect" session).

Sometimes for therapists who have reluctance around setting limits, the reluctance distracts from empathy. For example, if a beginning therapist who is reluctant, has to *make* himself apply necessary limits, he may have to work so hard to make himself do it that this "trying too hard" becomes a persistent distraction from empathy.

Whatever the reason, it is helpful to remind yourself that empathy and unconditional positive regard is the skilled therapist's *natural and constant mode*, and that limits serve to facilitate the child's reception of this empathy and unconditional positive regard.

## Too Many Limits

An opposite-seeming but related error to those above is setting too many limits. This error could be caused by a low tolerance for ambiguity in the therapist. It could be caused by a therapist's lack of trust that the child can find her own way or the therapist may be trying to use limits to teach a behavior or shape the child client's play. The error may come in response to pressure felt from administrators or other caring adults who want to see change quickly, so the therapist may be trying to hurry the child's process. Reviewing early chapters regarding what makes therapy possible and most efficient for children should help with this error, as well as our sections on helping administrators and other caring adults value and establish reasonable positive expectations from CCPT. In the extreme, therapists may need to find avenues such as supervision, consultation, and counseling to explore thoughts and feelings that seem to prompt an unwarranted need to control. Most therapists will have entered the helping professions out of a need to help others. But, ironically, when the need to help by teaching, shaping, and controlling is too strong, it is not helpful and can be harmful.

## Failing to Add a Limit Because It Was Not Previously Provided

Sometimes you will have to limit behaviors that you allowed before. You may realize that the noise level you allowed one day is not reasonable for your neighbors in the agency or school in which you work. You may discover that some behaviors are unreasonably hard on toys or the playroom. You may realize when reviewing your work that you were wincing around certain behaviors, that you didn't want to limit them, but they were negatively affecting your capacity for unconditional positive regard and your ability to be empathic and accepting of the child—in short, your therapeutic relationship. Although, in general, being consistent with limit setting is indeed important, failing to set a therapeutic limit just because one did not do so in the past ultimately inhibits the therapeutic process. The errant belief for some therapists is that the structure must be fair (with fair implying nonchanging). This is unrealistic. You will have to "backtrack" at times. While it is not preferable, it will happen.

## Failing to Make Limits Specific, Understandable, and Enforceable

Limits should always apply to specific, understandable, enforceable behaviors. To an inexperienced child-centered play therapist, this can sometimes seem impossible, but with practice and experience it is possible. In one of our supervision experiences, a supervisee was counseling a little boy who was stretching a rubbery lizard nearly to its breaking point, when he directed her to help by pulling its tail across the room to the doorway. The counselor knew this stretch would likely break the toy, so she said, "one of the things I cannot do is pull the lizard tail all the way to the door." To which he excitedly replied, "Sure you can, I'll help you!" As he began to stretch it out further and further, she quickly clarified the limit, by adding, "You want to see just how far it will go. One of the things you may not do in here is stretch the lizard all the way across the room." This limit named his behavior. He got the point and moved on. Often, you will have to try more than once to get the limit right. Early in your practice you will make errors with this. A good rule of thumb is to remember to name the specific behavior, rather than making broad statements; for example, if a child throws a block at you, the limit would be "You may not throw the block at me" rather than "You may not hurt me" or "You may not throw things at me." In cases where a child persists in, for instance, picking up different objects to throw, you might at that point generalize to "You may not throw things at me." Likewise, if a child is doing something unsafe, such as climbing on a table, the limit would be "You may not climb on the table" instead of "You may not do dangerous things in here." Other helpful practices are to get in the habit of gently saying the child's name first (to gain attention) and using the words "may not" instead of "cannot" when setting the limit. This can be especially helpful with anxious, high-energy, impulsive children. For instance, in another of our supervision experiences, a therapist was barely keeping up with highly energetic "Zach" during his first play session. The boy darted about the room, jumping over toys, somersaulting into the beanbag, crawling under the table, and then, suddenly, he was climbing up a shelf. Fearing for the boy's safety, the therapist quickly blurted out, "One of the things you cannot do is climb the shelf!" Mistaking this for a statement about his ability level, the boy smiled and began to climb quicker, while happily reporting, "Oh, yes I can . . . watch me!" The therapist first laughed, but then quickly added, "Oh! You want to show me you *can* do it . . . but Zach, climbing on shelves is something you may not do in here." This gets Zach's attention. Looking straight at the therapist with a good-natured smile, he remarked, "Why didn't you just say so!" and then climbed down!

Some errors are acceptable. Errors as you're learning are unavoidable. Sometimes the child you are helping in CCPT will take you by surprise and teach you something new! The goal is to state limits in specific, understandable, and enforceable ways.

## Thinking That Limits Can't Include Qualities of Behavior

A play therapist we worked with in a school setting had a little boy in therapy whose voice tone would get quite loud during his sessions. She realized it was unreasonable for her setting, since it would disturb others and might compromise the child's confidentiality in session as well. As she was taping her sessions with him, she studied the tapes to become clear as to the point at which or level in which his voice was *too loud*. She learned to limit his loudness at just that moment. Beginning with empathy for his experience in the moment, and as fitting for the mood of the moment, speaking quickly, she would say to him, "This is so exciting to you! But remember, I told you there were some things you may not do. One of the things you may not do is to be that loud in special playtime." He usually reacted with mild surprise and continued whatever he was doing with a little lower and softer voice. This had to be repeated a number of times. After the first couple of times, he would automatically lower his voice even before she could finish the first couple of words into the limit. When she noticed the change, she could stop her limit-setting statement and begin tracking with empathy, "You know, you are really fighting the tiger now—just not so loudly!" Soon he learned to moderate his voice tone, regardless of his level of force and intensity in play. In this case, the limit involved a behavioral quality. The limit set was due to practical requirements of the setting and would not have been set otherwise; nonetheless, the child benefited from the capacity for self-regulation learned in the playroom and started to moderate his voice in the classroom, where this was a problem. In short, although the therapist does not set limits to directly teach social skills or moral behavior per se, children learn many things when limits are set primarily to maintain safety of the child, therapist, and property, and for the therapist to maintain acceptance and empathy.

## Carrying Limits Over or Holding Previously Ignored Limits Against the Child—Realizing That Sometimes a Child "Wins a Round" of Conflict Around a Limit

It is important to note that no consequences of limits (e.g., being at the second limit level and risking an end to the session) carry over beyond the session at hand. It would be too hard for the therapist or child client to remember such specifics from one session to the next.

Knowing this brings up the common question, "What if a child knows that he can't break the limit again or his session will end, but then he breaks it—right at the last second—as his session would end anyway?" This is very rare, but it does happen. Children are great at outwitting adults, and some children in therapy are determined to keep a "safe distance" from the therapist for some time. Often out of fear of a relationship or deep beliefs of "I can't be liked" or "I will eventually be rejected or abandoned," a child will try to drive her therapist away. Such a child can teach you the most about your capacity for patience and will strengthen your capacity for unconditional positive regard. So, although very rare, it is helpful to be prepared for such situations.

When this happens, the therapist still ends the session, while also acknowledging the action by the child. For example, if a child was testing the limit of throwing blocks at the two-way mirror and had already done this twice and received a warning, but then, in the last minute, threw a block at the two-way mirror, the therapist would acknowledge, "You wanted to wait until our playtime was up to throw the block at the mirror because you don't want to lose playtime. Our session is over for today." But what if the child responds in a sassy, *I got one over on you* tone, by saying, "So what . . . our time was up for today anyway!" It is best to *always* respond with empathy. As you move toward the door and ending the session, you might say, "You're letting me know that it doesn't matter to you since our time was up anyway." Know that sometimes a child "gets one over on you" and try not to take it personally. With your empathy surrounding such behavior, he gets to learn what it feels like to behave in such ways. Your empathy will focus him on his choice and the internal prompts and reactions to his choice.

For now, it is important for the therapist to recognize the important therapeutic gain the child has made by self-controlling until the last second of the play session. He will eventually choose the more considerate, respectful path within your therapeutic relationship. Then he will begin to more consistently make such choices *outside of sessions* as well. Have faith in empathy and unconditional positive regard. The child that tests such limits is learning about being in a respectful relationship with someone else who is trying to understand him. He will come around. It happens every time!

## Not "Being There" Until the Very End (the Very Last Minute) in CCPT

It is important to be self-aware of your own feelings around endings during the ending phase or countdown sessions of CCPT. Well-intentioned therapists can become caught up in ideas like "throwing a party" or switching to a more directive, advice-giving mode, or even giving a departing gift to the child. If this is happening during ending phases for you, sit with yourself and reflect on it, and speak to your supervisor about your feelings around the endings. Do not become one of those well-intentioned therapists who, through your actions, indicates to the child, "You can't handle endings, so I'll throw you a party!" The child needs to process to the end and will want her therapist to remain consistent in providing deep empathy and unconditional positive regard while following her lead. We have often been touched and surprised by how children choose to use their time up until the *very last minute* of special playtime during a countdown of sessions. Let the child be in charge of the good-bye. This is what they will learn from, heal from, and take with them.

## Opportunities for Practice, Study, Skill Development, and Self-Supervision

### Consideration of Limit Setting for Children's "Free Play" in Noncounseling Settings

Observe children in relatively free play situations that are being supervised by adults (e.g., a playground, schoolyard, classroom, neighborhood). Notice how limits are set. Are the adults who are supervising attempting to direct, control, or limit the play with phrases such as "Wait your turn," "Johnny, be nice," "Remember to share," "Try it this way" "Slow down," and so on? These phrases, while meant to lead children toward prosocial and safe behavior, are examples of adult-centered supervision. As you watch, do you notice adults explaining why certain actions or behaviors should or should not be, and establishing an adult-driven, organized game that ends free play? Are there conflicts between some of the children? How are these being attended to? How often do you hear the adults use empathic phrases or allow the children to negotiate and take a part in problem solving? Create categories for the ways you see that behavior is limited. Note the usual reactions to each method for limiting behavior. Journal (describe and react to) or form your observations into an essay in which you advocate for more effective methods for allowing for free play, while keeping the play situation safe. Describe your vision of a more child-centered approach to supervision of free play. Please note that the purpose of this activity is to focus your attention to how limits are set for children's "free play" behavior, not to focus you on the ways parents and children should limit children's behavior, although additional understandings there may be a useful by-product. Keep in mind that different modes of limit setting are appropriate in different situations.

## Contemplation and Practice of Key Concepts

The key concepts of CCPT often present new ways of being. Contemplation and academic practice can help you develop depth of understanding and comfort with the skills. The following eight activities provide opportunities for contemplation and academic practice of critical key concepts. They can be completed alone or with a partner, or in a small group or classroom.

- *Activity A:* Use the following list of hypothetical child statements/ scenarios to test your skills in structuring and limit setting. Work with a partner or think through the scenarios suggested by the statements on your own.
  1. Child kicks Bobo (bop bag) and it accidentally hits you.
  2. Child pleads, "Please, can we leave early? I have a headache."
  3. Child says, "I want you to do a back flip! Do a back flip now!"
  4. Child asks, "Can I please take this home? I don't have any toys."
  5. Child throws a block at the two-way mirror.

6. Child grabs two big handfuls of sand and says, "Let's pretend we're in a sandstorm . . . I'll throw the sand!"
7. Child asks, tearfully, "Can I go see if my Mommy is here?"
8. Child starts to leave the room before the session is over.
9. Child asks, "Can my friend come in with me next week?"
10. Child loops a rope around his neck, and begins to tighten it.

- *Activity B:* Explain to a peer or write in your own words what is implied by the opening statement for CCPT about the structure of CCPT. Address things that are said and not said, and the importance of keeping it simple. Generate your own examples to illustrate these concepts. This activity can work just as well or better if you can make your explanation clear to a nontherapist.

- *Activity C:* Explain to a peer or write in your own words the therapeutic implications or effective differences of preannounced rules and limits that are given *only* as needed. How does limit setting "in the moment" or only as a behavioral boundary is reached help the child develop self-regulation and a sense of self-efficacy?

- *Activity D:* Journaling individually or discussing with a small group or partner, generate your own examples illustrating how limits in CCPT assure safety, promote self-responsibility and self-regulation, and serve to maintain the toys and equipment of the playroom.

- *Activity E:* Journaling individually or discussing with a small group or partner, describe the importance of neutral voice tone, body posture, proximity and movements, and the demeanor of the child-centered play therapist in limit setting.

- *Activity F:* Journaling individually or discussing with a small group or partner, give examples of how effective limit setting is conducive to therapy, and how therapy is hindered when the therapist is not able to maintain attitudes of acceptance, empathy, and unconditional positive regard for the child.

- *Activity G:* Journaling individually or discussing with a small group or partner, explain the therapeutic value of using the "empathy sandwich" model of structuring and limit setting in scenarios with a slow-to-warm-up child; a limit-testing, aggressive child; and a questioning, anxious child.

- *Activity H:* Journaling individually or discussing with a small group or partner, explain why the most important facet of using structuring and limit-setting skills is the therapist's self-awareness during play therapy sessions, and ability to know when something has gotten in the way of their remaining emotionally accepting and congruent while in play sessions with children.

## Mock Session Practice

An excellent way to develop your skills for service to children is to practice with a peer in mock sessions. Take turns in the roles of child and therapist. You will find that you'll learn from the role of the child, therapist, or, if you have the extra opportunity, as observer. We find 15 minutes to be a reasonable length for mock sessions. Longer sessions allow more time for practice, but it can get difficult to sustain the role of the child for very long periods. You can limit yourselves to small sets of representative toys at a table, or expand to a playroom. If you can establish mock sessions to follow most chapters, try to stay with the same partner to see how your relationship develops. The following practice set instructions can be taken together or separately:

- Engage in a mock session in which the person in the role of the child provides you with opportunities to use the opening statement and utilize structuring statements within the steady mode of tracking with empathy.
- Engage in a mock session in which the person in the role of the child provides you with opportunities to set limits. When in the role of the child, try not to be an impossibly difficult child before your partner has had at least one practice opportunity to develop her skills (a temptation is to play the worst-case scenario to see what happens). After your turn in the role of the therapist, ask for feedback on your voice tone (is it critical, questioning, apologetic, overly demanding, too loud, or too soft?) and your body posture, proximity, and movements and demeanor during the limit setting process.
- Engage in mock session(s) that push your skills beyond the minimum. For example, include experiences of children's disgruntled responses to limits (e.g., resistance, voicing anger or frustration, ignoring). Include a scenario in which the child acts out and limit-tests in "rapid fire" mode. Include a scenario where the child refuses to accept a limit and repeats the limit breaking.

## Informal, Nonclinical Practice with Children

If you have the opportunity to play with a child (your own child, niece or nephew, a friend's child) and allow yourself to be minimally directive, you will find opportunities to practice setting limits within empathy. This opportunity will help you hone your skills for play therapy sessions, but will also have the immediate payoff for you and the child by improving your relationship and increasing the child's sense of being understood and attended to with care. Journal, essay, and/or discuss your reactions to the experience with peers.

## Guidance for Clinical Practice and Review

If you are in practice, and able to video sessions, a great way to self-supervise, and/or work with an experienced CCPT supervisor, is to watch your own tapes and take note of your skills during the sessions. Review your opportunities to limit set and structure for common problems in application. Notice your strengths as well as error patterns. Especially in regard to errors, consider what you were thinking and feeling in that moment of the session. If working with a supervisor, mock role-play your trouble spots. Practice/pretend giving "perfect" responses to build good habits.

# Responding to Questions, Requests for Help, and Commands

*Most child therapists would readily state the development of children's self-responsibility as one of their major objectives in therapy, but in reality, many limit children's opportunities to assume responsibility by making decisions for children that foster dependence. This does not happen in some major catastrophic way but rather, in little, almost imperceptible parts of their interactions with children, by giving answers, making choices for children, helping when help is not needed, and leading children when they should be allowed to lead.*

*—Garry Landreth*

## Application Focus Issue

As you know, in the child-centered play therapy (CCPT) approach, a therapeutic relationship that fosters the child's self-expression and self-reliance are valued goals. In almost all cases, when the child asks a question—is wondering what, which, or who—or makes a request or demand in a therapy session, these opportunities for self-expression, self-reliance, and relational progress are at stake. A skillful or unskillful way of responding to questions, requests, and commands can progress or inhibit therapeutic growth.

So how should you respond when a child seems reticent and insecure and asks you to make choices for him: "What would you like to do today?," "Would you like me to paint?," "What should I draw?," "What color should I make this?" Before you know it, it can quickly become your session, and the focus is on your choices. You decide to draw a great-looking dinosaur. The child praises your hard work. It's fun for you, but not therapeutic for the child.

Or even more daunting, how do you handle it when the child expresses her own feelings and insecurities indirectly through questions directed to the therapist: "Do you like my drawing?," "Do you have any children?," "Have you ever hit your children?," "Have you ever used drugs?" Such questions are therapeutically loaded, and unskillful responses to them can open up a therapeutic "can of worms."

Or what about when a child who is anxious about separating from his mother and has started to play, but then suddenly remembers Mom, and his anxiety rapidly grows while he asks, "Where's my mom?" Becoming tearful, he asks, "Can I see her?" "Can I leave?" Such questions often are expressions of the central area of growth needed by the child and represent valuable opportunities to help the child process her inner world—if handled correctly.

Finally, what do you do when children express themselves through imploring requests for help—"Please tie my shoe for me"—or controlling demands—"Get that ball for me and get it quick!" Do you comply? Do you set limits? Guiding you through such dilemmas by preparing you to know which questions to answer, how to respond to the self-expression within questions, as well as how to productively respond to requests and commands is the goal of this chapter.

## Chapter Overview and Summary

In CCPT, when the child asks questions, makes requests, or issues commands, the therapist recognizes these as important forms of self-expression and valuable therapeutic opportunities to help the child develop self-understanding and to work on important therapeutic issues. Simply answering questions, or complying or not complying with requests/commands, often removes the opportunity to work with these valuable forms of self-expression. Instead, the therapist responds with the central skill of empathy so that the meanings behind questions, requests, and commands are surfaced and deepened for the child, and thus allows for a therapeutic working through of therapeutic issues to occur. Sometimes responding therapeutically to questions means answering the questions; other times not answering questions is the most therapeutic response. Informational questions and questions surrounding the structure of the therapeutic space (e.g., "How much play time do we have left?," "Can I play with this toy?," "Where did you buy this toy?") are generally answered. Questions surrounding the seeking of direction by the child (What do you want to do today?,"

"What color should I make this drawing?") are not answered but result in a response by the therapist that clarifies the role of the child in the playroom. Finally, questions that are of a minor personal nature (e.g., "What is your favorite color?") may be answered, but more deeply personal questions (e.g., "Were you sexually abused as a child?") result in the therapist's setting appropriate therapeutic boundaries.

The therapist must also know how to respond to requests and commands made by the child in the playroom. In many cases the therapist will comply with such requests and commands unless they trigger the need to set a limit. Compliance with requests and commands is seen as a valuable way in which the therapist can participate in helping the child work through issues of insecurity, need for control, nurturance, and attachment. In all cases, the first response to questions, requests, and commands is to empathically acknowledge the meaning and self-expression indirectly communicated by the child through the use of a question, request, or command. Only after "mining" them for their therapeutic value through the use of empathy does the therapist consider whether to respond to a given question, comply with a request, or alternatively clarify the boundaries existing within the playroom.

## Primary Skill Objectives

The following Primary Skill Objectives are provided to guide you through the chapter and for reflection and review after completing the chapter reading and exercises. Through reading and study with this chapter exercises, you will be better able to:

1. Understand therapeutic meanings that often underlie children's questions.

2. Maintain a disciplined approach to responding therapeutically to children's questions, including an initial response of empathy, assessment of the therapeutic implications of answering or not answering a given question, followed by either a skilled answer or setting of boundaries.

3. Effectively respond to common questions in which children seek information from the therapist either about basic factual information or about the therapist's personal life.

4. Effectively respond to common questions in which children seek to learn about the structure of the therapeutic experience (e.g., the

role of the therapist, the role of the child, the boundaries and opportunities for expression existing within the playroom) or to questions in which the child attempts to get the therapist to give direction to the child's activities.

5. Describe common mistakes that play therapists make when attempting to respond to children's questions.

6. Understand the therapeutic importance of requests and commands made by children.

7. Develop skills to effectively respond to requests and commands made by children, including the recognition of when setting of limits is necessary.

## Responding to Children's Questions: A Therapeutic Opportunity

In the context of a play therapy session, almost every question asked by a child is a therapeutic communication that expresses something of emotional importance to the child. Questions asked by a child provide the therapist with an opportunity to help the child develop expressive skills and self-understanding. Questions are often indirect forms of communication. For example, when the child asks, "How much time do we have left?," at the surface level he is expressing an intent to know how much longer he has to play in the playroom. However, at the deeper and more therapeutic level, the child may be communicating one or more of the following things:

"I really want to be able to finish my drawing."

"I am emotionally spent and want this session to be over."

"I have a birthday party to go to after my play session and hope it's over soon."

"I am anxious that my session may end soon. I love being here and don't want to leave."

"I am wondering whether I will have time to do all the things I want to today."

Therapeutically responding to questions means responding in a way that allows the time and space for the meaning underlying the child's question to emerge so that what is initially an indirect expression

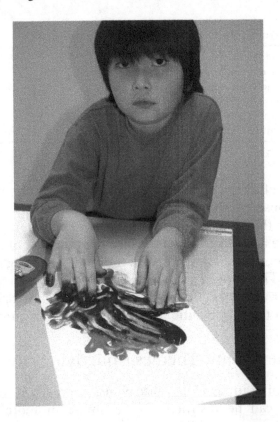

Figure 8.1

can enter into the awareness of the child in a more direct manner so it can be understood by the child and empathically validated by the therapist. Unfortunately, a common temptation of a beginning therapist can be to focus on the question as a request for information rather than a form of expression by the child. In such cases the therapist may immediately move into information-providing mode rather than moving into a receptive mode in which she is empathically open to the meaning communicated by the child. Even more unfortunate is that the quick move to answer a child's question has a tendency to end access to the therapeutic meaning underlying the question, since the child may simply move on.

For example, take the case of a child who has significant problems with transitions. When the child asks, "How much time do we have left?," if the therapist answers "20 minutes," the child may experience relief since the transition time is far away and no longer of concern. However, if the therapist says "2 minutes," the child may immediately experience a wave of anxiousness and run over to the shelf to get

Table 8.1 **Questions Generally Appropriate to Answer**

Informational-factual
Example: "Where did you buy this toy car?"
Informational-mildly personal
Example: "What is your favorite color?"
Structuring-parameters of therapy
Example: "How much time do we have left?"

another toy before the end of the session. In either case, the therapist's abrupt response eliminates the ability to work with the emotional experience in the present since in the first case the therapist's response eliminates the anxious feeling by indicating that a lot of time remains, and in the other case makes access to the anxious feeling more difficult since the child has moved on to trying to alleviate the anxiety by trying to fit in other activities. In either case, a therapeutic opportunity for working with the therapeutic issues underlying the question is lost.

## Central Therapeutic Themes Underlying Questions

Before beginning to develop a disciplined approach to responding to questions, it can be instructive to examine in more depth some therapeutic issues that children express through common questions asked in the playroom. Such an examination will help reinforce the fact that seemingly "tame" and matter-of-fact questions often not only reflect significant therapeutic issues of the child, but also have important implications for the developing relationship with the therapist. As you review the questions and the possible "underlying issues" listed below, we encourage you to deepen your own understanding of the complex and rich meanings that questions may communicate by speculating alternative "underlying issues" of your own for each example before moving on to the next.

Question: "What happens when children break the rules in here?"

Underlying Issue: I want to know that I am safe in this room.

Question: "Can I really say anything I want? Even bad words?"

Underlying Issue: I am still not sure that I can really trust the therapist and really express what I need in here.

Question: "Why do you have the stupid rule that I can't throw the block at the window?"

**Underlying Issue:** I wish I could do *anything* I want . . . be in complete control.

**Question:** "Can I please, please, please stay for more time in the playroom?"

**Underlying Issue:** I really love being in the playroom with you. I am sad when I have to leave.

**Question:** "Did you like school when you were young?"

**Underlying Issue:** I am wondering whether you know how difficult school is for me and whether you would be upset with me if I told you I don't like it.

**Question:** "Do you have any children?"

**Underlying Issue:** I hope that you see me as special.

## The Variance and Frequency of Children's Questions in the Playroom

As noted earlier, a central belief of the CCPT approach is that a child's questions express a part of his interior psychological life. Accordingly, although there are some questions that are more commonly asked by children, there are many others that are unique to a given child. And so, although you will hear some questions come up frequently, you may also hear a new question many years from now as you complete the last play session of your career. Children vary considerably in their frequency of asking the counselor questions. Some ask a number of questions within minutes of entering the playroom for the first time, while others may ask only a handful of questions throughout the entire course of therapy. Children also vary in how questions are dispersed across sessions. One child may ask many informational questions in early sessions in an attempt to gain clarity about her and the counselor's role in the playroom, whereas another child may ask only personal questions of the therapist in later sessions after a relationship has developed.

Now that we have noted the great variability across children in terms of frequency of questions and dispersal of questions across

Table 8.2 **Questions Not Generally Appropriate to Answer**

Structuring-directive
Example: "What do you want to do in here today?"
Informational-highly personal
Example: "Were you sexually abused as a child?"

sessions, we also want you to keep in mind that your skills of responding to questions will be a small percentage of therapeutic total number of responses you make in a given session or across sessions. In this regard, the play therapist skill of responding to questions is similar to the therapist skill of limit setting in that the need for both skill sets vary across children and across the course of therapy, but when the need for either skill arises, important therapeutic issues are at stake and a skillful response is required.

If you are fielding a great many questions from a child, the questions may be a part of that child's unique way of approaching life, anxiety, and new relationships. But if you are experiencing a great many questions throughout your work, you should look for errors in your work. For example, if you are indefinite in the structure you provide, including your way of being, this would prompt many children to greater anxiety and to question you and the structure you provide.

## The Two Major Types of Questions and Their Subtypes

At this point, the counselor new to CCPT may feel a bit apprehensive in the face of questions, given that children's questions can be so varied, can spring up at anytime, and yet are therapeutically important. The purpose of this chapter is to give you a predictable and effective process for responding therapeutically to children's questions. The first tool we provide in creating a predictable process of responding to questions is to categorize the infinite variety of questions children can ask into a few easy-to-recognize categories to guide your responses. Although all questions at the broadest level are a request for information, we classify children's questions into two major categories: (1) informational questions and (2) structuring questions.

Informational questions can be broken into two subtypes: (a) factual questions and (b) questions pertaining to personal information about the therapist. Examples of factual questions include: "Where did you get this toy?," "How much is 12 plus 6?," "Can penguins fly?" Questions pertaining to personal information about the therapist range from mildly personal (e.g., "What is your favorite color?") to moderately personal (e.g., "Do you have children?") to deeply personal (e.g., "Did your dad ever hit you when you were a child?," "Do you use drugs?").

Structuring questions can also be broken down into two types: (a) questions about the parameters of therapy and (b) questions in which the child is seeking direction from the therapist. Questions about the parameters of therapy include: "Can I play with this toy?," "How much time do we have left?," "Can I take this drawing home?," "Will you come to my birthday party?" Questions pertaining to the child's seeking direction from the therapist include: "What do you want to do today?," "What color should I make this drawing?"

The division of the immense variety of children's questions into two major categories and their subtypes is, of course, artificial, but it allows for the development of some basic guidelines for consistently responding therapeutically to children's questions.

## General Guidelines for Responding to Children's Questions in the Playroom

The following guidelines pertain to "responding" therapeutically to children's questions, not simply "answering" them. The play therapist ultimately provides the child with what is deemed to be therapeutically most beneficial to the child. Therapeutic responses generally include the following four options:

1. Simply making an empathic response (or series of empathic responses)
2. Empathy followed by clarifying the child's freedom to make decisions
3. Empathy followed by setting a boundary/limit on providing certain types of personal information
4. Providing the requested information.

Note that all cases of responding to children's question will begin with an empathic response that captures the significant meaning of the question for the child, but in some cases (option 1), empathy is all that will be needed by the child. Clarifying the child's freedom to make decisions (option 2) will often be the response utilized when children ask the therapist to give them some form of direction. Setting boundaries or personal limits around providing certain information (option 3) will often be the response utilized when children ask the play therapist personal questions deemed to be therapeutically inappropriate to answer. Providing the child with the requested information (option 4) is usual in cases where the child requests factual information, personal information about the therapist deemed appropriate to provide, and information about the parameters of therapy.

We will now give an example for when each of these specific response options is most appropriate. Again, it is important to note that the play therapist should always begin their response to children's questions with empathy, regardless of what other types of responses they may give.

## Option 1: Empathy Is All That Is Needed

*Situational context:* Tommy has been actively building a tower of blocks.

> **Tommy:** *[Asks anxiously] How much time do we have left?*
> **Counselor:** *You really want to finish your tower and are concerned you won't have enough time.*
> **Tommy:** *[Nods] This is the biggest tower I have ever tried to build!*
> **Counselor:** *You are proud of how big it is and hope you will be able to finish it.*

Tommy, with clear satisfaction, continues to build, no longer concerned about the time. *Note:* If Tommy had asked again about the time, the counselor would have provided the information to him.

## Option 2: Empathy Followed by Clarification of the Child's Freedom to Choose

*Situational context:* Rosa is a child who is anxious to please the therapist.

> **Rosa:** *What do you want to do today?*
> **Therapist:** *You would like for me to decide what we do today.*
> **Rosa:** *Yes, pick something that you would like to do. I don't want you to be bored.*
> **Therapist:** *It is important to you that I like the things that we do. But Rosa, in your special time you get to choose what we do in the playroom.*

## Option 3: Empathy Followed by the Counselor's Setting Boundaries About Sharing Personal Information Deemed Inappropriate to Share

*Situational context:* Georgia is a little girl who has been sexually abused. The case has been duly reported to Child Protective Services and she is now in treatment. Georgia begins to play with the dollhouse and starts a role-play where the dad figurine engages in aggressive sexualized behavior toward the baby.

> **GEORGIA:** *[With a frightened tone in her voice] My daddy used to do this to me, and it hurted me.*
>
> **COUNSELOR:** *That was very scary for you and it really hurt you.*
>
> **GEORGIA:** *Yes, did your daddy ever do that to you?*
>
> **COUNSELOR:** *You are wondering whether other daddies do that, and whether it happened to me.*
>
> **GEORGIA:** *I hope it didn't happen to you.*
>
> **COUNSELOR:** *You are hoping that I wasn't scared and hurt by my daddy.*
>
> **GEORGIA:** *Yes, were you?*
>
> **COUNSELOR:** *You would like to know if we were both scared and hurt by our daddies, but in the playroom it is your life that is important.*
>
> **GEORGIA:** *Yes, but were you?*
>
> **COUNSELOR:** *It is important for you to know whether I was hurt by my dad, but that is not a question I will answer in here.*
>
> **GEORGIA:** *Well, I hope you were not scared and hurt like I was.*
>
> **COUNSELOR:** *That was really, really scary for you and really, really hurt.*

## Option 4: Empathy Followed by the Therapist's Providing the Requested Information

*Situational context:* Alex enters the playroom and notices a set of army men and equipment with which he is delighted.

> **ALEX:** *[Excitedly] Look at this! There are two sets of army men, and tanks, and even jeeps!*
>
> **THERAPIST:** *You are surprised and excited to see all these army men and equipment.*
>
> **ALEX:** *Yes, where did you get them? These would be great to play with at home.*
>
> **THERAPIST:** *You would like to have some like this for yourself at home.*
>
> **ALEX:** *Yes, where did they come from?*
>
> **THERAPIST:** *I believe that they came from Walmart.*

# Responding to Children's Questions: Common Misconceptions and Mistakes Made by Beginning Play Therapists

Skillfully responding therapeutically to children's questions is a complex process that requires a solid understanding of theory that guides the application of techniques and strategies. In this section we will explore some common misconceptions and mistakes often made by beginning therapists in order to improve your understanding of the theory underlying choices made in responding to questions.

## Mistake/Misconception 1: The Play Therapist Believes the Goal Is to Avoid Answering Questions Altogether

This goal is to respond therapeutically. In practice as a play therapist, you will ultimately answer the majority of children's questions, but you will answer after responding with empathy to help the child become aware of the meanings, feelings, beliefs, or intentions underlying the questions. A child-centered play therapist will develop a profound trust in children's ability to tackle their important therapeutic issues in the playroom. Responding to the meanings behind questions is one among many opportunities in CCPT to help the child express and process an aspect of meaning in her psychological life.

It is also important to recognize that although children's questions inevitably relate to important therapeutic issues and goals, it does not follow that answering questions will always further therapeutic growth. When a child asks a question like "What do you want to do today?" and ultimately gets a response by the therapist, "In here, you get to decide what you would like to do," the child may indeed grow in the areas of self-expression and confidence. However, if the question regarded the location of a toy that was left in a hard-to-find place, and you know where it is but don't answer, that probably results in frustration, but not growth.

## Mistake/Misconception 2: The Play Therapist Believes That the Goal Is to Delay as Long as Possible in Answering Questions

This is a variant of the first mistake/misconception. Although the use of empathy may seem like a delaying tactic, its purpose is to help both the play therapist and the child to gain better understanding of the child's psychological life. As has been mentioned previously, abruptly answering questions frequently makes the underlying therapeutic meaning of questions inaccessible. So, although the play therapist will nearly always use empathy prior to answering a question, the skilled play therapist is seeking a balance between responding therapeutically to questions without being seen by the child as nonresponsive or to the point of frustrating the child. The following example illustrates a *failure* to skillfully balance the need to work therapeutically with a question with the need to be responsive to the child and is to be avoided by the therapist.

### Example 1: Delaying Too Long in Responding to a Question

**TRENT:** *Where is the deck of cards?*

**THERAPIST:** *You want to play with them.*

**TRENT:** *Yes, I like the game of ''Go Fish.'' Where are they?*

**THERAPIST:** *You are afraid you won't be able to play your game if you can't find them.*

**TRENT:** *[Getting frustrated] Yes, where are they?*

**THERAPIST:** *You really want to find them.*

**TRENT:** *[Angrily] Can't you tell me where they are?*

**THERAPIST:** *You are getting mad and you want me to help you find them.*

**TRENT:** *Oh, forget it. I will play something else.*

### Example 2: The "Right Balance" of Empathy and Responsiveness

**TRENT:** *Where is the deck of cards?*

**THERAPIST:** *You want to play with them and you want my help finding them.*

**TRENT:** *Yes, I like the game of ''Go Fish.'' Where are they?*

**THERAPIST:** *They are on that table over there.*

## Mistake/Misconception 3: Seeing Questions as a Teachable Moment

There are certain types of questions that tempt the play therapist to adopt a teaching role rather than to remain true to the CCPT method and trust it to provide the vehicle for children's healing. Consider the following questions asked by hurting children:

"I always get into trouble, do you think my dad left my mom to get away from me?"

"No one wants me. Why can't I come live with you?"

"My dad hits me in the face when I am bad. He says I deserve it. Do you think I am bad? "

In the face of such questions, some play therapists may feel a strong desire to reassure the child or to engage in psychoeducation. Although it is quite permissible to engage in other therapeutic methods after the session is complete, it is important to resist such temptation during the play session and instead to make use of such skills as extended empathy and the types of responses suggested in this chapter in order to help the child work through such issues. Switching to the role of teacher, although motivated by good intentions, will make the role of the therapist unpredictable to the child and prevent the child from developing the resources of resolving these painful issues for themselves.

## Mistake/Misconception 4: Inappropriately Answering Personal Questions Because the Play Therapist Believes She Can Truthfully Give the "Right" Answer

First, it is important to emphasize that it is vital to be authentic when answering children's questions. This means that when you deem it appropriate to answer a personal question, then you should honestly answer the question. For example, if the child asks, "What is your favorite football team?," then, if you decide that the question is within appropriate therapeutic boundaries to answer, you should not create an answer that is not true simply because you think that it will please the child.

However, even more importantly, you should not deem a personal question "appropriate to answer" simply because it might give comfort or reassurance to the child or because it would set a good example for the child. For example, if the child asks, "Do you use drugs?," your decision about whether to answer this question should be based on whether this is an appropriate area of your personal life that should be shared with any client (adult or child), not on whether your ability to say "no" would establish you as a good role model for the child. It is helpful to gain self-clarity about what areas of one's life are appropriate for sharing with children before such questions emerge in play therapy session. Although there is some room for disagreement about where to draw the line in self-disclosure, some fairly common boundaries are drawn around areas such as drug use, history of physical or sexual abuse, sex life, and personal religious beliefs (although some therapists may share that they believe in God, sharing one's theology is generally off limits).

## Mistake/Misconception 5: Giving Too Much Detail When Answering a Factual or Personal Question

When you decide that an answer to a child's question is warranted, it is important to be sparing in your response. As has been noted numerous times, when a child asks a question in a session, it is a therapeutic opportunity to respond to the issue underlying the question. Extended and detailed answers have a tendency to either end the opportunity for careful therapeutic work with the child's issue or to open up other therapeutic issues that were not originally ones the child was focused on. For example, if a girl client asks, "Do you have children?," after responding empathically to her, your answer of "yes" may be warranted. This allows for her to inquire further, "Do you have a daughter?," which may then result in her working through issues surrounding whether she is special to you. However, if your initial response is, "Yes, I have three daughters," or even worse, "Yes, I have three daughters whom I am so proud of—they are each honor roll students," one can easily imagine how this might not only prevent further therapeutic work on the initial therapeutic issue of wanting to feel special, but also bring the issue of the child's difficulties in school to the forefront, even though this was not originally the issue underlying the question.

## Mistake/Misconception 6: Failing to See the Most Central Underlying Meaning of the Question for the Child and Giving a Less Effective Response

In many cases it is possible to readily identify the underlying meaning of the child's question, and to both classify the question by category and subtype and follow up with an appropriate response. However, in some cases there may be some ambiguity in terms of the meaning communicated by a question, and this means that you have to decide between two types of responses. For example, if the child who is drawing a picture of a duck anxiously asks, "Does a duck have wings?," the therapist may realize that the child is asking a question that fits in the category/subtype of "informational-factual" and thus merits an empathic response followed by the answer "Yes." However, it may be just as clear that this child is worried about "doing things wrong" and does not yet understand that in the playroom the child can make decisions for himself without a need to "get everything right." This realization would justify the question's receiving the category/subtype classification of "structuring question—request for direction" and would mean that you should clarify for the child that in the playroom he is free to make decisions for himself. Instead of simply responding "Yes," you would instead reply, "In here, you can decide whether your duck should have wings or not."

## Models of Responses to Common Informational and Structuring Questions

We have attempted to make the process of responding to questions manageable by organizing questions into two categories: informational and structural. We have also distinguished two subtypes of informational questions: those requesting factual information and those requesting personal information about the therapist. We have also distinguished two subtypes of structuring questions: those requesting information about the parameters of therapy and those in which the child requests direction from the therapist. In addition, we have provided four specific therapeutic strategies or "options" for responding to children's questions and noted when each is most commonly used.

To further your skill development, we will provide additional examples of how to respond to common questions asked by children in the playroom. We will then give you an opportunity (with a partner in the role of the child, if available) to practice the knowledge and skills that you have learned so far.

## Common Question 1: "Can I Play with These Things?"

**Category:** Structural

**Subtype:** Request for direction

**Usual response:** Empathy followed by clarification of child's freedom to make decisions

> CHILD: *[Tentatively] Can I play with these things?*

THERAPIST: *You are not quite sure what you can do in the playroom. In here, you can play with almost anything you want.*

## Common Question 2: "I Am Going to Make a Drawing. What Do You Want Me to Draw?"

**Category:** Structural

**Subtype:** Request for direction

**Usual response:** Empathy followed by clarification of child's freedom to make decisions

CHILD: *[Excitedly] I am going to make a drawing. What do you want me to draw?*

THERAPIST: *You want to draw something that I would like. But during your special time you get to draw things that you would like to draw.*

## Common Question 3: "Can I Stay for Just 5 More Extra Minutes?"

**Category:** Structural

**Subtype:** Parameters of therapy

**Usual response:** Empathy followed by answer

THERAPIST: *We have 1 more minute left for our playtime today.*

CHILD: *[Pleadingly] Can I pleeeease stay for 5 more minutes?*

THERAPIST: *You are really having fun and don't want our time to end.*

CHILD: *No, I like it here. I wish I could stay here all day! [Child continues to play]*

Note that in this case the therapist does not have to answer the child's question, since the therapist's empathy helps the child to have self-understanding and allows the child to have some resolution related to this issue of transition and/or attachment.

## Common Question 4: "Can I Take This Toy Home with Me?"

**Category:** Structural

**Subtype:** Parameters of therapy

**Usual response:** Empathy followed by answer

> CHILD: *Can I take some of these crayons home and bring them back next week? I don't have any at home and want to be able to draw.*
>
> THERAPIST: *You really wish you could borrow some crayons; however, all of the toys have to stay in the playroom.*
>
> CHILD: *[Disappointedly] Why? There is a whole bunch of them. No one would miss just a few.*
>
> THERAPIST: *You really want to have some crayons; that doesn't make sense to you. But all toys stay in the playroom.*
>
> CHILD: *Well, I will play with them first thing when I come next week.*

Note that in this case the therapist gives empathy and then answers the questions; however, this results in the child's asking another question, and the therapist then gives empathy and answers the second question; this results in the child's working through the disappointment that comes with acceptance of the limit.

## Common Question 5: "Can You Come to My Birthday Party?"

**Category:** Structural

**Subtype:** Parameters of therapy

**Usual response:** Empathy followed by answer

> CHILD: *I am going to be 5 on Saturday! I am having a big party. Can you come?*
>
> THERAPIST: *You are really excited about turning 5. You are going to have a special party and everything and hope I can come.*
>
> CHILD: *Yes, we are going to have chocolate ice cream! Can you come? The party is at 2 o'clock.*
>
> THERAPIST: *You are really looking forward to your party and would like me to be there, but the time we get to spend together is only in the playroom, so I won't be able to be there.*

## Common Question 6: "How Do You Spell the Word *Astronaut*?"

**Category:** Informational

**Subtype:** Factual information

**Usual response:** Empathy followed by providing requested information

> CHILD: *[With uncertainty] How do you spell the word astronaut?*
> THERAPIST: *You are not quite sure how to spell it. In your special time you can decide how it is going to be spelled.*
> CHILD: *But I want to spell it the way it is in the dictionary.*
> THERAPIST: *So you want to make sure that it is spelled the ''right'' way. A-s-t-r-o-n-a-u-t.*

Note that in this case the therapist first interprets the question as being one in which the child is seeking direction and answers accordingly. Once it is clear that the child is seeking information, the therapist answers.

## Common Question 7: "What Is Your Favorite Color?"

**Category:** Informational

**Subtype:** Personal information

**Usual response:** Empathy followed by providing requested information

> CHILD: *What is your favorite color?*
> THERAPIST: *You want to know what color I like. Red.*

## Common Question 8: "Have You Ever Used Drugs?"

**Category:** Informational

**Subtype:** Personal information

**Usual response:** Empathy followed by setting of boundary/ personal limit

> CHILD: *My dad uses drugs. Do you use drugs?*
> THERAPIST: *Your dad uses drugs; you are wondering whether I might use drugs, too.*
> CHILD: *Yeah, everyone I know uses drugs. Do you use them, too?*
> THERAPIST: *You are wondering whether I am different from other adults you know. In here, however, it is you and your life that is important, not my life.*

CHILD: [Insistently] But I really want to know!

THERAPIST: For you it is important for to know whether or not I use drugs. But that is a question I will not answer.

CHILD: My dad hits me when he gets mad and is high on drugs. Would you hit me if I do something bad?

THERAPIST: You are worried that I might get mad at you and hit you if you did something that's wrong. I will not hit or hurt you in the playroom.

# Responding to Children's Requests and Commands

During play sessions it is common for children to make a wide variety of requests or commands directed toward the therapist. Such requests or commands are a vehicle for the child to express and work through important therapeutic issues. Requests/commands can be made in the context of the child's solitary role-play or in the context of interactive role-play.

## The Many Meanings of Children's Requests and Commands

Requests and commands can represent a wide range of therapeutic issues for children:

**Desires for control:**
  "I am going to do some target shooting and you have to pick up all the darts and bring them back really quick!"
  "I am going to be the king and you will do everything I say!"

**Attachment:**
  "You need to stay close to me no matter where I go in the room."
  "You have to stay far away from me the whole time I am here."
  "I am going to be a baby and get lost and you will search all over for me."

**Dependency:**
  "Please tie my shoe for me."
  "Please help me pull the trigger of the dart gun back."

**Nurturance:**
  "You are going to play my mommy and you will feed me cake."
  "Whenever the animals fall down, you pick them up and put bandages on them."

### Safety:

"You are going to play my dad and sneak into my bedroom and touch me here (pointing to genitals)."

"If I miss the target when I shoot the dart gun, you throw a block at me."

"You are going to pretend to be a baby and cry, then I will whip you with this rope."

### Boundaries:

"I want to take my clothes off." or "You take your clothes off."

"I want to wrestle with you."

"Give me a kiss." or "Let me kiss you."

As can be seen from these examples, requests or commands by the child are rich with meaning. And you can see from these examples that play therapists need criteria for deciding how to respond to such requests and commands. Our criteria and guidance follow.

## Responding to Children's Requests and Commands

The major decision to be made is where to draw the line in setting a limit or complying with a request. Within the CCPT community, there is some variation concerning where this line is drawn. We believe that the therapist's willingness to comply with requests and commands (as well as to engage in role-play that is a special form of request/command) expands the ways in which the child expresses himself and works through therapeutic issues. Therefore, we generally advocate complying with children's requests/commands unless: (1) the child asks you to violate a general playroom limit, (2) the child is intending to violate a general playroom limit, or (3) honoring the child's request would be so aversive physically or emotionally that you would not be able to maintain unconditional positive regard for the child.

The general process of responding to children's requests/commands has three steps:

**Step 1:** Identify the therapeutic issue underlying the request/command.

**Step 2:** Make an empathic response to the child utilizing the understanding developed in Step 1.

**Step 3:** Comply with request/command or set a therapeutic limit.

Following are examples to illustrate the process of responding to requests and commands:

*Example 1*

**Type:** Request
**Theme:** Control issue

> CHILD: *[Throws a deck of cards in the air, smiling] You have to pick them all up now.*
> THERAPIST: *You like the idea that you got to throw them all over, but that I have to clean them up.*
> CHILD: *And you have to pick them up quickly!*
> THERAPIST: *[Begins to pick cards up] You like being in charge and want me to do it really fast.*

*Example 2*

**Type:** Request/Limit Necessary
**Theme:** Competence

> CHILD: *Let's play ball. You throw the ball at me so hard that I can't catch it.*
> THERAPIST: *You would like to see if you can catch it even when I throw it really fast, but one of the things I won't do is hit you with the ball.*

In cases where limits need to be set, the therapist uses the standard limit-setting process. However, in some cases, the therapist may deem it acceptable to offer to honor the child's request in either a more limited way than requested by the child or through offering the child the option of "pretending" to honor the child's request.

*Example 3*

**Type:** Request/Limit with "Pretended" Compliance

> CHILD: *You be a robber and rob the bank, then I will shoot you with the dart gun.*
> THERAPIST: *You would like to be able to shoot me since I am robbing the bank; but one of the things you may not do in the playroom is to*

*really shoot me. If you want to, you can pretend to shoot me and I will pretend I am shot.*

In cases where the child requests physical help from the therapist, the therapist may assist the child, but should be open to the child's willingness or desire to switch back to doing the task by himself.

*Example 4*

**Type:** Request for Help
**Theme:** Dependency

> CHILD: *[Tries to set dominos up but they keep falling. Sounding discouraged] Oh, they are never going to stay up. [Pleadingly] Can you help me?*
> THERAPIST: *You are trying so hard to get them to stay up. You are tired of them falling and want some help.*
> CHILD: *Yes, it's impossible. Can you try?*
> THERAPIST: *You are hoping I may be able to do it. I can help if you want me to. [Therapist begins to slowly set them up, but is always open to the child's taking over the process.]*

Occasionally, a request may be made in a nonverbal manner. In such cases the therapist would respond empathically, and if the actions of the child still indicate the child desires help, the therapist would reply with this nonverbal request.

*Example 5*

**Type:** Request for Help/Nonverbal
**Theme:** Dependency

> CHILD: *[Straining to get top off of a jar of paste] It won't come off.*
> THERAPIST: *You want to be able to use the paste but the top is stuck.*
> CHILD: *[Hands jar of paste to therapist]*
> THERAPIST: *You want me to open it for you.*
> CHILD: *[Nods]*
> THERAPIST: *[Loosens lid, while keeping jar close enough for child to reach, and is open to the possibility the child may take over once the top is loosened.]*

Although a therapist will generally comply with most types of requests or commands the child makes, you would not comply with a request or command that turned over decision making in the play session to you. In short, although requests for help and commands made of you may allow the child to work on a wide variety of issues, you should be careful to avoid violating Axline's principles of accepting the child completely, establishing a feeling of permissiveness, letting the child lead the way, and using limitations wisely.

*Example 6*

**Type:** Request/Violation of Principles of Letting the Child Lead the Way

> **CHILD:** *Today, you get to decide what we do in our playtime.*
> **THERAPIST:** *You think I should get to choose this week, but during our play session, you get to choose all the time.*
> **CHILD:** *[Firm and commanding] I know, but I choose that you get to choose today!*
> **THERAPIST:** *You really want me to choose, but in our playtime I will not choose what we do.*

# Concluding Remarks Regarding Requests and Commands

Therapists who are new to CCPT often find the freedom granted to the child difficult to understand. Common questions or concerns expressed include:

"If you allow him to be bossy in the playroom, won't he be bossy in other places?"

"If you help the child with things, won't she become more dependent?"

If one were utilizing a behavioral approach to addressing the child's problems, then indeed the therapist would attempt to discourage such behaviors through having negative consequences for such behaviors and/or reinforcing alternative desired behaviors. The child-centered model, however, like many personality-centered methodologies, sees such behaviors as an opportunity for therapeutically working with the child's inner world to promote healing and growth.

Nonetheless, even when a therapist understands the importance of allowing children to play out themes of control and dependency, she may still have her own negative reactions to children's exertions of control or dependency toward her. Such reactions can be mild or very strong and may affect the unconditional positive regard, and thus her ability to be accepting and empathic toward the child. If you find yourself reacting strongly to children's play that is very controlling or very dependent, don't be discouraged; this is simply part of the learning process many child therapists and counselors go through. If this remains a significant problem over time, formal supervision will help in working through this and enhancing your skills in this area.

# Activities and Resources for Further Study

## Contemplation and Practice of Key Concepts in Responding to Questions

The key concepts of CCPT often present new ways of being. Contemplation and academic practice can help you develop depth of understanding and comfort with the skills. The following activities provide opportunities for contemplation and academic practice of critical key concepts. They can be completed alone, with a partner, in a small group or classroom. The answers for Activities A and B are found at the end of the book in Skills Support Resource D.

- *Activity A:* Use the following list of hypothetical child questions/ scenarios to test your skills in responding to questions. Work with a partner or think through the scenarios suggested by the questions on your own. For each of the following questions, identify what category and subtype it most likely fits into:
  Category: Structuring    Subtype: Parameters of therapy
  Category: Structuring    Subtype: Request for direction
  Category: Informational    Subtype: Factual information
  Category: Informational    Subtype: Personal information
    1. "What is your favorite football team?"
    2. "Let's play cards. Which card game do you want to play?"
    3. "Can I come back again tomorrow?"
    4. "Let's see who won. How much is 12 plus 9?"
    5. "Does your husband hit your kids?"

6. "How many legs does a spider have?"
7. "What is your favorite type of pizza?"
8. "What color should I make this doggy?"
9. "Will you tell my mom that I created a mess in here?"

- *Activity B:* For each of the questions listed in Practice Exercise 1, identify which is the most likely response option that would be utilized, then give a possible response by the therapist. Remember, your options include:

   Empathy followed by providing requested information
   Empathy followed by clarification of child's freedom to make decisions
   Empathy followed by the setting of a boundary/personal limit

*Note:* In actual play sessions, it is also possible that the therapist giving an empathic response (or series of empathic responses) will result in the child's no longer desiring or needing an additional response. However, we will assume for these practice activities that more than just empathy will be required by the therapist.

## Contemplation and Practice of Key Concepts in Responding to Requests and Commands

Answers for Activity C are found at the end of the book in Skills Support Resource D.

- *Activity C:* Use the following list of hypothetical child scenarios involving requests and commands to test your skills in responding. Work with a partner or think through the scenarios suggested by the questions on your own. For each of the children's requests and commands, please note whether you would (a) comply with the request or (b) set a limit, and explain why.
  1. "After I shoot the darts, you have to run and pick them up and return them to me."
  2. "I am going to be a doctor. You need to take your shirt off so I can examine you."
  3. "Oh, my poor tower of blocks fell over. Can you please help me get it back together?"
  4. "Let's do an art project; you decide what it will be."
  5. "You have to stand on your head for 10 minutes!"

## Activity D: Mock Session Practice of Responding to Questions, Requests, and Commands

An excellent way to develop your skills for service to children is to practice with a partner in mock sessions. Take turns in the roles of child and therapist. You will find that you'll learn from the role of the child, therapist, or if you have the extra opportunity, as observer. We find 15 minutes to be a reasonable length for mock sessions. Longer sessions allow more time for practice, but it can get difficult to sustain the role of the child for very long periods. You can limit yourselves to small sets of representative toys at a table or expand to a playroom. If you can establish mock sessions to follow most chapters, try to stay with the same partner to see how your relationship develops. The following practice set instructions can be taken together or separately.

- Engage in a 15-minute mock session in which the person in the role of the child provides you with opportunities to respond to questions, requests, and commands. Stop and allow the person in the role of the child to give feedback. Ask your partner how it *felt to be in the role of the child* in the mock interaction. Switch roles and repeat this exercise, with you now playing the role of the child.

## Return to and Review the Primary Skill Objectives

- *Activity E:* Revisit the Primary Skill Objectives for this chapter and see if you have mastered them to your satisfaction at this time. If not, seek additional readings, practices, and discussions for clarification, and in order to master them to your satisfaction.

# Role-Play: The Therapeutic Value of Taking Part in Dramatic or Pretend Play During Child-Centered Play Therapy Sessions

*The child may use the therapist to symbolize the good or bad parent, the benevolent or tyrannical despot, or the possessor of magic to cure. These shifting roles, which the child assigns to the therapist, who holds steadily to his real role, spring from the heart of the child's turmoil and represent his efforts to find a solution for his difficulties.*

—*Frederick H. Allen*

*Imaginative play is fun, but in the midst of the joys of making believe, children may also be preparing for the reality of more effective lives.*

—*Dorothy G. and Jerome L. Singer*

## Application Focus Issue

Six-year-old Darin begins his sixth play therapy session by immediately dashing over to the dress-up trunk in the playroom. Pulling out the long black cape, he holds it up and smiles. "Now, where's that other thing I need? . . ." Darin talks to himself as he dumps out the contents of a toy tool box and quickly locates the wooden hammer. Holding it up triumphantly, he looks at you and declares, "I'm doing just like last time . . . so you better watch out, Missy!"

This is your sixth session with Darin, and you know by now that he will likely continue a role-play scenario that began 3 weeks ago. He is the "all and powerful judge" and you are assigned the role of "the frightened little girl" (and, at times, "the girl's little brother"), who both have to testify in court. You match his tone of excitement by responding, "You're getting everything you need, and letting me know I'd better be ready!" Darin requires some help from you getting the cape on and adjusted just right. Watching his face, you can see that this is serious business, and every detail is important. Darin looks in the mirror and adds a finishing touch. He flips his shirt collar up and asks that you tie the cape "just so" to ensure that the collar stands straight up. With another check in the mirror, Darin takes a long, stern look at himself. He is smug and obviously pleased with the result. Hurrying now, Darin grabs a book, some paper, and a pencil and sits down at the small art table. With an official beckoning wave to you, he motions that it's time to come over and sit down directly opposite him. He bangs the hammer down hard three times—BAM-BAM-BAM.

> **DARIN:** *[Speaking in a low, gruff voice] Order in this court!*

So, the scene is set, and Darin is the scriptwriter, director, and star. You know that he needs you both as his therapist and as a "cast member," so how then do you confidently proceed? It is obvious that dramatic role-play is Darin's chosen mode of self-expression, so how can you maintain therapeutic perspective, empathically respond, and best take part?

Preparing you for such questions and situations—for taking part in role-play with confidence, self-awareness, and enjoyment—is the goal of this chapter.

## Chapter Overview and Summary

Dramatic or pretend play comes naturally to most children, so it is no surprise that role-play is a frequently chosen mode of self-expression in child-centered play therapy (CCPT) sessions. Role-plays can be of three main types: (1) solitary role-play, in which the child plays all the roles; (2) therapist role-play, in which the child asks the therapist to play the role or roles while the child observes and directs the role-play; and (3) interactive role-play, in which the child assigns roles to both himself and the therapist. When a child realizes the therapist *can and will take part in dramatic play*, an invitation to act out roles often follows. When a child feels safe to play and freely express at the dollhouse or in the sand tray without intrusive questions or interruptions, the stage is set for self-generated activity. With great exuberance and spontaneity, a child will offer her own vivid and symbolic scenarios. Confidently, the child will often invite the therapist to take part in scenes, with instructions beginning with "Make believe . . . " or "Let's pretend. . . . "

How can you, as a skilled play therapist, ready yourself to respond to this invitation and take part in pretend play during CCPT sessions? Many child play therapists and counselors struggle with this question, and as a result, "to role-play or not to role-play" and the skills necessary are often discussed and debated. While most CCPT specialists would agree that the therapist is never to be considered simply a "playmate" in therapy sessions, or to follow the lead of the child without regard for realistic boundaries and safety, there are varying opinions about how active a role the therapist should take when assigned a character or a role to play in a dramatic scenario.

Although some practitioners of CCPT choose not to participate in role-play with children, those trained in Louise Guerney's model (Guerney, 1983b, 2001) have embraced the participation in role-play when requested by the child. Criteria have been developed to help therapists and counselors develop self-awareness, understanding, and skills necessary to make sure that the child leads the way; that is, the child maintains *control of the direction and the contents of the scenario* as it unfolds during role-play. The training model also recognizes that role-play can take a variety of forms and that different skills can be enhanced and developed to help the counselor recognize the type of role-play (solitary, therapist oriented, or interactive) and utilize skills to take part without interrupting the process, or restricting or adding unnecessarily to the child's play. This chapter will illustrate that taking part in role-play while also maintaining therapeutic perspective is not only possible, but also often is the "golden road" to providing empathy, unconditional positive regard, and support as the child leads the way. Role-play vignettes, demonstrations, and skill practice exercises are provided to help you better understand the therapeutic value of pretend play, and enhance and hone your own skills in CCPT role-play situations.

## Primary Skill Objectives

The following Primary Skill Objectives for this chapter are provided to guide the reader through the chapter, and for reflection and review after completing the chapter reading and exercises. By reading and working through the chapter exercises, readers will be better able to:

1. Explain and/or demonstrate within role-play the necessary skills of the therapist as "confident companion" in a role-play:
   - "Asides" or "the stage whisper" for guidance and clarification from the child
   - Temporarily suspending action for necessary limit setting within a role-play
   - "Playing the part" with enthusiasm without taking over the narrative
   - Making process and reflective statements within role-play without interrupting, and while also playing your assigned role
   - Tracking with empathy while "witnessing" solitary role-play wherein the child plays multiple characters
   - "Witnessing" and observing without comments, questions, or interruptions that introduce non-child-centered elements
2. Provide examples of solitary and interactive role-play in CCPT.
3. Explain and provide examples of therapist responses in solitary and interactive role-play scenarios in CCPT.
4. Explain and give examples of the importance of pretend play in children's emotional and moral development.
5. Demonstrate the different types of role-play and therapist responses in mock sessions with a partner.

## The Therapeutic Value of Role-Play in CCPT: Being a "Confident Companion" to the Child in Therapy

In our practice and supervision of CCPT, we have found that role-play enhances the therapist-child relationship and allows children to create their own metaphors and lead the way. We feel that when a child chooses role-play, it is because it is his quickest path to healing. In order to better understand the therapeutic value of role-play, it is helpful to first consider Carl Roger's description of "empathic understanding" and "confident companion" in the following passage:

> The third facilitative aspect of the relationship is empathic understanding. An empathic way of being with another person means entering the private perceptual world of the other and becoming thoroughly at home in it. . . . It includes communicating your sensing of the other person's world as

you look with fresh and unfrightened eyes at elements of which he or she is fearful. It means frequently checking with the person as to the accuracy of your sensings, and being guided by the responses you receive. You are a confident companion to the person in his or her inner world.

In order to strike a balance between offering "empathic understanding" while remaining a "confident companion" during role-plays in CCPT, it is necessary that the counselor be self-confident and prepared to accompany the child in this "private perceptual world" without "getting lost" in it. The child who chooses pretend or dramatic play has likely chosen this as a mode of self-expression because it is his own path to healing, and therefore, as stated before, likely the *quickest and most efficient* way for him to work through the interpersonal and intrapersonal issues causing distress. In a sense, the role-plays are the child's *own metaphors* by which she begins to lead the way and create corrective experiences. In addition to providing such corrective experiences, children often experiment in role-play—trying out new behaviors and skills—and work to master overwhelming situations to establish a sense of security and control. By role-playing, the child is able to set up and experience scenarios that come from within and explore ways in which she can function in a healthier, happier, and age-appropriate way.

## Play and Child Development: The Value Inherent in Pretend Play

To highlight the importance of pretend play in a child's development, let's return to the scenario from the beginning of this chapter and the role of the therapist in assisting this child in benefiting from the therapeutic value of dramatic or pretend play. According to Piaget

Table 9.1  **Reasons Why Role-Play Is Important and Powerful Within CCPT**

1. It is a golden opportunity to be a child's "confident companion" into frightening places that a child may not process fully and heal from when playing alone.
2. It can help imaginative and therapeutic play go places that it could not go alone.
3. It can provide a deeply shared experience—deep empathy and connectedness.

(1951), children in their play assimilate reality to their wishes. Children have many powerful wishes that cannot be adequately expressed with words, as well as fears and anxieties that can overwhelm and seem unmanageable or, at the very worst, unbearable. To escape this predicament, children will often "play out" feelings in dramatic scenarios. In this type of play, they can reconstruct the scenario and "be" the doctor giving the shot, "be" the teacher grading the paper, or, as in the case of little Darin, "be" the judge banging the gavel. By assuming a fictitious role (a stern and powerful judge) and creating his own scenarios (court scenes where children must answer questions), Darin develops a tool for managing and expressing a range of emotions resulting from his requirement to testify in court. The scenario—completely within his control—makes bearable what previously may have seemed unbearable. Consider the therapist's responses to Darin as the scene unfolds below. Note how the therapist accepts Darin's position as scriptwriter, director, producer, and star of the role-play scenario, and is also careful to stay "right there with him"—to not get too far ahead or to lag too far behind. In other words, the therapist avoids adding non-child-centered elements such as questioning, interrupting, or adding her own perspective. Asking for clarification and guidance along the way, the therapist is ready to accept direction and take a role; however, she is also sensitive to Darin's need to process on his own and be the one "in control" of his own metaphor or story. Within the scene of the role-play, notice that the therapist uses a "stage whisper" or "aside" to briefly step outside the scene for clarification. While questions are generally off limits in CCPT, this use of the "stage whisper" is allowed in the context of role-play, and is a skill that is used sensitively to allow the child to lead without too much interference with the child's process and action of the role-play.

> **DARIN:** *[Speaking in a low, gruff voice] Order in this court!*
> **THERAPIST:** *[Quickly sits up straight as if in an immediate obedient* response *to this demand]*
> **DARIN:** *Now then . . . [tapping his pencil] . . . little girl . . . what is your name? [Before the therapist can respond, Darin comes out of character, and in his natural voice, adds] No . . . wait a minute. I'm not the judge now. Act like I'm a man who gives you some money.*
> **DARIN:** *[Quickly grabs a fistful of pretend money from a toy bin, and hurries back to the table] Here . . . [hands the money across the table] . . . little girl . . . quick . . . take this money!*

THERAPIST: *[Seeking direction from the child, the therapist leans in and asks as an aside, quietly in a ''stage whisper'']* What do you want me to do?

DARIN: *You take it and put it in your pocket.* [*The therapist complies, and quickly puts the pretend money in her pocket. Darin gets up and looks in the mirror to adjust his collar to make sure it is straight up, and then sits back down. He bangs the gavel three times, and in his ''official judge'' voice bellows*] Order in this court!! Okay, little girl . . . do you promise to tell the truth, the whole truth, and nothing but the truth?

THERAPIST: *[Leans in and again asks quietly as a ''stage whisper'' aside]* What do you want me to say?

DARIN: *Say ''I do.''*

THERAPIST: *[Speaking in a quiet, ''little girl'' voice]* I do.

DARIN: *[Sternly]* You'd better speak a little louder, Missy. This is a courtroom! Now . . . I want you to try to remember . . . did you take . . . any money? Think very carefully before answering . . . I need you to remember and tell the truth.

THERAPIST: *[Leans in and again asks quietly as an aside]* What do I say now, Darin?

DARIN: *[Thinks for a second before responding]* You start to say yes . . . but then you start crying.

THERAPIST: *[Back in character, in a soft ''little girl'' voice]* Umm . . . yehhh. . . . *[Puts her head in her hands and pretends to sob quietly. Darin watches in silence for a moment, and then begins to scribble ferociously, flipping the pages of a spiral notebook, frowning as he ''pretend writes'' page after page after page.]*

DARIN: *[Loud and stern]* You see this, Missy? *[Holds up all the ''pretend scribbles'' in the notebook, pointing to them line by line.]* All this is what I'm writing about you and your brother, so you better stop crying, sit up straight, and tell the truth!

By "reversing" the situation in a make-believe courtroom, and placing himself as the powerful judge, little Darin is able to feel in control while he works through many feelings regarding having to testify in court. As Piaget (1951) points out, make-believe and pretend play is much more than simply a way for children to express their interests. It also serves the emotional function of *liquidating* conflicts to lessen the intensity of bad (or stressful) feelings. During role-play, children are able to experience within a make-believe scenario what it feels like to bring certain feelings to the surface, and "work through" conflicts in a quest for mastery.

# Different Types of Dramatic Role-Play Situations: Skills for Participating in Interactive and Solitary Role-Play Scenarios

## Interactive Role-Play

When a child chooses interactive role-play, in which the therapist is asked to play or act out roles or characters, the following skills allow for active participation that ensures that the child leads and is in control of the narrative or scene. The therapist, as "character," is required to:

1. Check in with the child first to establish the basic parameters from the child as to how to act out the roles. For a simple example, consider the following. A child is walking a little plastic dog figure along her side of a row of blocks that she has arranged apparently to represent a wall or fence. She says to her therapist while gesturing to a cat figure, and then motioning to the other side of the wall, "You be that cat." It's fairly obvious what she wants, so the therapist responds while picking up the cat figure and moving it along the other side of the wall, "So, I'm the cat and I walk along this other side."

2. Step outside the role (use the "stage whisper" as an aside when needed) to ask for clarification when uncertain as to how to proceed. Following in the example above: The dog and cat get to the end of the "wall," each apparently having not known the other was on the other side, and the dog barks ferociously when seeing the cat. It seems obvious that the cat is supposed to be scared and run—that's what most cats would do in that situation, but the therapist stops to ask (quietly, using the "stage whisper" with her hand cupped to one side of her mouth in an "aside" gesture), "What is the cat going to do now?"

3. Once these parameters are set, the therapist is expected to use some acting talent to "bring life" to the assigned character without taking over the lead, but feeling free to add behaviors expected of

the role assigned by the child. Following from the example above, the girl made her dog back up while her therapist asked for directions above. So, her therapist made her cat character back up at the same time, and in the same way. The scene plays forward again, with the dog and cat coming to the end of the wall without knowing they are about to run into each other. This time they are both surprised. The dog barks ferociously. The cat yells, "Aaaaagh," as she runs away.

4. The therapist remains acceptant to the child's corrections and changes in the direction of the role-play at all times, unless a limit is needed to keep the session safe. The child is allowed to be the scriptwriter, director, producer, and star. Following from our example above, the girl laughs and corrects, "Cats don't say 'Aaaagh!' Cats say 'reeoooow!'" To which her therapist responds, sharing the laugh, "Oh, I didn't get that right, the cat should have said 'reeeooow!' as it ran away."

5. If, within the context of a role-play, playroom or personal limits are necessary, the therapist temporarily suspends the role-play in order to set the limit. In such cases, it is again important to remember the empathy sandwich model in limit setting to avoid startling the child or making the child feel possible guilt or shame or that he is being scolded. For example, in the midst of a very active cops-and-robbers role-play, a little boy is enjoying arresting his counselor by "slapping on the handcuffs and tightening them up good!" His counselor notices that the little guy is highly excited by this playful drama and is very likely not meaning to tighten the handcuffs so terribly tight; however, each time, the cuffs get a little tighter! The counselor temporarily suspends the play and gets the boy's attention, saying (in an even, matter-of-fact tone): "(Child's name), you're having lots of fun playing this game, but I need to let you know . . . one of the things you cannot do is make the handcuffs that tight. You'll need to leave them a little looser on my wrists when you arrest me."

## Therapist Role-Play

In therapist role-play, the child asks the therapist to play the role or roles while the child observes and directs the role-play. For example, little Julie asks her therapist to stand up, and she gives her a microphone with the instructions to "sing a song." Instead of singing an aria

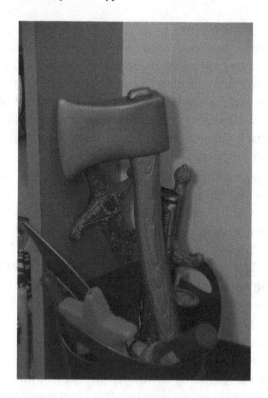

Figure 9.1

in a beautiful, operatic voice, or telling little Julie " . . . Oh, one of the things I can't do is sing," the therapist would ask for some guidance. The interchange might then follow like this:

> **THERAPIST:** *[Quietly, as an "aside"] Julie . . . how do you want me to sing?*
>
> **JULIE:** *Ummm . . . very loud . . . and not too good!*
>
> **THERAPIST:** *[Loudly and off key] DO . . . RE . . . MEEE . . . FA . . . SOOOO . . . LAAAA!!!*
>
> **JULIE:** *[Laughing] That's awful! Sing a real song, like Happy Birthday!*
>
> **THERAPIST:** *Oh . . . you mean a real song! [Loudly and still off key] HAPPY BIRTHDAY TO MEEEEEE!*
>
> **JULIE:** *[Laughing even harder now] BOOOOOO! Get off the stage!*

In therapist role-play, the idea is to seek guidance in order not to take over the role-play. It may also involve a need to balance some limit setting, for instance, if in a challenge little Julie then instructs:

JULIE: *Get back up there . . . on stage now . . . and hop on one foot until I say stop.*

If the therapist is unable to do this, she might need to respond with a limit such as:

THERAPIST: *Oh! You want my next challenge to be hopping on one foot! That would be a great challenge! Julie, one thing I cannot do for the challenge is hop on one foot.*

JULIE: *Okay. Let me see then . . . I want you to dance real silly until I say stop!*

THERAPIST: *[Begins a silly dance] Okay! Here goes!*

In general, the therapist must always balance her ability to maintain empathy, genuineness, and unconditional positive regard when responding to requests and commands during therapist role-play. For more on the skills of responding to questions, requests for help and commands, refer to Chapter 8.

## Solitary Role-Play

In solitary role-play, the child conducts the narrative and scenario on his own. A child may request that the therapist engage in a role-play without his own participation, or a child may ask the therapist to *take a stance* of onlooker or "witness" to a role-play wherein the child acts out multiple characters. When a child engages in solitary role-play, the therapist engages primarily in tracking and empathic responding; for example, consider the following:

Using small stones, shells, and Popsicle sticks, 8-year-old Luis spends 20 minutes quietly building an underground fortress in the corner of the sand tray. He then methodically sets up two long rows of army men. His counselor consistently offers support with his solemn attention and facial expressions, and verbally acknowledges how important it seems for Luis to get "everything set up just right." Luis nods in agreement. He is somber and very serious. His counselor respects this overall tone that seems to "hang in the air" by not interrupting, but still offering nonverbal support and serious attention. Luis periodically stops, stands up, and surveys the scene from above. He scratches his head. He takes a small truck and turns it over on top of a small plastic cow. He scatters a few small plastic trees and stones and shells around the scene. He sits down and sighs. He then begins to knock over the first line of army men, making quiet "pistol shot" sounds as they fall. He sits again in silence. Then he carefully moves one army man from the back row slowly in advance toward the fortress.

> COUNSELOR: *The whole first row is down . . . now one from the back row moves carefully forward. . . .*
>
> LUIS: *[Quietly] Uh-huh, he's the one to . . . his job is to check things out.*
>
> COUNSELOR: *He moves forward to check things out. . . .*
>
> LUIS: *He's sees all these ones . . . all dead.*
>
> COUNSELOR: *He sees they are all dead.*
>
> LUIS: *The trees . . . all burnt . . . fell down . . . and this truck over . . . on a cow.*
>
> COUNSELOR: *Uh-huh, I see that.*
>
> LUIS: *It is getting dark now, so he is going to try to go to the underground hide-out. He tries for all the others.*
>
> COUNSELOR: *He'll try for the others . . . to make it to the underground hide-out.*

In solitary role-play, the child often requires attention and non-verbal support (facial expressions) balanced with tracking that does not interfere with his process. While this can require patience, it also may be likened to a meditative and quiet stance that simply and empathically lets the child know, "I'm right here with you."

## Balancing "Playing the Part" or Improvisation With Taking Directions

To help a child effectively self-express in interactive role-play, a play therapist has to be able to *play* the role as assigned by the child. Generally, but not always, the therapist is a supporting actor, and the child is the lead actor, star, and the all-powerful director. If you are too careful as an actor, in need of so much direction that you are completely unable to make the role come to life, unable to improvise in even obvious ways, then you are of no use to your director. In such instances, the child will sometimes simply eliminate your participation and engage in solitary role-play.

However, if you go too far in interpreting and implementing your role, you can take the play in directions completely alien to your director, destroying the role of the lead actor, the star of the show, and frustrating the intentions of your director. Remember that there is a

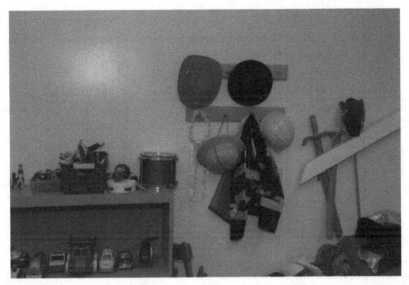

Figure 9.2

huge power differential between you and your child client. Our director–supporting actor metaphor breaks down in that while your client may act like a surly, demanding director, in reality, he is a child in your playroom, as well as a child who is likely vulnerable to insecurities. If you begin to play your role in an overly dramatic way and make unwarranted assumptions, you will call too much attention to yourself and exceed what is desired by the child. The danger in such cases is that it becomes your play with his support vs. the other way around.

Remember the honor of participating in your child client's private world. You must enter sensitively. You must be a good actor who can improvise, or the two of you will never get his private world out in the open for him to experience at a higher level of awareness. The following scenarios of therapists' participations in role-plays are provided to help highlight the skills necessary for engaging in CCPT role-play.

### Scenario 1: Terrance the "Tentative and Caring Doctor"
Terrance has been sitting with his back to the therapist quietly sorting through the doctor's kit. He places the stethoscope on his neck and turns to his therapist.

> **Terrance:** *I'm gonna play like a doctor.*
> **Therapist:** *You're gonna play like a doctor.*

> TERRANCE: *Uh-huh . . . now where's that hammer thing . . . and where's that shot thing? [Continues to sort through until he finds the toy hammer and syringe.] Aha!*
>
> THERAPIST: *You found what you need!*
>
> TERRANCE: *Okay . . . put out your leg.*
>
> THERAPIST: *[Quietly and as an aside] You want me to do something . . . can you tell me more?*
>
> TERRANCE: *When I hit it on here (points to therapist's knee), you kick your leg out. [Terrance taps the therapist just below the knee. The therapist kicks his leg out to simulate a ''reflex kick'' as instructed. Terrance giggles, obviously pleased with the play.] And now the other one. [They repeat the reflex test with his other leg. Terrance giggles again.]*
>
> THERAPIST: *[Smiling] You like being able to make my leg kick out.*
>
> TERRANCE: *[Taking a more serious tone] And now for your shot.*
>
> THERAPIST: *[Quietly] Terrance, what do I do? Do you want me to act happy or sad about the shot?*
>
> TERRANCE: *You cry just a little. [Shifting back to his ''official doctor'' voice] Now roll up your sleeve. [Gives shot, looking intently at his therapist's face as he does.]*
>
> THERAPIST: *[Pretends to begin to whimper quietly.]*
>
> TERRANCE: *Shush now . . . it's okay. [Pats his therapist's shoulder] I'm gonna give you candy and a sticker.*

### Scenario 2: Kayla the "Evil and Demanding Doctor"

Kayla excitedly dumps the contents of the toy doctor's kit out on the table in front of her counselor. She leans in and stares at her counselor. Then she let's out an evil-sounding "Heee-Heee-Heee!

> COUNSELOR: *Oooooh . . . [feigning a slight startled reaction to match the intention of the child] you're looking like you have an idea for those things.*
>
> KAYLA: *I do . . . you know what's gonna happen now. It's time to have your doctor appointment! [Picks out a toy syringe and some large plastic tweezers and waves them menacingly in front of the therapist's face.]*
>
> COUNSELOR: *[Shrinking back a little, in order to begin participation in the role-play that is developing] Oh . . . and you have something in mind for those.*

Since Kayla's counselor is fairly sure that this child wants her to "be afraid" in the role-play, the counselor could simply act afraid, or if the counselor wanted to be extra sure, she could ask for clarification by asking in a "stage whisper" as an aside, "Am I going to be scared?"

> KAYLA: *Yes! Now be quiet and pull up your sleeve!!*
>
> COUNSELOR: *[Quickly pulls up sleeve]*
>
> KAYLA: *[Starts to give shot, then steps out of character, and directs] . . . Now you turn your head away not to look . . . 'cuz you really don't want it.*
>
> COUNSELOR: *[Turns away as Kayla pretends to give a shot.]*
>
> KAYLA: *[Pushes the plastic syringe down forcefully and hard on her therapist's forearm.]*
>
> COUNSELOR: *[Temporarily suspends play and in a calm tone sets a limit] Kayla . . . you're wanting to give me a shot, but I need to let you know pushing down hard on my arm with the pretend shot is one of the things you may not do. [See Chapter 7 for more on limit-setting procedures and qualities.]*
>
> KAYLA: *Okay . . . I didn't mean to . . . and now I'm going to do some . . . surgery!*
>
> COUNSELOR: *You didn't mean to . . . and now you've got another idea for . . . surgery!*
>
> KAYLA: *Yep! [Kayla steps out of character as she rummages through the toy doctor's kit supplies.] Hey . . . do you have a knife in this kit? Or is there something I can use to cut . . . never mind these will do just fine! [She holds up some large plastic tweezers with a big smile.]*
>
> COUNSELOR: *You found something that will work just fine.*
>
> KAYLA: *Yeh . . . now pretend that I leave . . . and when I come back in the room, you see these [holds up the tweezers] . . . and you scream, "Noooo! Not surgery!" [Kayla walks to the back of the room behind the counselor, and then comes back around and pretends to enter the room holding up the tweezers.]*
>
> COUNSELOR: *[Giving her best horrified look and scream] Noooooo! Not surgery!*

The similarities in the scenarios provide a comparative example to highlight how the therapist must be sensitive to the overall tone and emotion conveyed, and, at times, not proceed until given some extra direction for guidance and clarification. The therapist must also be perceptive to subtle cues of the child's self-expression. Limits, when set, need to be stated in a calm, nonjudgmental, matter-of-fact tone, with your own voice and not "in character." Remember that children can become very caught up in their role-plays, and in the midst of high

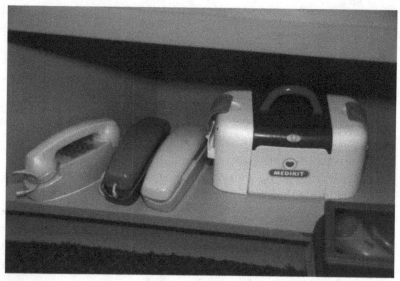

*Figure 9.3*

activity may become overexuberant. When setting limits is necessary during role-play, the therapist must be ready to temporarily suspend the action, using the three-step empathy sandwich method when possible, and then return to role-play. Being able to step smoothly in and out of role-plays may take some practice; however, this ability is a reassuring reminder to the child of the structure and safety that the adult therapist is there to provide.

## Themes in Roles Assigned During CCPT Role-Play

### Common Themes in Role-Plays: The "Good vs. Evil" Theme or "Powerful and Powerless" Themes in Aggressive-Regressive Stage Play

A 10-year-old boy's "vicious beatings" of Bobo for seven sessions seem to end abruptly when, during session 8, he jumps in the sandbox and begins "planting a garden." An 8-year-old girl's "crying baby" is ignored and denied food for part of the session, and then, toward the end of the session, is held, rocked, and given a bottle. Trying on different roles in CCPT allows the child a safe experiencing—a back and forth of feeling "evil" and "good"—"vulnerable" and "safe"—"all powerful" and "totally powerless."

Children use CCPT to ponder the existential questions of meaning and choice: "Who am I?" "Who do I want to be?," "What ways of being in life *feel* right to me?" These important questions are often most evident in the back-and-forth role-plays commonly seen during the Aggressive and Regressive stages (see Chapter 10) of play. While a therapist should never over-interpret any single action in play, and while we know interpretation is of little value (see the problem of interpretation in the Common Problems section near the end of this chapter), the overly simple "interpretations" of a child's actions in play therapy below may help illustrate what we mean by the "good vs. evil" struggle for choice.

In one 5-year-old boy's play, a large T-rex dinosaur devours the helpless baby doll. This is a highly detailed, visceral, graphic experience. The little boy experiences it, in the role of the dinosaur, with great relish—ending with a loud "GULP" and then smiling and licking his lips. Perhaps the self-defining self-statements understood out of assuming his identification with each character would be, "I am small and power-less—a victim—in some situations. I might like to be all-powerful. I might like to victimize. What does that feel like?" Later, after time has passed (which can be mere seconds or many sessions) and the manifes-tations of his first self-statements have been experienced or tried out, the baby is rescued. The baby rides on the big dinosaur's back and is protected from other predators. The assumed self-defining self-state-ments would be, "I need, want, like, and deserve to be protected, cared for, and nurtured. It feels good. And I can grow to rescue and nurture. I can protect others and seek the protection and nurturing of others."

## The Importance of Recognizing and Respecting the Child's Thematic Metaphors

In our experience in practice and supervision of CCPT, when children utilize dramatic or pretend play, roles assigned typically represent two broad categories: those of antagonists to the child's "character" or those of a supporter, fan, or assistant. Family roles, teacher/student, or doctor/patient roles are the most frequent choices in our experience, but all-powerful heroes and "super evil" villains are also very common. Animals, cars, and Play-Doh figures, as well as action figures, dolls, and puppets, are used as characters in expressive scenarios.

It is important to remember the general storyline and themes, to "stay on track" from week to week. We suggest that you note the outline and important *qualities* of the role-play within your session notes (e.g., stage the child is in, tone of the session, demeanor [emotional qualities] of the child, and general themes that are important). Then, review these notes before your next session. Your main purpose here is to keep track of the themes, qualities (tone), and characters from week to week—to not *have to be reminded*—which shows respect for your client's inner world and mode of expression. Another purpose is to remind yourself of the child you are preparing to be with for a play session. Some children require more patience and structuring than others, but all are deserving of the core conditions of empathy, genuineness, and unconditional positive regard from the play therapist.

It is not necessary or advisable to write down specific details of the role-play, as this poses the risk of tainting the enduring client record in a way that could create problems if the file is reviewed by parents, lawyers, or even other mental health professionals who do not understand play therapy. (For more on record keeping, you may want to refer to Chapter 12.) In mid-therapy, or Aggressive-Regressive Stage play (see Chapter 10), it is not unusual for children to pick up where they left off from one session to the next, even if unusual amounts of time have passed between sessions (e.g., sessions were missed due to illness or breaks in the school schedule when counseling is provided at school). At other times, children will leave a theme for weeks, then come back to it and expect the therapist to fall right back into the role when that mode of self-expression is needed again and there is "unfinished business." Still other times, a child may discontinue a role-play or repeat the same role-play over and over for some time. Still other children will never use role-play as a mode of self-expression. Therefore, what is perhaps most important is that the therapist remain open to the possibility of the child's therapeutic progress, which *results in both subtle changes and sometimes significant changes to the role-plays in which they engage*. Indeed, it is often subtle changes that will allow the therapist to know that the child is not "stuck" but instead is advancing and working on different aspects of a given therapeutic issue. This is covered in detail in Chapter 10.

## Common Problems Regarding Engaging in Role-Play

### Balancing "Playing the Part" With Taking Direction

The novice play therapist must learn to be a good enough, self-directed enough supporting actor to play the part, while also taking direction well and not taking over the play. We find it more common, at least among our students and supervisees, to err on the side of being too careful, and we encourage taking risks and being oneself within the role. We think that overly tentative beginning play therapists err this way out of a conscientious desire to facilitate the child's self-expression and a fear of wrongfully, unsupportively shaping the child's self-expression. We find it helpful to remember what a strong force a child's self-expression is once it has begun within a therapeutic relationship. If you have established an atmosphere that allows a child's self-expression; if you maintain an attitude of interest, valuing, and honoring a child's self-expression; if you are empathically attuned such that you will see a child's reaction when you are "off" or going in the wrong direction (all of which are core aspects of CCPT and should be qualities that you have been developing prior to and throughout your study of role-play skills), then when you are occasionally off, or you overplay a role, there will be no serious lasting consequence for being wrong, since you will pick up your mistake or the child will correct you. In short, such rare lapses in attunement with the child are preferable to being a chronically poor supporting actor in the child's role-plays.

We have also seen novice therapists err on the side of overacting or becoming overly dramatic within a role-play. Usually, this is a result of not cultivating, not deeply contemplating the qualities creating an atmosphere that allows, maintains interest, values, and honors each child's self-expression. Another possible reason for such an error is that the therapist is working out his own "stuff" in the child's session. Consider the following fictitious and exaggerated example.

> JOHNNY: *These dinosaurs are going to fight. You be that one [handing the therapist the larger one]. He's the daddy.*
> THERAPIST: *[Asks in an aside] So, I'm the daddy and we fight?*
> JOHNNY: *Yeah . . . you have to make him really fight.*
> THERAPIST: *[Shortly after fight is engaged, he pins boy's dinosaur down with the larger dinosaur, then picks the smaller dinosaur up and pounds him down repeatedly.]*
> JOHNNY: *[Shocked and obviously disempowered] But . . . they were . . . they were just play fighting . . . like wrestling for fun.*

This therapist may have thought he saw an opportunity to "help" Johnny express the abuse that he knew or believed had been a traumatic part of his life. This well-intentioned therapist may have forgotten that the core purpose is for Johnny to express what he needs

*Table 9.2* **Role-Play Reminders**

Remember to avoid the following problem areas or errors that can occur for novice play therapists engaging in role-play:

- Balancing "playing the part" with taking directions
- Interpreting vs. connecting and processing through self-expression
- Questions and/or questioning tone in role-play (unless as an "aside")
- Taking the role-play personally when placed in a "powerless" role
- Taking the role-play personally when from a "demanding director"
- Forgetting to express empathy in the context of role-play
- Skipping a necessary limit for fear of interrupting the flow of the story
- Underestimating the importance of role-play

to express and in a manner that is safe and not too intense for him, and that the CCPT process will help Johnny ready himself to express and heal as quickly and efficiently as possible. He may have forgotten that "slow is fast" and "haste makes waste." He may have been purely playing out "stuff" from his own childhood, or maybe just having "too much fun" there for a moment! Probably none of you would err so far as in this story, but hopefully you get the idea of how even less dramatic errors by the therapist in role-play can happen and why.

## Use of Supervision

Qualified supervision from an experienced CCPT supervisor is incredibly helpful in establishing the balance discussed earlier, as well as overcoming errors in that area and those described below. Role-play, especially interactive role-play in CCPT, is a complex, subtle, and difficult skill set for play therapists to master, but well worth the effort. Videotaping CCPT sessions, and reviewing these tapes with an experienced CCPT supervisor, will assist the novice therapist in honing the skills necessary to engage in role-plays when this is chosen for self-expression by the child.

## Questions and Questioning Tone

It is helpful to remember that questions or a questioning tone are rapid methods of squashing a child's self-expression, even in role-plays. If questions are meant for you to figure out why things are happening—to interpret—this is not your primary and critically important role. If the questions flow from your lack of understanding of what the child wants your role to be in an interactive role-play, it is better to ask for direction and get clarity than to imply questions out of a lack of certainty.

## Boredom with or Worries over Repetition

Some role-plays are repeated quite a long time with only slight variation each time. This can get boring to some therapists and worrisome to others. We find keeping descriptions of role-plays in session notes helpful in that there is almost always change occurring, even if gradual, and being able to reflect on previous notes may help you see that. Some boredom is understandable in that the role-plays are the child's primary experience and only secondary to the therapist. Plus, at some level, *the child knows where he is going*, but the therapist does not.

Regarding worries over repetition, the authors have learned over the years to find a way of reminding one another of the importance of this notion that *the child knows where he is going*. Earlier in our careers, we often sat out on the porch at night, with one of us saying to the other, "He's (referring to a child one of us was counseling) just stuck. He's so demanding and aggressive in his play. I've decided it's unhealthy, and I'm going to have to intervene to help him move forward or move out of this repetitive role-play." The other would respond something like, "Why don't you give it one more session first, and see if change doesn't begin, or see if you aren't thinking about it and feeling differently?" Interestingly and inevitably, this always seemed to work! After the very next session, it always seemed that either the child would have shifted significantly, sometimes dramatically, and/or the one of us who was that child's therapist would be seeing the situation significantly differently! We've come to think of this phenomenon this way: As the therapist is thinking, "I just about can't tolerate this role-play any more," in his own way, the child is feeling this too, and this feeling in the therapist is empathy. A parallel might be when one persists in doing a negative behavior long enough, at some point in the light of deep self-reflection and self-awareness, he finally decides that it doesn't feel good or right anymore, and chooses to move on. The playroom and therapeutic relationship provide a safe place to do just that.

We sometimes ask ourselves, if an adult is telling the same story over and over, perhaps a painful story of the loss of a loved one when grieving that loss, what is the purpose? We think there can be two purposes. The person may be repeating the story because somehow no one has heard, deeply understood, and connected with what that experience is like for her, and she longs for that. The person may also be repeating the story as she is trying to make sense of it, trying to see how it fits within her view of self and others. A "bearing with patience," caring attentiveness, and deep empathy during this repetition is needed. A child is often accomplishing these same tasks in repeated role-plays, and the same is needed from his play therapist. Even in such "repeated" role-plays, there are subtle changes in both the behavior of the role-play participants, and in the meaning of the role-play for the child. Often, subtle changes are occurring and therapeutic progress is being made, which can be difficult, especially for the therapist new to CCPT to see or for the impatient seasoned therapist to notice.

## Taking It Personally

It can be important to remember that actions in role-play, even *pretend hurtful* or *demanding and scornful* actions directed at you as the therapist, are not real. If in role-play you are continually scorned and scolded, it can actually come to hurt, especially if rejection is a sore spot for you, as it is for many of us. So, for many therapists, it is necessary to remind oneself that (1) this is a drama and it isn't real; (2) it is not personal but about a character I'm playing for the child, and the child must have a deep trust and security with me in order to risk bringing this "not so positive" side of herself out; and (3) the child needs this role-play in order to change and to work through obvious conflicting feelings, and she's not likely to get it anywhere else. If these centering thoughts are not enough to help you gain perspective, as was mentioned in the chapter on limit setting, it is more important to set personal limits on how you can participate in role-play than to risk losing unconditional positive regard for the child.

## Taking Direction from a Really Demanding or Cantankerous Child in Role-Play

A supervisee of one of the authors was hugely and roundly criticized by her disgruntled play therapy child client for her "lousy work" as the actor in his role-play. It seemed that whatever the therapist did, it was never quite what the child wanted to see. It helped the therapist (in contemplation outside the session with her supervisor) to realize that this was this child's general approach to life, if perhaps acted out to the extreme in his sessions. It seemed to be exactly what the child needed to "try out" and to exaggerate in role-play in order to contemplate and make new decisions about his approach to life outside of sessions. Indeed, this child's relentless rejection and evaluation of the therapist's acting talent became a role-play within a role-play. The therapist's acceptance of her "cantankerous" director was a great trust builder and profoundly strengthened the relationship.

## Forgetting to Express Empathy in the Context of Role-Play

It helps to remember that being empathically attuned to the child is your constant mode of being present to the child. Being an actor in the animation of a child's internal world is a deep form of empathic, shared experience. But basic empathy for the child is your primary and constant mode. So, for example, if you are "off" in how you play a role, empathic attunement should help you realize this as you experience the reaction of the child as to how you are playing a role. As the child experiences your empathic attunement, when the rare mistake in playing a role occurs, even the most shy and reserved child will feel comfortable in correcting your error. Empathy is not simply conveyed through the verbal acknowledgment of the child's internal state, but also behaviorally communicated by how you perform your role to meet the needs of the child. For example, in response to a child who is hurrying to finish before time is up for today, you can respond to the child by saying, "This is important to you! You want us to work fast to get it done today!," even while, at the same time, you obviously "speed up" your part, which *really communicates* that you get it.

## Skipping a Necessary Limit for Fear of Interrupting the Flow of the Story

It is important to always keep in mind that the need to set limits always overrides the continuing to play a role. Although this is a common temptation of novice play therapists—to let the breaking of minor limits within role-plays "slide"—this is not advisable. For example, if a child is playing "cops and robbers" and shoots his therapist with a dart, it is important to stop the role-play long enough to make the child aware of the limit of not shooting darts at the therapist, and then returning to the role. Remember, it is one of your primary roles and duties to provide the structure, including keeping the child safe. If you abandon that role in any significant way, self-expression is limited. Within the structure that you provide, the drive to self-express is a powerful force that can easily survive necessary interruptions.

## Laughing Inappropriately

Sometimes the things children do in play therapy, especially in role-plays, are very creative and are just plain "funny." But, if they aren't meant to be funny, the therapist's laughter could be restricting or, at worst, humiliating. Sharing a good laugh when the actions are *meant to be funny* can be a shared, empathic experience, but there is a difference when the counselor is laughing inappropriately at the actions of the child as being "cute" and "silly" if the child is serious in the role. It often helps us to remind ourselves in a split-second thought in a session, "I'm gonna laugh with this as a memory *later.*" Then return to the present moment and the task at hand!

## Expectations That the Child "Should" Engage in Role-Play

Some children will engage in solitary role-play or interactive role-play regularly. Pretend play seems a natural "voice" for them. However, some children will not engage in role-play often or at all, and will instead opt for solitary activities (drawing pictures, building with blocks) or interactive activities with the therapist (playing card games with the therapist) or in parallel with the therapist (working side-by-side with Play-Doh). While certain children seem to enthusiastically engage in role-play from the start, others also may assign roles to the therapist in a more subtle or indirect manner. For example, a child who is shooting the dart gun at a target begins by simply asking the therapist to retrieve the darts, but soon begins to sternly command the therapist to get the darts "faster." This results in an implied "servant" role which, if the therapist realizes has been informally assigned, allows the therapist to better meet the child's needs.

When children do engage in role-play, the assumption of CCPT is that the role-play represents an important issue in the psychological life of the child; however, children will vary in terms of the directness or indirectness of how real-life issues are symbolically represented in the playroom. For example, for a child whose parent has died, one child may do a very direct symbolic role-play of a funeral scene; another child may instead do a role-play in which an animal family is walking through the forest and the largest animal gets lost and the rest of the animal family is worried and sad; and still another child may repeatedly order the counselor to hold his hand and to follow him all over the room (indirect symbolism in which the child is trying to exert control over the adult counselor and reestablish a sense that the world and significant attachment figures are not completely unpredictable). In any case, in CCPT, the counselor allows the child to choose the level of directness/indirectness of self-expression in role-plays, and understands that some children choose not to engage in role-plays at all.

## Interpreting or Attempting Diagnosis vs. Connecting in the "Here-and-Now"

It is important to remember not to use role-play within sessions as an interpretive, investigative, or diagnostic tool. Role-play used for these purposes is not curative or healing, can be potentially damaging to the child, and can lead to false conceptualizations of the child's experience. Items and actions in role-play can be about the child's external life (e.g., a family fight in a role-play may represent an actual family fight), or may represent a more symbolic and internal-to-the-child process. By this we mean that a conflict in a role-play is more likely to be a conflict between a child's internal constellation of thoughts, feelings, urges, and inclinations than a direct statement about his external world. It may help to remember that the key healing factors are the deep, shared experience of being invited into the depth of a child's internal world, of having him share that with you.

That being said, the therapist is always careful to formulate any interpretations of the meaning of the play after the session—never during it. The obligation of the therapist is to stay in the "here and now" with the child through the use of empathy and tracking and direct participation in the role-play at the request of the child. Attempting to interpret during the session, even if it is kept to oneself and not shared with the child, takes the therapist out of the immediate and present therapeutic relationship with the child.

It is also important to remember that even after the play therapy session, it is often difficult to make literal interpretations from the child's thematic play. For example, a child experiencing the divorce of her parents may be playing at the dollhouse and exclaim, "I hate you, Mommy; I want to be with my Daddy!" In such cases, the child may be expressing anger at her mother for leaving her father, even though the case history reveals that the father was abusive to both the mother and the child. In this case, the child may be expressing the desire for an

intact family, and that she misses her father; however, a literal interpretation that she doesn't want to be with her mother and would prefer
being with her father would be erroneous. It is important to realize that
a role-play may represent a single aspect or many aspects of important
issues in the child's internal world and psychological life.

# Taped Supervision to Enhance and Develop the Necessary Role-Play Skills of a "Confident Companion"

Engaging in role-play without losing therapeutic perspective, if not a
strength for the therapist, can be a focus of the training and taped
supervision. In our classes and trainings, role-play—once practiced and
supervised—is possible for those who are at first uncomfortable with
this CCPT skill. In fact, many who are new to CCPT find that the ability
to role-play and be more engaged in the child's play "frees" them up as
therapists, and brings them to a deeper level of empathy for the child.
By engaging in role-play, many therapists report feeling much better
able to sense the child's inner experience, and build a stronger relationship with the child.

In supervising novice play therapists, these authors have found
mock demonstrations and practice of role-plays, along with discussions
concerning the therapeutic value of dramatic play, helpful in assisting
these therapists to become more comfortable and skilled with role-play.
As the therapists' skills improve, it is possible to help them in their
ability to make empathic statements within the context of role-play,
and also effectively—and with empathy—use "asides" smoothly to gain
clarification when needed and to set limits when necessary.

# Opportunities for Practice, Study, Skill Development, and Self-Supervision

## Contemplation and Practice of Key Concepts

The key concepts of CCPT often present new ways of being. Contemplation and academic practice can help you develop confidence, depth
of understanding, and comfort with newly acquired skills. The following activities are provided for this purpose. They can be completed on

your own, but most are designed to be completed with a partner, or in a small group or classroom.

- *Activity A:* Childhood memories—what do you remember playing as a child? With a group in class or a group of friends (or family members), discuss the play activities you remember from childhood. What function or purpose do you imagine this play served? Do you remember enjoying or having time for make-believe play?

- *Activity B:* Select a pretend activity (family/house play, cops and robbers, superhero saves the day, school teacher and student) and write a short story using this as a theme. After writing the story, try to develop it as a dramatic role-play. How many characters are needed? What do the characters say to each other? Select one partner or classmate, and without using notes, attempt to "act out" your story with you as director assigning roles to your partner. What was this experience like for you? What was it like for your partner? Switch places and take part in another partner's story/role-play.

- *Activity C:* Imagine, for a moment, you're in a play session with a child. It's early on—either you've just met this child or it is within the first few sessions. After surveying you, the room, and toys, the child seems to suddenly "light up" with enthusiasm and exclaim:
  1. "Hey, can we pretend this is a schoolroom and I'm the teacher?"
  2. "I know, we can make believe this is a castle! I'm the queen and you're the princess! Here . . . (hands you a crown) Put this on and go sit on that beanbag chair—it's your throne!"
  3. Child picks up a foam sword and waves it in the air. "ARRRGH! Let's play pirates! Quick . . . get a sword and follow me!"
  4. "I got a good idea! Pretend I'm your mommy. You stay here alone while I go get groceries." Child opens the door and actually starts to leave the playroom.
  5. Child picks up handcuffs with a smile. "That's it . . . put your hands behind your back! You're under arrest!"
  6. Child sits down in the therapist's rolling office chair. "Today we're gonna do things a little different . . . I'm gonna be you, and you're gonna be me!"
  7. "Let's be ghosts! I'll be invisible, and you act like you don't know why things keep getting moved around the room!"
  8. Child starts banging chalk erasers together and spreading chalk dust around the room with abandon. "Act like you're choking . . . hey, this is just like smoke!"

In each instance, how did you first imagine your response? Because this is the beginning of a role-play, are there possible structuring instructions that would be helpful for the child? Do any of the scenarios require an "aside" for clarification or a limit for safety? Do some scenarios seem to more easily allow for you to simply follow the instructions and start playing the role? Compare your answers or responses to those of a partner or others in the class. Are there differences? What do you think accounts for these differences?

## Mock Session Practice

- *Activity A:* Use the following list of hypothetical child statements/scenarios to test your skills in role-play situations. Work with a partner to "play out" the scenario, or think through and respond to the scenarios on your own. What considerations come to mind as you role-play and discuss each situation? What type of skill was needed ("aside" for clarification, limit setting, structuring, or simply taking a role in response to the request) to best respond? (If you get "stumped," you may want to review Chapter 8 while contemplating these).
    1. "I'm a cowboy, and you're my horsey! Hurry! Get down . . . down there and crawl around, so I can jump on your back!"
    2. "Shhhh . . . be very quiet now and close your eyes and go to sleep. REALLY . . . close your eyes tight so you can't see anything!"
    3. "Hands up . . . NOW!" Child points play gun at you. "Don't move an inch or I'll shoot you dead!"
    4. "You're a singer, and I'm the judge." Child hands you the microphone. "Now sing a song!"
    5. "This is slimy, dirty, dog-poo soup." Child hands you a bowl of sand mixed with water. "Now eat it all . . . or else!"
    6. Child hands you a doll. "This doll is the neighbor and she comes over to my house to visit."
    7. "Pretend I kidnap your baby when you aren't looking. Go ahead . . . turn the other way and I'll grab the baby, and then you start screaming for help."
    8. "Act like you're the policeman, and you catch me when I try to sneak out the back!" Child hands you a toy gun, and then starts tiptoeing toward the back of the playroom.

9. Child starts playing contentedly with matchbox cars in a far corner of the room. "You stay over there at the table, and work on that puzzle for me. I want you to finish it, too!"

10. "Let's pretend we're in a contest. It's called 'who can take it the longest?'" Child hands you a pair of large brass cymbals. "Here . . . you bang these together real close to my ear until I say to stop!"

## Concluding Thoughts

The hypothetical child statements are provided to give realistic examples, and for you to use in your practice exercises. If you are in a class, practice and discussion with others will reveal that first responses to these sample scenarios will differ to some extent from one therapist to another based on personal boundaries and individual style. However, as you hone skills in CCPT, you will find that your responses will come to have much in common with others studying CCPT and that responding and engaging in role-play comes much more naturally.

In conclusion, it is helpful to remember not to underestimate the importance of role-play in CCPT as serious, purposeful business. Role-play has significant therapeutic value in conveying faith in the child's ability to tap into inner resources and resolve interpersonal and intrapersonal conflicts. Role-play gives the child in therapy abundant opportunities to solve his own problems and exercise self-control. For example, after 20 minutes of quiet play with family figures at the dollhouse, an otherwise withdrawn child might stop, come out of the role that is being played, and very seriously tell the therapist how she feels about her parents' divorce—something that seems to have suddenly "come to mind." And even in the midst of a fast-paced "cops-and-robbers" chase, an otherwise impulsive and sometimes aggressive child playing the "cop" might temporarily step out of role-play to (with genuine concern) ask his therapist, "I didn't get those handcuffs too tight, did I?" Role-plays are not random, and often the themes are associated with issues that children are working on during a given stage of play. Some children use role-play to self-express throughout all stages of CCPT, and others use little or no role-play as a means of self-expression in CCPT. In Chapter 10, we will continue to explore unique and powerful curative benefits of role-play as seen throughout the typical stages of CCPT.

# Recognizing Stages: Understanding the Therapy Process and Evaluating Children's Internal Progress

## 10
### Chapter

> *. . . As Dibs stood before me now his head was up. He had a feeling of security deep inside himself. He was building a sense of responsibility for his feelings. His feelings of hate and revenge had been tempered with mercy. Dibs was building a concept of self as he groped through the tangled brambles of his mixed up feelings. He could hate and he could love. He could condemn and he could pardon . . . Yes, Dibs had changed. He had learned how to be himself. Now he was relaxed and happy. He was able to be a child. . . .*
>
> —Excerpt from Virginia Axline's classic book, Dibs: In Search of Self

## Application Focus Scenarios

During her first two play therapy sessions, Nikki spent the entire time exploring the different toys in the playroom and frequently switching from one activity to another. Dan, her therapist, is wondering whether Nikki has attention deficit/hyperactivity disorder (ADHD) and because of her lack of focus is wondering whether the child-centered play therapy (CCPT) model is appropriate for her. A solid understanding of the stages of the play therapy process would allow the therapist to realize that this is one of a number of common approaches that children adopt to the early Warm-up Stage of the CCPT process.

In his most recent play session, Troy spent the first part of the session doing role-play in which he was the policeman and the therapist was in the role of a prisoner. In the role-play he repeatedly prevented the prisoner from escaping—often resorting to the use of pretend violence to reestablish control of the prisoner. In the second half of the session, Troy spent time making elaborate lunches containing all of the prisoner's favorite foods. His counselor is not sure what to make of what he considers "ambivalent" feelings of the child. With a solid understanding of the stages of the play therapy process, his counselor would understand that Troy is demonstrating a transitional stage between the Aggressive Stage and the Regressive Stage of the CCPT process.

For the past five sessions, Felipe's play has included almost exclusively violent fantasy role-play. He spends time stealing animals from the zoo and then performing painful experiments on them in his "secret" laboratory. In the sixth session, Felipe enters the playroom, puts a plastic bottle in his mouth, and begins to crawl around on the floor whimpering and cooing like a baby. Understanding of the stages of the CCPT process would allow the therapist to recognize that Felipe has entered the Regressive Stage of the play process, and while he is engaging in behavior that is unusual, it is not extremely rare during this stage.

For the past three sessions, Darnella's play has included role-plays in which she becomes a ride operator at an amusement park and enforces rules to keep all the riders safe. This contrasts considerably with play from earlier sessions in which she made animals her slaves and whipped them for the slightest disobedience. In her recent sessions, she has also been showing her counselor how far and high she can jump, how she can hit the target with the dart gun, and other successes with physically challenging tasks. Darnella's mom is wondering how much longer her daughter has to come to play therapy sessions. Knowing the stages of the CCPT process and the improvement seen by mom and teachers, her counselor decides it would be a reasonable time to consider beginning the termination process.

## Chapter Overview and Summary

Although each child could be said to have his own "therapy print"—a unique path to healing within the playroom, nonetheless most (but not all) children will also travel through some clearly identifiable stages commonly observed with the majority of children participating in CCPT. The four commonly observed Stages in the CCPT process include the Warm-up Stage, Aggressive Stage, Regressive Stage, and Mastery Stage. Children tend to progress through these stages in a sequential manner in the order listed. However, depending on a child's therapeutic needs, the time spent in any specific stage will vary considerably. Each therapeutic stage is often associated with specific types of behavior, therapeutic themes, and advances in the development of the therapist–child relationship. Each stage also presents unique challenges for the therapist (e.g., child refuses to enter the playroom in the Warm-up Stage).

Although for a given play therapy session, a therapeutic stage can appear in its discreet "pure" form in which 100% of the behaviors/themes are associated with a specific stage, in most cases at least some behaviors/themes associated with either the preceding and/or the next therapeutic stage are also present, but not focal to the session. When a child's play in a given session displays about an equal amount of the behaviors/themes associated with two separate stages, the child is said to be in a "transitional" stage.

Knowledge of these stages of the CCPT process empowers the therapist to know what things are to be expected, what things are unusual, and what things are sources for concern. Knowledge of the stages can also help the therapist track therapeutic progress and to make decisions about termination. In short, an understanding of the stages of the play therapy allows the therapist to experience some degree of commonality across the truly unique therapeutic journey of each child. It is the goal of this chapter to help you develop this understanding of therapeutic process.

## Primary Skill Objectives

The following Primary Skill Objectives for this chapter are provided to guide you through the chapter, and for reflection and review after completing the chapter reading and exercises. By reading and working through the chapter exercises, you will be better able to:

1. Describe the behaviors and themes generally associated with the four stages of the CCPT process: Warm-up Stage, Aggressive Stage, Regressive Stage, and Mastery Stage.

2. Recognize the three major transitional stages: Warm-up/Aggressive, Aggressive/Regressive, and Regressive/Mastery, which may appear between major stages of the play therapy process.

3. Understand atypical situations when tracking progress via therapeutic stages is difficult or not possible.

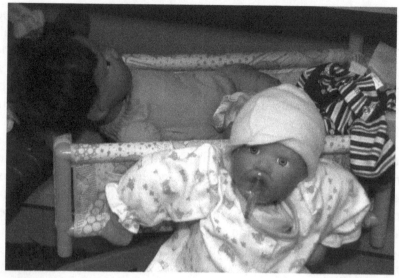

Figure 10.1

4. Understand the meaning of movement backward from advanced stages of the play therapy process to earlier stages of the play therapy process.

## The Stages in the Play Therapy Process: Introductory Remarks

Each child has a unique way of engaging the CCPT process. Given that children have maximum freedom to make decisions about how to express themselves in sessions, and given that the content of play sessions is determined by the child and not the therapist, it might seem that there would be no uniformity or predictability within the therapeutic process. It is therefore often surprising for therapists or counselors to learn that there is a significant amount of uniformity and even predictability within the diverseness of children's play sessions.

To see this uniformity when it is encountered in play sessions takes a trained eye. The purpose of this chapter is to sensitize you to the patterns or stages often seen in CCPT play sessions. Such stages have been noted by researchers (Hendricks, 1971; Withee, 1975) and recently given more elaboration by CCPT play therapists (Nordling & Guerney, 1999). This is an important development since the identification of stages with the CCPT process allows you to track therapeutic progress in a complementary but independent manner, from reports of parents and teachers. Given that therapeutic progress noted within sessions often precedes progress made on treatment goals for a child outside of sessions (e.g., symptom reduction), being able to identify movement within therapeutic sessions allows a therapist or counselor to have confidence that change outside the session will eventually follow.

We have still not answered the big question: "Given that child-centered play therapists follow the child's lead, and children approach the CCPT process in their own unique way, why is there any uniformity at all?" Although the CCPT session content is unique to each child, a number of things are uniform across all play sessions and for each child. First, the role of therapist is uniform across sessions and across clients. The therapist establishes a permissive, accepting environment that fosters self-expression, but is always balanced with limits to promote safety and responsibility in relationship. Second, the therapist utilizes a small set of therapist skills (e.g., empathy, limit setting, role-play) in a consistent manner; in short, if the child has been assigned to a different

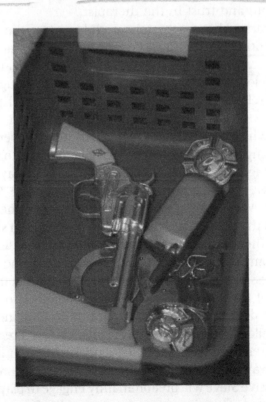

Figure 10.2

CCPT therapist and had done the exact same things in the playroom, the "alternative" therapist would have responded to each action of the child in a roughly similar way. Third, it is important to recognize that although children bring their unique circumstances to the playroom, each child is a human being, and therefore shares some common universal issues and developmental challenges with other children: the desire to express oneself, the desire to have self-control, the desire to connect and relate to others in a positive manner, the desire to view oneself as good, and the desire to feel capable and competent. Therefore, although each child may have a unique pattern of strength and deficits in these areas, it is also true that they ultimately share much in common with other children who enter the playroom, as well as those considered healthy and not in need of treatment. Finally, all children entering the playroom encounter a common set of challenges unique to being a play therapy client: developing an understanding and comfort with their role in the playroom, developing an understanding of the therapist's role in the playroom, needing to test limits and discover the boundaries of the playroom, and acquiring a feeling of safety in the playroom and trust in the therapist.

In summary, when each unique child enters the playroom, she shares with all other play therapy clients a common therapeutic milieu (e. g., common therapist role and skills employed), the human condition and universal developmental challenges, and the challenges of forming a therapeutic relationship. It is the convergence of all these common factors that we believe produces some uniformity in the pattern or sequence in which behavior and themes emerge over time in play sessions. Nordling & Guerney (1999) have given names to four sequential patterns or stages commonly seen in children's play sessions: the Warm-up Stage, the Aggressive Stage, the Regressive Stage, and the Mastery Stage. We examine each of these stages of the CCPT process in detail and in the order in which they tend to appear. In should be noted that the stage theory offered by Nordling and Guerney is an attempt to organize the complexity of what is typically seen throughout the course of a child's play sessions. Children will vary in the length of time they spend in each stage of the process. For example, children with problems with opposition and defiance will tend to spend more time in the Aggressive Stage than children not having problems in this area. In addition, although children tend to progress sequentially through the four stages, they do not always do so in a "pure" manner. In other words, a child who is in the Aggressive Stage will predominantly engage in play behaviors and themes associated with that stage, but may also focus on therapeutic

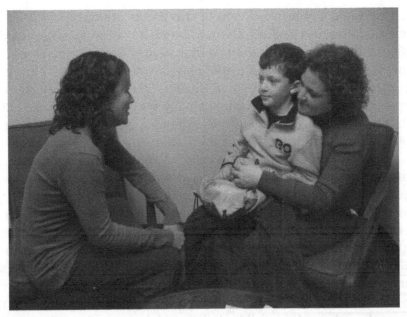

Figure 10.3

issues/themes/behaviors associated with an earlier stage (i.e., Warm-up) or the next stage (i.e., Regressive) for a minority part of the session. At times a child may engage in play associated with two different stages about an equal amount of time in a given session; in such sessions the child is said to be in a "transitional" stage. Transitional stages will be discussed after our discussion of the four basic stages of the play therapy process.

## The First Stage of the Play Therapy Process: Warm-Up

The first stage of the CCPT process is the Warm-up Stage. Although children vary in how they first react to the therapist and the playroom, all children face common tasks that must be achieved in order for the central therapeutic work to begin. These tasks include orienting oneself to the playroom space (and toys); discovering the opportunities for self-expression and freedom to make choices; understanding the role of the therapist as facilitator and not leader; developing trust that the therapist values them and that it is safe to bring out who they are in the session without fear of physical punishment, shaming, or loss of relationship; and testing limits in order to understand what is and is not acceptable in the playroom. In the Warm-up Stage, children will often examine toys and use them for a variety of purposes, including engaging in activities that they do in everyday life (e.g., playing cards, drawing), test whether aggressive play is acceptable (e.g., hitting the bop bag, playing with army men, firing a dart gun), and engaging in regressive behaviors (e.g., feeding a baby with the baby bottle). However, in the Warm-up Stage, these behaviors often do not contain the projective material, intensity, and duration that will be present when the child is working therapeutically on issues in later stages. For example, a child may hit a bop bag around for a while in Warm-up, whereas in the Aggressive Stage he may identify the bop bag as "my brother" and with great intensity engage in all kinds of contests for much of a session as he works on sibling rivalry issues. In addition, in the Warm-up Stage, children also tend to test limits in order to see what the therapist's reaction is and through this process learn about boundaries of the playroom. By testing limits children also learn that the therapist consistently sets limits in a firm but empathic way that affirms the values of the child's desires and does not shame the child or threaten the relationship. Such experiences allow the child to clearly differentiate the therapist from other authority figures and communicate that this is really a "special room."

Children will show considerable variability in terms of how long they need to spend in the Warm-up Stage in order to orient themselves to the playroom, their role, and the role of the therapist, and to develop the necessary trust in the therapist and comfort in adopting a leadership role in the playroom. Some children will enter the playroom with a basic positive attitude toward the therapist and confidently begin exploring and learning about the possibilities of the playroom. Such children may complete the therapeutic "work" of the Warm-up Stage in one or two sessions and then move quickly into typical therapeutic work seen in the Aggressive Stage. However, some children will spend a much longer time in the Warm-up Stage. Often, but not always, these include children who are very anxious (e.g., separation anxiety), children with a high level of oppositional behaviors (especially those who are very resistant to coming to the agency where they are being seen), and children with a long history of rejections and failures in attachment relationships. Occasionally, such children present significant challenges in Warm-up. While this is rare, we describe some of these difficulties in the latter part of this chapter as a way to introduce seldom needed but possible variations in therapeutic procedures for children who are struggling to warm up in unusual ways.

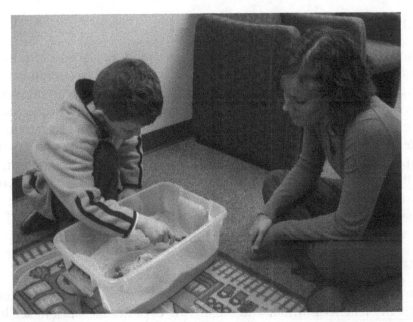

Figure 10.4

## Illustrations of Normal Variety in the Warm-Up Stage

Before moving to a discussion of the second stage of the play therapy process, we share the following illustrations of the Warm-up Stage, which demonstrate the wide variety of ways children initially engage the therapeutic process.

### Illustration 1

Terrell rushes into the playroom and, with a smile on his face, immediately begins to check out all the toys. First, he begins to knock the bop bag all over the playroom. Next, he picks up the baby doll and pretends to feed it, but quickly moves on to setting up army men on opposing sides and having them battle. He tries to shoot the therapist with a dart gun and learns that is a limit. He delights when he says the word *butthole* and finds that the therapist is accepting of this, and no limit is set. He finishes the session by drawing a picture of himself.

## Illustration 2

Kathy enters the playroom tentatively. She stands in place looking at all the toys, clearly hesitant. The therapist is accepting of her anxiousness, using empathy to note her uncertainty about what she can do in the playroom. The therapist is also comfortable with Kathy's quietness. After 5 minutes, the therapist gives the opening statement again in its extended form. Kathy begins to walk cautiously over to the toys. By the end of the session Kathy is much more comfortable; she has tried three additional activities, and although she is still clearly trying to avoid doing anything that would be considered "wrong," she is also beginning to take over the lead in the playroom.

## Illustration 3

Martin enters the playroom and announces, "I shouldn't have to come here. My teacher is unfair and mean!" He eyes the therapist to see her response and seems surprised when the therapist gives empathy. He begins to talk more about how he hates school and how his parents are on his case. After an extended period of his complaining and receiving empathy from the therapist, he asks whether he can play with the toys. Upon an affirmative answer, he begins to use the dart gun to shoot the bop bag, which he identifies as his teacher. He then tries out other toys. By the end of the session he seems considerably more relaxed and clearly views the therapist as being very different than his parents, teachers, and other authority figures.

# The Second Stage of the Play Therapy Process: The Aggressive Stage

Children emerge from the Warm-up Stage with a clear understanding of their role and the therapist's role in the therapeutic process. They have developed a basic sense of trust in the unconditional nature of the therapist's positive regard for them, confidence and comfort in the permissiveness of the playroom, and their ability to make decisions and choices—while also having an idea of what boundaries and limits are present in the playroom. It is from this comfort zone that children feel and are more able to begin working on additional therapeutic issues associated with the Aggressive Stage. Typical therapeutic issues and themes worked on by children in this play therapy stage include desires to exert control over others, to be invulnerable to others' attempts to control or hurt them, the desire to be the "best," getting revenge, and learning to accept controls/limits placed on them. In the Aggressive Stage, children develop increasing capacities for emotional awareness, constructive self-expression, frustration tolerance, and self-control—in short, they make great gains in "emotional intelligence" and in self-regulation.

Often, children's play can contain considerable fantasy-based aggression. Although there can be considerable variation in content of role-plays, common ones include ones with authority figures in which domination can be exerted: slave–master, battles between opposing armies, teacher–student, policeman–robber, powerful witch or magician, big animal–small animal, stronger vs. weaker human figure. In interactive activities, such as playing games with the therapist (e.g., cards, ring toss, target shooting with dart gun), the child may "cheat" by changing rules or seeking advantages so that they can win. Children may also seek to directly control you by issuing commands for what they want you to do, where to sit/stand, or even to "shut up."

It should be noted that, unlike the Warm-up scenario with the attachment-aversive child in which the child may make some personal attacks meant to prevent a relationship from developing with the therapist, in the Aggressive Stage much of the confrontation is fantasy-based. Even in the case where the child exerts direct control over you (e.g., "Go get that ball, slowpoke!" or "You have to 'shut up' when I tell you to"), it is only in the context of her clear trust that her relationship with you is strong and that your unconditional positive regard for her is unshakable, that she feels secure in bringing such negative aspects of herself out in her therapeutic work.

A major challenge for a counselor or therapist in this stage is to develop comfort with remaining accepting and empathic toward sometimes amazing displays of control and aggression present in the many children's fantasy play. This can be especially challenging when a child assigns you role-plays in which you are controlled (e.g., assigned role as a "slave," subjected to verbal abuse, given the role of a student and the child is in role of abusive teacher) or asked to do strenuous activities (e.g., continuously retrieve the child's darts as he rapidly fires a dart gun at a target). Another challenge faced by a therapist or counselor in this stage is growing comfortable with the anger, resentment, and pain that some children display in their play. The authors remember a case in which a child spent a number of sessions angrily pretending to burn the limbs off a male puppet with acid. The counselor tended to think that the boy was working though his anger and pain resulting from his father's slow death from cancer. Nonetheless, the intensity and pain of such types of play can take an emotional toll on you. In cases where a child's demands of you become too exhausting physically or emotionally, you may need to consult a supervisor, and/or set a personal limit in order to maintain the therapeutic relationship.

## Illustrations of Variety in the Aggressive Stage

The following is a small sample of illustrations of Aggressive Stage play, exemplifying the wide variety of ways that the elements of this stage can be exhibited.

## Illustration 1

Drew assigns the therapist the role of slave and, as the "master," commands the therapist to move all the toys to different places in the playroom.

## Illustration 2

Sally asks the therapist to play the card game "battle" with her. Whenever the therapist turns up a high card, Sally looks through her deck to find a card that can beat it. She then exclaims, "I am the best card player in the world. You will never win!"

## Illustration 3

Jose sets up the army men into two sides. He asks the therapist to "be the general of the other side." Throughout many battles, Jose's soldiers dominate the battlefield. His soldiers have more powerful weapons and all attempts of the therapist's troops to sneak up on Jose are soundly defeated.

## Illustration 4

Lamar identifies himself as "Batman" and the therapist is assigned the role of "Robin." Batman and Robin spend the session responding to crimes committed by puppets assigned the roles of various super villains. They battle the super villains, defeat them, lock them up in prison, and prevent various escape attempts.

## The Third Stage of the Play Therapy Process: The Regressive Stage

The next stage of the CCPT play therapy process is the Regressive Stage. In this stage, children work broadly on therapeutic issues related to relationship and attachment with other people. More specifically, children work on issues related to closeness and connection, dependency, boundaries, nurturance, protection, grief, and loss, viewing attachment figures as positive and benevolent, and viewing oneself as likable and lovable. Although these therapeutic issues can be casually listed, it is important to note that these are among *the most central and profound aspects of self* that either children or adults work on in therapy. Exploration of such issues requires a child to develop extraordinary trust in the therapist since the issues involve considerable risk of rejection, shame, and threat to sense of self.

Therapists and counselors who are new to CCPT may wonder why there tends to be such order in the play therapy stages. One reason may be that children must learn and experience through the Aggressive Stage that the therapist–child relationship and unconditional positive regard of their therapist can endure in the face of their "darker" side, which can come out in controlling, aggressive, vengeful play in the Aggressive Stage. It may be that children must see that their therapist will not reject these negative aspects of themselves before they can develop confidence in entrusting the vulnerable and "softer" sides of self that are present in the Regressive Stage.

In the Regressive Stage the content of play sessions can be quite varied but tend to fall into predictable themes and patterns. Common role-plays centering on nurturance include doctor taking care of patient, parent feeding/comforting/caressing a baby, and parent cooking special meals for the child. Common role-plays centering on protection include parents protecting the child from intruders, big animals protecting smaller animals, police catching criminals who try to harm others. Attachment-oriented role-plays may include birthing scenes, being tied up or handcuffed together, and the foiling of plots of "bad" characters trying to separate therapist and child. It should be noted that a child may desire to be the recipient of such nurturance, protection, or attachment, or may be the one who occupies the role of nurturer, protector, and sustainer of attachment. Other children may want the therapist to engage in role-plays which have these themes and either be an observer or assign themselves a role that requires less direct participation and more opportunity to observe.

It should be noted that during the Regressive Stage children may demonstrate some actual behavioral regression. This behavioral regression, when present, is most commonly seen in role-plays but may also be present in non-role-play situations such as interactive play with the therapist. For example, a child may be drawing a picture and ask in a regressed tone of voice for the therapist to get "cwayons" (i.e., crayons) for them. Another child may ask his counselor to tie his shoe or help him get up when he is quite able to do these things on his own. A less common, but more intensive form of behavioral regression is seen in role-plays in which a child may adopt and play out the role of a much younger child—newborn, infant, toddler. In such regressed states, children may crawl around the room talking baby talk, suck on a baby bottle or pacifier, pretend to sleep in a cradle, and want the therapist to be in the role of nurturer. In such cases, it is not uncommon for a child who is crawling to "grow himself up," saying to the therapist while standing first on knees, and then fully up, "Now, I'm 1 . . . 2 . . . 3 . . . 4 . . . I'm 5 again!"

## Illustrations of Variety in the Regressive Stage

The following is a small sample of illustrations of Regressive Stage play, exemplifying the wide variety of ways that the elements of this stage can be exhibited.

### Illustration 1

Gabriel came into the playroom and began playing with toy cars, which he then crashed into each other. He then rushed them to the hospital and took the role of a doctor who had to bandage them up, sometimes having to do operations to bring them back from the brink of death.

### Illustration 2

Beth entered the playroom and set up a role-play where the therapist was to be the chef at a restaurant and she would be a customer. The therapist in role of chef had to make all of Beth's favorite dishes. Many times these dishes were not quite to Beth's liking and were sent back until they tasted exactly the way that Beth wanted them.

## Illustration 3

Charlie had been involved in fierce role-play battles between opposing armies during the previous two sessions. In this session he entered the playroom, fell to the ground, and began crawling around. He then rolled over on his back at the therapist's feet and said, "Mama, feed baby." An implied role-play was developing, and the therapist got a baby bottle, which she handed to Charlie, who immediately popped it into his mouth. He continued to spend the rest of the session wanting the therapist to feed him, "burp" him, sing lullabies, and put him to bed.

## Illustration 4

Catherine began a role-play in which she distributed a gun to her therapist and kept a play knife for herself. She then instructed the therapist to get behind a chair with her and to try to hide from the "boogie man" who was trying to kidnap her. Hiding was unsuccessful, and Catherine squealed as the boogie man (represented by the bop bag) approached. The therapist was instructed to attack the boogie man and do anything to keep it from taking her away.

In the Regressive Stage, it is important for therapist or counselor to be comfortable and accepting of the regressive behaviors of the child. At times, depending on the rules of their setting and own comfort level, the therapist may decide or need to set limits during Regressive Stage play around a child wanting to sit in her lap or be held. However, in such a situation, you should be accepting of the regressive intent of the child. Although rare, during the Regressive Stage a child may also exhibit some regressive behavior at home. If parents note this, you should reassure them that this is a natural occurrence in the therapy process, like pulling back a little before going forward in normal development, that it should not be discouraged, and that they can expect it to be short lived.

## The Fourth Stage of the Play Therapy Process: The Mastery Stage

Will play therapy ever end? Yes, the play therapy process does have an ending. The Mastery Stage of the play therapy process signals the counselor that a child has moved on to work on the final therapeutic tasks. The psychological work of the Mastery Stage is twofold. First, the Mastery Stage represents a period in which the positive changes of the earlier stages can be integrated more solidly into a child's personality structure. During the Mastery Stage, it could be said that a child develops "integrity." The child is now able to be emotionally self-expressive, able to exhibit self-control and make choices, accept limits and boundaries, view self and others as good, and cooperate with and be responsible in and valuing of relationships with others. Second, and related to these accomplishments, the Mastery Stage represents an opportunity for the child to develop a sense of competency. This sense of competency is founded on the successful working through of the issues of dependence/ independence and autonomy in the Regressive Stage and the issue of self-expression and self-control in the Aggressive Stage. However, this emerging sense of competency is also something more in that it reflects the child's confidence that she can be effective in the world and that she can exert control that can best be described as leadership. Such control is not merely self-centered but is also wielded in a socially responsible and relationship-valuing way. In the Mastery Stage, children will display this integrity and sense of efficacy and competence in a variety of ways. Some children will be quite involved with role-plays in which the themes of positive sense of control and competency are demonstrated.

### Table 10.1  Basic Therapeutic Tasks of the Four Stages of the CCPT Process

**Stage 1: Warm-up**

Develop comfort with and trust of the therapist; feel free to express, give direction, and make choices; discover limits and boundaries of the playroom and therapeutic relationship.

**Stage 2: Aggressive**

Work on issues related to desires to control others; work through feelings of hurt, anger, resentment, and desire for revenge; learn to self-control in response to limits.

**Stage 3: Regressive**

Work on issues related to attachment and connection to others, including giving and receiving of nurturance; viewing oneself and others in a more positive way.

**Stage 4: Mastery**

Integrating growth of other stages into the child's personality structure; developing a positive sense of self-efficacy and competence; having greater capacity for responsible relationship with others.

## Illustrations of the Mastery Stage

The following illustrations exemplify variety in and the relationship of the Mastery Stage to earlier stages.

### Illustration 1

In the Aggressive Stage, David spent much time telling the therapist what to do and berating him for doing things too slowly and not in conformity with his demands. When he entered into the Mastery Stage, David announced that he was a ride operator at an amusement park. In this role-play he would calmly, but authoritatively, lay out all the rules to keep the people who would be riding safe (e.g., "walk, do not run, to your seat; keep your hands and feet in the ride at all times"). He would emphasize that everyone can have fun, but they need to follow the rules to stay safe. He enforced these rules in a nonhostile way, giving riders "another chance" if they violated the rules.

### Illustration 2

For a number of sessions in the Regressive Stage, Anna engaged in a role-play in which she was captured by bad guys, who handcuffed and imprisoned her. She would pleadingly yell for her dad to come rescue her, but her dad never came. When she entered the Mastery Stage, she repeated the beginning parts of the role-play, but then discovered a way to escape the prison on her own, saying, "I've found the key to the handcuffs by myself." She then evaded the "bad guys" and escaped the prison on her own.

Other children will communicate their sense of self-mastery by engaging in challenging physical tasks or engaging in elaborate games that they make up. Unlike what is seen in Aggressive Stage play, children in the Mastery Stage will seldom "cheat" in order to win and at times even emphasize the importance of following the rules. They are more able to lose and are often gracious winners. They take pride in their achievement but do not have the need to put others down in order to feel good about themselves.

### Illustration 3

In the Mastery Stage, Annette wanted to play bowling with her therapist, a game that she had played earlier in the Aggressive Stage.

In her Aggressive Stage, she stood much closer to the pins than the therapist and, when she missed the pins, would make excuses for why she got to take a turn over. Often, she would either set the pins up to make it harder for the therapist to hit them or sometimes blatantly would stick her foot out to deflect the bowling ball after the therapist threw it. In the Mastery Stage, she set the rule that both she and the therapist had to take turns trying to hit the pins from the same distance and, when she was successful, even moved the starting line further back to make it more challenging. At one point, the therapist actually stepped over the starting line and Annette, with a smile on her face, announced, "Sorry, that throw doesn't count since you crossed the line. Everyone has to play by the rules." Amusingly, in a later session, Annette was aware of how poorly the therapist was doing in bowling that day and stated, "You are not doing very well today; you can have an extra turn so you can catch up to me."

Some children in the Mastery Stage will not only demonstrate their competence and confidence in themselves but will verbally, physically, and symbolically illustrate how much better they feel about their psychological lives.

## Illustration 4

Danny entered the playroom and with great insight demonstrated how much he had grown while in therapy. He said to the therapist, "When I first came here, my hands were like this." He then, with feigned anger, wildly flailed his hands in an out-of-control manner, striking out at everything around him. Then, he smiled and said, "Now my hands are like this." He then proceeded to calmly hold his hands in front of himself, proudly communicating symbolically how he was now the master of not only what his hands did but also of his emotional expression and interactions with others. Although many children will often demonstrate their newfound competence and emotional self-mastery through fantasy role-play or through challenging physical feats, and will continue such play until therapy is terminated, some children's play may at some time during the Mastery Stage resemble play seen in the Warm-up Stage. For such children, it is as if once they have worked through the psychological issues of the Aggressive and Regressive Stages, they no longer have the need or internal emotional motivation to maintain such types of highly emotionally laden and energetic play. In such cases, it is clear that the child continues to value the relationship with the therapist, but the urgency and central importance of the therapeutic play in their lives has diminished.

## Illustration 5

Marcos's play was filled with dramatic role-plays since early in the Warm-up Stage. He continued use of role-plays to work through control/dominance themes in his Aggressive Stage and through nurturance/protection themes in his Regressive themes. Toward the end of one of the sessions in which Regressive Stage themes were dominant, he suddenly asked whether he could play cards with the therapist. In the sessions following, he continued to play card games and draw pictures of cars but never returned back to the dramatic role-plays of earlier sessions.

## Transitional Stages

As mentioned earlier, although children may engage in play that is "pure" and nearly 100% associated with a given stage of the play therapy process, often movement from one stage to the next is not completely abrupt. It is not uncommon for a child to have gradually increasing ratios of behaviors and themes associated with the next stage of play as they work through issues associated with the current stage of play. For example, if a child enters the Aggressive Stage in the fourth session, the ratio of Aggressive Stage play to Regressive Stage play (i.e, the next stage in the play process) may be as follows: 4th–6th sessions (100% Aggressive Stage/0% Regressive Stage); 7th session (90% Aggressive Stage/10% Regressive Stage); 8th session (80% Aggressive Stage/20% Regressive Stage); 9th session (65% Aggressive Stage/35% Regressive Stage); 10th session (55% Aggressive Stage/45% Regressive Stage); 11th session (50% Aggressive Stage/50% Regressive Stage); 12th session (40% Aggressive Stage/60% Regressive Stage). We would call these sessions in which the balance of one stage of play to the other is roughly 60%/40% or 40%/60% (i.e., sessions 10–12) "Transitional Stages." Logically, then, there are three possible types of Transitional Stages: Warm-up/Aggressive Transitional Stage, Aggressive/Regressive Transitional Stage, and Regressive/Mastery Transitional Stage.

## Illustrations of Transition Sessions

Below are illustrations of how such stages may appear in the playroom.

## Illustration 1: Warm-Up/Aggressive Transitional Stage

In her second play session, Marta spent the first 30 minutes trying out a variety of activities in rapid succession. In the last 20 minutes of the session, she began a role-play in which she said she was the parent and the therapist was a little girl. She then spent the remainder of the session with her as mom catching the little girl doing things wrong and then sending her to her room without supper.

## Illustration 2: Aggressive/Regressive Transitional Stage

Ben started his fifth session with a role-play that he did in earlier sessions. He would pretend to be a policeman who would arrest the therapist, who was in the role of a criminal. In past sessions he would think of "mean" things to do to the criminal in prison. However, in this session, after putting the criminal in jail, he would ask the criminal (i.e., therapist) what she would like to have for lunch. He would then make elaborate meals for the criminal. Next, the criminal would escape from prison and he would recapture her, only to repeat the meal-making role-play.

## Illustration 3: Regressive/Mastery Transitional Stage

Inez began her ninth play session as she had earlier sessions. She did a role-play in which a mom and dad dinosaur had to protect their baby dinosaur from other dinosaurs, lions, bears, and other animals. Around 25 minutes into this role-play she stated she wanted to play something different. She established that she was going to be a teacher and teach her students, which included all the dinosaurs and animals, how to spell words. She enforced proper classroom etiquette, requiring the students to raise their legs/paws before answering the teacher's questions. She had a patient, positive attitude when animals did not know the answer and drew gold stars on a dry erase board when they did get the answers right. She spent the last 5 minutes of the session showing the therapist how she could juggle three balls.

   It should be noted that some children will continue to do some of the play of earlier stages throughout the course of therapy. So we would still categorize as a "Regressive/Mastery Transitional Stage" a session with the following ratio (5% Aggressive Stage/40% Regressive Stage/55% Mastery Stage).

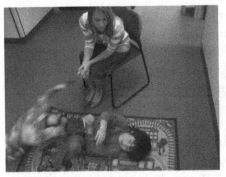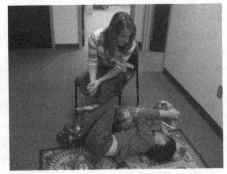

Figures 10.5 and 10.6

## Atypical Responses of Children to the Play Therapy Process

Although most children will go through the stages of the play therapy process (including transitional stages) in an identifiable way, some will not. We will refer to these children as "atypical." This designation is not meant to imply that these children's approach to the playroom is deficient in some way or that it will prevent therapeutic progress from occurring. It is simply meant to indicate that their approach to the therapeutic process is infrequently observed—perhaps less than 10% of the time—and that in some cases, but not all, makes it more difficult to track progress from in-session behavior alone.

One such group of "atypical" children will work on therapeutic issues related to two or more stages simultaneously from early play sessions, often needing little if any Warm-up Stage. These "atypical" children differ from children who are going through transitional stages in that they do not go through purer forms of a given stage prior to entering a mixture of two stages; instead, they move directly toward engaging in behaviors/themes of both stages.

### Illustration 1

Sam entered the playroom for his second session. After 20 minutes, he began to play with the dollhouse. He did role-plays in which the parents locked the "bad" children in their rooms and implemented a whole series of punishments. In the last 15 minutes of the session, Sam did another role-play in which a mommy fed and nurtured a baby. This blend of aggressive/regressive role-plays continued throughout the next 10 sessions until Sam began to include some Mastery Stage play. Eventually, Sam's play became primarily Mastery Stage play.

Although it is clear that Sam did not need much of a Warm-up Stage, he is also atypical from most children in that he never engaged predominantly in Aggressive Stage or Regressive Stage play alone anytime during the course of therapy. Functionally, he could be described as skipping the Warm-up Stage and moving to an Aggressive/Regressive Transitional Stage, followed by a pure Mastery Stage. In short, we can describe Sam's progress in terms of the stages and understand that progress was being made, but his journey through the therapeutic process was different than most children—effective for his healing, but still unusual.

A small percentage of children go through the Warm-up Stage and then move directly into the Regressive Stage, apparently bypassing the Aggressive Stage and the typically occurring intervening transitional stages. In some cases, careful examination of these children's play sessions will often reveal that they did actually go through an Aggressive Stage of very short duration; nonetheless, even in such cases it is clear that for these children the major focus of therapeutic work has to do with Regressive Stage issues, and that the Aggressive Stage issues are much less central. In the infrequent situations where children "skip" a stage, the therapist is not alarmed, but simply understands that this child's path to healing is different from that of other children.

Finally, another group of "atypical" children are those who do not appear to go through the stages of the play therapy process at all. They may not engage in projective solitary role-plays or interactive role-plays with the therapist. They will also often not include projective material in any of their drawings. Such children may appear to be in a continuous Warm-up Stage even after a number of sessions. Sometimes the therapist may be able to identify clear gains in the relationship quality between himself and the child, but sometimes even this is not discernable. Since the therapist may not be able to track progress via the method of identifying stages of the play therapy process, she may have to depend on parent and teacher reports in order to track therapeutic progress. In the majority of such cases, even though the therapist cannot observe in-session progress in terms of stages, nonetheless, progress is being noted by parents and teachers. However, in rare cases in which the therapist cannot track progress from in-session movement through the stages and no progress is being reported by parents or teachers after 10 or 15 sessions, the therapist may experience considerable concern from parents, and even experience self-doubt about the effectiveness of the CCPT method for this particular child. Although continuing on with play sessions may eventually yield progress, it is also possible that the CCPT method may not work for this child. It is therefore reasonable for the therapist or counselor to consider adding an additional treatment intervention or switching to an alternative therapeutic approach such as parent skills training (Guerney, 1995) or filial therapy (Chapter 13; Guerney, 2000).

## Special Problems: Examples of Types of Child Clients Who Have Unusual Struggles in Warm-Up and Potential Variations in Therapeutic Procedures

The following examples of very rare struggles in the Warm-up Stage are helpful to consider in that they bring up the possibility of varying therapeutic procedures in rare but realistic situations.

### Potential Challenges in Helping a Child With High Anxiety to Warm Up

Often, children who have problems with high anxiety, such as perfectionism or severe lack of confidence, may be very tentative in the initial play therapy sessions. Such children may be reluctant to engage in the typical exploratory play seen in the Warm-up Stage because they are afraid they might "do something wrong" and thus risk condemnation by their counselor. Such a child may be reluctant to take the lead in the playroom, but instead will look to his counselor to give him direction. His discomfort may leave you with a strong urge to encourage and reassure him or to attempt to make the situation easier by suggesting possible things for him to do. In short, he may pull you to do exactly what he *does not* need if he is to experience growth in the therapeutic experience. In such cases, you need to be able to be comfortable with his anxiety, make empathic responses about his lack of confidence (e.g., "you are not sure what to do"), but continue to communicate the nature of his role in sessions (e.g., "you would like me to decide what we do, but in here you are the one who gets to decide what we do"). If a child is especially quiet and inactive, you must be comfortable with silence, and if appropriate "normalize" his inaction through an empathic response (e.g., "you are not sure what this place is like or what you can or want to do"). As has been indicated in a previous chapter, you may also decide to restate the opening statement in a more extended format as a way of making the nature of the playroom more apparent (e.g., "In this special room you may say anything and do almost anything you want. You can use the toys and materials in many of the ways you would like, you can do things alone or ask me to join in, or if you like you may choose to do nothing at all." If the therapist is comfortable with silence, makes occasional empathic responses, and does not try to rescue the child by giving structure, in most cases the child will eventually begin to "warm up," and this will represent true therapeutic gains.

In the case of a child with separation anxiety, the child may refuse to enter the playroom without her parent. Although ultimately you will want to be able to work with her alone, allowing the parent in the initial session may be required in order to honor the principle of "accepting the child where they are at" and to provide support to the warm-up process. It is generally advisable to ask the parent to bring something to read into the playroom and to coach the parent to emphasize to the child that this is a time for the counselor and the child. You may implement a "systematic desensitization hierarchy" in future sessions with the parent sitting right outside the playroom with the door open for session 2, then sitting right outside the playroom with the door closed for session 3, and finally the parent sitting out in the waiting room with the child being able to check on the parent as frequently as desired in session 4. In very rare situations, a more gradual process of helping the child separate from the parent will be required. In an extremely rare situation in which there appears to be little progress either toward the child's allowing the parent to be outside the play-room, or at least the child's appearing to make therapeutic progress with the parent present in the playroom, you may wish to consider switching to the filial therapy or parent skills training (Guerney, 1995).

## Potential Challenges in Helping a Child Warm Up Who Is Passive Oppositional

Although in almost all cases we find the Warm-up Stage for children with opposition/defiance problems to be unremarkable, there are times when some such children will enter the playroom during the first session and passively refuse to engage the therapist or the playroom. Such a child may become a bit more direct and vocalize that he "doesn't know why he has to be there," and may be critical of the playroom and its toys, and maybe even you and just the whole situation in general.

In a situation where a child is simply quiet, you must be comfortable with this silence and try to empathize with what appears to underlie this silence (e.g., "you don't like it that your parents brought you here," or "you don't think there is any reason for you to be here"). Much like the anxious child mentioned in the previous section, an oppositional child may attempt to evoke a response from you that initiates a pattern of interaction with which he is comfortable (e.g., adult tries to get him to do something and he resists.) The key to success with such a child is to maintain comfort through the silence and lack of action, to use empathic responses to bring to the surface his anger and frustration about being brought to the playroom, and to demonstrate unconditional positive regard in the face of passive opposition. Although it may take a session, or even a few sessions, pretty much every time he will come to experience you as being very different from parents, teachers, and other authority figures, and come to recognize the opportunity offered in the playroom to express feelings more directly and to exert control actively through fantasy play.

## Potential Challenges in Helping a Child Warm Up Who Seems Attachment Aversive

It is a sad truth that some children have experienced abandonment and rejection, and have otherwise not received warmth and affirmation in their attachments to parents and other significant adults. We find that the vast majority of such children readily engage in CCPT, but in some situations children with such backgrounds may initially engage the therapist and playroom in a manner similar to the oppositional and defiant children noted above. In such a situation, a child who is attachment aversive may express opposition that is much more overt. Such a child may verbalize insults toward the therapist that come across as quite personal and are meant to push the therapist away and to avoid the establishment of a relationship. Alternatively, such children may simply fail to engage the therapist, much like the anxious child; however, the failure to engage is not so much related to the possibility of doing something that would earn the disapproval of the therapist, as in the case of the anxious child, but for the purpose of avoiding the establishment of a relationship. Needless to say, building a relationship with such children is a challenge that requires perseverance in maintaining unconditional positive regard, empathy, and in dealing with the rejection that the child engages in toward the therapist. Progress is often slower than with many other problems children experience. The consolation for the therapist is that the CCPT methodology, if adhered to, will reach such children and over time allow them an opportunity to have trust and be willing to gradually develop what may be for them the first "secure" relationship they have experienced. Being able to work with and be part of the incredible transformations that such children experience in the playroom is unforgettable, and although sometimes an ordeal, also a precious and profound privilege.

## Concluding Thoughts

What we hope you have learned from this chapter is that although each child is unique and is allowed to craft their own psychological work space in the playroom, nonetheless, the therapeutic climate established by the therapist often results in the child's moving through the play therapy process in four identifiable and sequential stages: Warm-up, Aggressive, Regressive, and Mastery. Each stage presents an opportunity for the development and advancement of the therapeutic relationship. Each stage is also associated with work on specific psychological issues and areas of growth, as evidenced by the behaviors and themes present in the child's play. As children move from one stage to the next, they often move through transitional stages, which contain significant elements of the stage to which they are moving as well as the stage that they are leaving. A minority of children move through the stages in an atypical manner. However, in the vast majority of cases, the therapist can use knowledge of the play therapy stages in order to understand the play therapy process and to track in-session progress.

## Activities and Resources for Further Study

### Activity A: Practice Makes Perfect

A major premise of this chapter has been that in spite of the unique content of a child's play sessions, there is nonetheless some common identifiable stages within the play therapy process. Learning to identify the four major stages of the play therapy process (e.g., Warm-up,

Aggressive, Regressive, and Mastery), as well as transitional stages, will allow you as a therapist to track therapeutic movement from within-session behaviors. In turn, this will give you confidence that progress is occurring independently of the parent and teacher reports. This is important because often therapeutic progress may be seen within the playroom prior to improvement in the child's behavior and emotional functioning outside the playroom. In order to help you improve your skill in identifying the stages of the play therapy process, we provide the following activity with scenarios. After working through the activities on your own, compare your answers with the stage assessment answers provided in Skill Support Resource Section E.

# Activities for Practice and Review on Stages of CCPT

## Activity A: Identifying Stages of CCPT

For each of the descriptions of a child's play session, identify what stage (e.g., Warm-up, Aggressive, Regressive, Mastery, or Transitional) the child appears to be in and give a rationale for your answer:

1. Kenesha spends the session participating in a variety of types of play including ring toss, drawing, hitting a bop bag, and a role-play where she pretends to be a cook and feeds some animals. She spends about 5 minutes in each activity before switching to a new activity. She is initially tentative in her play at the beginning of the session but becomes a bit more confident in her choices as the session unfolds, even testing a limit by shooting a dart from the dart gun at the therapist.

2. Kenesha identifies herself as the queen of the world. She places a crown on her head and gives commands to the therapist who plays various members of her royal court. Occasionally, when the therapist does not comply quickly enough with her commands, he gets sent to the dungeon.

3. Kenesha spends the first part of the session in role-play where she is queen of the world. She then switches the roles and the therapist becomes the queen of the world and Kenesha becomes the royal maid, who is ordered by the queen to clean the whole castle. When she does not clean fast enough, the queen sends Kenesha to the dungeon.

4. Kenesha spends the first part of the session in a role-play locking up the therapist, in the role of the royal maid, for not cleaning fast enough. In the second part of the session, while the maid is in the dungeon, the queen comes to visit the maid and orders the royal cook to make all of the maid's favorite meals. Occasionally, the queen will order the cook to take away one of the maid's favorite dishes before she can eat it, but predominantly the maid dines on most of her favorite meals.

5. In the first part of the session, Kenesha, in the role of the queen, is informed by the royal maid that her daughter, the princess, has been kidnapped. Extremely worried, Queen Kenesha travels around her kingdom looking everywhere for her daughter, offering a million-dollar reward for anyone who finds her. In the second part of the session, Queen Kenesha finds her daughter, the princess, and a royal feast is given where the royal cook serves the princess all of her favorite foods.

6. In the early part of the session, Queen Kenesha hears of a plot to kidnap her daughter, the princess. She pretends to be asleep in her daughter's room and surprises the kidnapper as he tries to capture her daughter. The kidnapper is sent to the dungeon, escapes, and tries to kidnap the princess, only to be captured. In the latter part of the session, the queen goes on a royal hunt where she tries to shoot various animals (puppets) placed all around the room. She takes great joy when she is able to shoot with precision and hit an animal that is far away in the room.

7. Kenesha enters the session and says she would like to use the bowling pins. She sets the rule that both she and the therapist have to stand 7 feet away from the pins with their back to the pins. The two of them can look briefly to see where the pins are and then have to throw the bowling ball between their legs without looking at the pins. When she misses the pins, she says, "Oh well, I will have to aim better next time."

## Activity B: Compare and Contrast Therapy to Nontherapy

Observe and contemplate, then journal or discuss the likely meanings and functions of aggressive and regressive play outside of CCPT. What roles might it play in children's and families development? What roles might it play for the human species' maintenance and development?

Reflect on how it feels to you to master a new skill set, challenge, situation, or stage. From your reflection, consider the meanings and implications of how you respond to a child's sense of growing mastery in play therapy.

## Activity C

Review journals and publications, and share your findings on past or current research and writings relating to the stages and process of play therapy.

# Helping Parents, Teachers, and Principals Understand and Support the Child's Work in Play Therapy

| 11 |
|---|
| Chapter |

*It seemed to me that it would be more helpful for [the mother] to have learned in this interview that she was respected and understood, even though that understanding was, of necessity, a more generalized concept which accepted the fact that she had reasons for what she did, that she had capacity to change, and that changes must come from within herself. . . .*
—*Excerpt from Virginia Axline's classic book,*
Dibs: In Search of Self

## Application Focus Issues

The following application focus issues are among the hurdles that play therapists overcome in order to reach child clients in need. This chapter explains and illustrates how to get beyond impasses, as well as preparatory work that serves to prevent conflicts, interruptions in therapy, and parent/teacher factors that can inhibit a child's progress in child-centered play therapy (CCPT).

## Application Focus Issue A

You are all set to begin play therapy with 8-year-old Nita. Her father, Carlos, is seeing another counselor at your agency. He was referred to you to counsel Nita because Nita is having anxiety-related difficulties, including being terrified to leave him for her classroom weeks into the school year. Nita and Carlos have separated from her mother, who from Carlos's description seems to be suffering from a personality disorder, but refusing treatment. Carlos seems ready to go along with whatever you recommend for Nita, as he is very worried and hurt for her. It seems that all is settled and set to proceed, when Carlos seems to have a sudden pang of fear and asks, "But how will I know what is going on with her? (He hesitates for a second of thought but, before you can respond, continues.) If you and Nita meet alone, I'm going to need you to report to me after each session."

You begin to explain about confidentiality, but Carlos interjects, sounding afraid, "Look, Juanita is my daughter and I do not know you." Beginning to raise his voice, he continues, "If you expect me to just turn Juanita over to you"—at this point, he stops short, exasperated—"I just don't know if it will work." He becomes adamant and begins to refuse services, threatening to leave the agency altogether.

So, you are at an impasse. You see that Nita is suffering from anxiety that is hindering her functioning and development in severe and persistent ways. Her difficulties have not subsided in reasonable time since the separation, even though her sibling's difficulties have. Nita's difficulties warrant individual counseling, and CCPT seems ideal for her—many school adults, including well-meaning counselors, have certainly tried guidance approaches, such as reassuring her, rewarding her, and helping her take reasonable perspectives on what is asked of her, but she has been unresponsive, shutting down further in response to each attempt. So, what do you do? If you can't get past the impasse with her father, you can't reach Nita. This scenario illustrates the quandary of needing to reach agreement with a parent in order to have the parent support the child's work in CCPT.

## Application Focus Issue B

By all reports, 10-year-old Cole is a "holy terror" in the classroom. The principal explains that she had thought to refer him for counseling off campus, but that his mom (who is parenting alone) seems so disorganized and overstressed that she doubts that she would or could follow through. Mom gave permission for your counseling services, and his teacher reportedly wants the help, too. However, Cole's teacher has not returned the behavior rating scale you've requested twice. When you ask to meet with her, she puts you off for other tasks. When you explained that you want her input into Cole's difficulties, she responded that Cole has become "her worst nightmare" and that if it (assumedly, she means Cole's misbehavior) continues much longer, she'll refer him for special education. She has also been difficult to schedule sessions with—first saying Cole is too far behind to miss instructional time, then insisting on scheduling during Cole's only opportunities to be physically active at school or during "fun times" in the classroom. When you mention play therapy, she chortles sarcastically in frustration, "Oh, he *knows* how to play." So how can you respond? It seems that you must somehow turn things around with Cole's teacher in order to reach Cole.

## Chapter Overview and Summary

The initial meetings with parents, teachers, and other caretakers lay the groundwork for cooperative and warm working relationships that will not only be very helpful in the beginning of CCPT, but will make the intervention more effective. Most parents, teachers, and other significant adults in a child's caretaking want to feel *effective* and *able to help* when a child is emotionally distressed. When a child is no longer able to function in a happy, well-adjusted manner, a mother may become highly frustrated and angry. When a teacher is not able to help a child learn or behave well in the classroom, she may become determined to point out fault with the child. Listening with empathy in consultation with parents and teachers is the key to gaining their support. Providing information as needed about the value of CCPT is vital to gaining understanding and support. Most parents and many teachers naturally want to know more about the counseling process and the meaning of "play" in a child's development and therapy. A common question from parents and teachers alike involves wonder at how "play" is helpful to the child's learning and emotional well-being. This chapter explains and illustrates what every referring parent should know about CCPT and your work with the parent and child, what teachers need to know, and key principles for parent and teacher consultation regarding CCPT.

## Primary Skill Objectives

The following Primary Skill Objectives are provided to guide you through the chapter and for reflection and review after reading the chapter. By reading and working through the chapter exercises, you will be better able to:

1. Understand the importance of the child-centered therapist's role—that is, as someone who is relationship-based—both in counseling

the child and in consultation with parents, teachers, and other significant caretakers.

2. Be able to explain what every parent should know in getting started with CCPT and why.

3. Explain the primary and secondary goals in getting started with a parent in an agency or school setting, as well as with principals and teachers in school settings.

4. Describe the principles of feedback sessions with parents, what usually happens, how and why, as well as how these same principles can apply in feedback sessions with teachers and principals and how the principles can vary.

5. Explain how the five things that every parent should know when getting started with CCPT also apply in working with principals and teachers.

6. Give examples of the service contexts (i.e., the set or array of services) that can surround CCPT in agency and school settings.

7. Describe the common problems in working with parents, teachers, and principals and how they can be overcome.

8. Understand basic explanations of CCPT and consider how explanations may be customized.

## Working With Parents

As parents are critically important in each child's life, your primary goals in an initial meeting should be to make a personal connection through empathy, to hear the problem in the parent or parents' own words, and to convey that you understand the problem—not that you understand every detail of how the problem works or why the problem developed, but that you get the level of difficulty and the nature of the problems that parent(s) or their child is experiencing. Secondarily, you can often provide an initial, small but helpful intervention by addressing the underlying positive message in their description of the problem to you. Once your primary goals are met, you can consider what treatment options seem to make sense, including CCPT, and explain the options to the parent(s). In the following sections, we walk you through the process as it typically unfolds in an agency setting, then a school setting. In these sections, we will refer to the mental health clinicians in the agency setting as "therapist" and in the school setting as "counselor." This is not meant to denote degree backgrounds, as degree backgrounds vary in both settings. Rather, it follows our practice of varying our use of the terms and, in this case, we are dividing our use by the terms that seem more commonly used in the two setting types.

## What Every Parent Should Know in Getting Started With CCPT

There are five things that every parent should understand before leaving an initial meeting with you from which you intend to provide CCPT for her child.

1. **A parent should know that you care for him and his child.** Perhaps this sounds obvious, but as a child advocate, it is easy to slip into the common error of seeing the parent as an enemy against you, who is trying to help the child. As a counselor or therapist specializing in children and/or family services, you have or will have encountered many parents who have been neglectful or abusive and some who begin in a hostile posture toward you and sometimes in a hostile posture toward their child. You cannot let this get in the way of your caring for the parent (even through an abuse report, if warranted). It may help you to remember that the parent is critically important to the child, and, in spite of all his past mistakes, can become a very helpful therapeutic agent for his child.

2. **A parent needs to know that you understand her and her child's situation in order to trust you with her child.** If you don't understand her situation, why would she see you as credible in offering services for her child. Plus, understanding leads to goal agreement and alliance.

3. **A parent needs to know that you see the underlying positive in who he is as a parent.** However misguided or seemingly absent, a parent's love for his child is almost always there. A longing for his child to succeed is almost always there. A part of your job is uncovering that truth, so that you and he have an opportunity to see him as a parent in that light, and to build on that bare basic strength.

4. **A parent needs to know that you have a plan, that you know what you are doing, and can follow procedures known to work.** By the time of accepting help, many parents

often are or feel desperate. They need to know that you are solid and confident in the services you offer. This does not mean that you are guaranteeing specific outcomes, but that you know that the CCPT that you offer will bring about positive results.

5. **A parent needs to know that follow-up communication will be a part of your work.** We recommend that instead of explaining confidentiality of the child's sessions from the parent, which can be explained if needed, you first explain that you will want regular feedback from her, in most cases you will set up periodic meetings for this, and/or you may use other formats such as regular ratings and comments sheets regarding goals that you decide on together (see Chapter 12). You should also explain that you will update her regarding her child's progress at these preset meetings as well as other times, if needed. While some parents may ask what was said and done in sessions, most simply want to know that their child is progressing well, that the services are working in the ways you expected, and that their child is okay.

There are several logistical pieces of information to provide most parents as well. We find that this information can be provided in verbal explanation or illustrated in a booklet that provides information that parents may need to understand and support their children's work in CCPT:

- The fact that children in CCPT can be loud, that if a parent hears loud, exuberant, emotional sounds from her child in session (e.g., while parent is in the waiting room), these are expressions of emotion that are quite normal and a good thing.

- Play therapy can be active and messy, so children should come dressed to play actively and to be moderately messy, so not in their best dress clothes.

- Because her child's work and language of therapy is play, he might likely reply if asked what he did in sessions, "Just played." Such an evasive seeming response to an innocent, simple question from a parent is normal in that the question requires the child to explain in words *work that he cannot explain in words*.

- Importantly, some sessions may be ended early. So, in agency settings, the parent will need to be in the waiting room during sessions.

Table 11.1  **The Five Things Every Parent Should Know in Getting Started With CCPT**

1. You care for her and her child.
2. You understand her and her child's situation.
3. You see the underlying positive in her as parent.
4. You have a plan for helping, you know what you are doing, and can follow procedures known to work.
5. Follow-up communication will be a part of your work.

- Also importantly, the CCPT session is the child's hour, so you will not be giving information or receiving feedback about the child before and after sessions. To do so would suggest a lack of privacy for the child and inhibit necessary expression. The two of you will need to talk in the regularly scheduled feedback sessions or in additional meetings as needed.

We find that most parents are okay with not getting reports of their child's actions in play as long as: (1) you have connected with him empathically, understood his situation, and know what you can do to help; (2) he knows he will get progress reports from you and that you will be sure he gets the information about his child that he needs; and (3) that you have at least an implied alliance in that you are working in an agreed way of helping his child improve and grow into a closer relationship with him.

## Getting Started in an Agency or Private Practice Setting

In agency settings, initial meetings are often referred to as "intakes." When conducting an intake, therapists usually have certain pieces of information that are required by the agency and may be needed by the treatment team. As long as it is allowable in your setting, we recommend that you complete information-gathering tasks after you have completed your primary goals of making a personal connection through empathy, hearing the problem in the parent's words, and conveying that you understand the problem.

In most settings, you must establish informed consent for the consultation you are providing, including confidentiality and its limits. This is often addressed through a written document that the parent, who at that time is the primary client, would read and sign, indicating that she understands. Often, therapists follow up verbally to check that the form is understood.

## Primary Goals

With the initial business of informed consent taken care of, you can continue with your primary goals. We find that an opening statement that warmly structures the meeting time is a most helpful way to start: "Thank you for coming, Ms. Smith. What I'd like to do in our time this evening is to get a sense from you of what brings you in and what the difficulties are that you and Johnny are experiencing. Following that, I may need to ask for some specific additional information. Then I can suggest options for how we can best help you." Ms. Smith may respond explaining that Johnny has become very hard to control at home, that they argue a lot. She may describe some of his misbehaviors, perhaps aggression toward her or siblings. It is critically important that you let her talk, let her tell you how she sees it from her unique perspective, and respond with empathy. Many parents will feel defensive and embarrassed in such a moment. Many see themselves to blame as failed parents, even when they defer the pain of admitting this thought by blaming their child. Your empathy is needed to help her tell you what is happening and how she is reacting to it. You need to listen therapeutically, warmly reflecting the key aspects of her situation and strongly stated or implied emotions and thoughts. She will need you to meet her with unconditional positive regard in order to be open and honest with you. We see it as both an honorable and brave step for a parent to admit the need and to ask for professional help. We consider it a privilege to be asked and to be able to help. Be sure to respond to how she feels, not just what has happened.

## Addressing the Underlying Positive

We find that there is almost always an initial positive underlying the parent's problem statement and her action in seeking help. A therapist's statement following in the example above for this could be, "I get that these difficulties, his behaviors, and the fix you are in are driving you away from him. I see how you are hurting with that. I see that it is not what you want. You want him to thrive at school and be happy at home."

## Proceeding to Ongoing Treatment Arrangements

Once you have listened well to the parent's reason for coming in and responded therapeutically with genuine, deep empathy and unconditional positive regard, we suggest that you proceed to gather the additional intake information that was not provided in the more naturalistic process of therapeutic listening. We sometimes ask questions during the primary goals (listening, connecting, and demonstrating understanding), but more often we find that all or almost all of the intake information we need is naturally provided within the therapeutic process of listening and responding empathically.

Having the business of intake information-gathering taken care of, and benefitting from the information gathered, you should be able to suggest treatment care options. The options we normally include are CCPT, parent consultation regarding parenting skills, individual counseling for the parent, couples counseling if there is a parental dyad, and possibly filial therapy.

We would normally offer CCPT in all cases where the child seems to have experienced significant trauma or when the child's difficulties have proven severe and persistent so far. We make this recommendation in most cases when the child's difficulty does not seem likely to be lifted by a minor or simple change within the parent—as in most situations that have gotten dire enough for the parent to seek professional help. Even the most well-meaning parents tend to find it harder to change than their children do. Additionally, we believe that when a child has experienced a significantly negative situation for a prolonged period, or a significantly painful short-term trauma, the child deserves and usually needs the focused opportunity to integrate or make meaning of the experience in her mind-set, as well as to correct mistaken beliefs prompted by the prolonged negative situation or trauma, and to redefine who she is and who she wants to be.

We normally explain this to the parent, saying something like, "Ms. Smith, one of my primary recommendations is for you to have me proceed with individual counseling for Johnny." In the case of oppositional defiant behavior implied above for Johnny, we might add, "Johnny's behavior has become a serious problem for him, as well as for you and your family. The mode of counseling that I will suggest for him is child-centered play therapy. In short, what that means is that he will use play in the specialized playroom and structures of child counseling in much the same way that an adult would use talk in her counseling. In this work, he will gain and be prompted to rethink troubled choices and ways of being; he will be helped to choose more mature behaviors." As with any such explanation, (1) your words should be tailored to this parent and child's specific situation; and (2) as soon as you say it, you should be ready to listen to the parent's reaction and respond with empathy, as well as answering informational questions, before providing additional information. A common error is expecting parent resistance and trying to explain too much while listening too little.

Parent consultation or parent skill training is often an effective addition to CCPT, but is rarely sufficient in and of itself. It is very hard to change a parenting style, which is a product of one's personality style, developed over years, if not generations, and shaped in systemic interactions with the child and others, unless the child is engaged in a powerful, independent path to positive change.

Individual counseling for the parent can be an excellent option in addition to CCPT. Usually, the parent is deeply hurting as well before seeking professional help for the child. If both parent and child are moving in new directions, based on carefully thought through and self-aware decisions made in individual counseling, the two will come together in harmonious ways.

If there is a parental couple, we would very strongly recommend couples counseling to support the strength of the couple while the child moves in mature directions through use of CCPT. In agreement with many approaches to family therapy, we believe that a strong parental dyad should be the key to a strong family, when available. We advocate and use the relationship enhancement model of couples counseling, which is a communications-based model that helps couples develop empathic listening and expressiveness skills that they can use to make parenting decisions, manage couple and family problems, and to maintain a close, loving relationship at the core of the family (Ginsberg, 1997; Scuka, 2005).

## An Example of Getting Started in an Agency Setting

> **THERAPIST:** *Thank you for coming in, Ms. Smith. What I'd like to do in our time this evening is to get a sense from you of what brings you in and what the difficulties are that you and Johnny are experiencing. Following that, I may need to ask for some specific additional information. Then I can suggest options for how we can best help you.''*

**Ms. Smith:** *[Speaking haltingly] I . . . I sure do hope you can help, because I don't know what to do anymore [begins to cry].*

**Therapist:** *This is very hard for you. Seems like it's very scary for you to say you may not know what to do anymore.*

**Ms. Smith:** *[Pulling herself back from tears, so that she can continue] I think Johnny may be becoming just like his father always was. . . .*

**Therapist:** *I know you let me know on our confidential intake questionnaire that Johnny's father beat a man very badly while drunk one night, and was also very violent with you before being sent to prison. That kind of violence is what you fear for Johnny, too.*

**Ms. Smith:** *Yes. The school says Johnny has no more chances. He's always been a handful, but this year he argues with his teacher all the time. She hates him. He spends most of his time in the office. They say the other day he pushed her. I know he's bad [starts to cry again], but I don't think he would've done that if she didn't do something to him first. They say he can have one more chance if I get him professional help, but that's it. They've already fixed up the papers to have him expelled—for the year. What will I do with him if he can't go to school?*

**Therapist:** *You seem desperate, really worried for his future at school. You don't know what to do for him, but you know you have to do something. Sounds like you don't think it's all his fault, but you know that he has to take some of the responsibility for his behavior.*

**Ms. Smith:** *He's not a bad kid . . . he gets angry fast, though. It's just that damn teacher!*

**Therapist:** *So you think a lot of this school problem is her fault.*

Ms. Smith vents for a few minutes about the teacher and how she is unfair to Johnny. The therapist goes with this empathically, continually responding to her strongly stated thoughts and feelings expressed in wordings like, "You are just so frustrated with her!" "You see that this is completely unfair to Johnny," and "You're thinking that if it just weren't for this really bad teacher, Johnny would be just fine!" Hearing this last quite accurate statement of empathy seems to strike Ms. Smith. She seems to realize how far she's gone in blaming Johnny's teacher and stops. She continues:

**Ms. Smith:** *. . . Well, it's not just her . . . it can't really just be his teacher, but she doesn't help much. I have this other problem, too. I can't really control Johnny at home like I used to. Used to be if I just* *got real strict with him, threatened or maybe took a little swipe at him, he'd fall in line. But now he's started getting hard on his little sister, and well . . . well. . . .*

**THERAPIST:** *There is something that's hard for you to say. You seem almost about to cry.*

**MS. SMITH:** *He reminds me for all the world of his father! When I get after him because I have to, he gives me this look of hatred—like he's disgusted with me. It's just like his father in the worst times. [She starts crying hard now. Therapist waits for her to continue, feeling her pain and having a hunch that she's going somewhere important to her] . . . It's like he hates me. . . .*

**THERAPIST:** *That's hard for you. To get that feeling that he hates you.*

**MS. SMITH:** *It is! After all I do for him. He used to be so sweet. As a little boy he always wanted me to lie in bed with him, so he could tell me all about his day. Well, he still wants that sometimes, but then when I have to go, or don't have time to listen, he's so hateful about it. He says horrible things. Calls me the same things his father did.*

**THERAPIST:** *That's one of the things that hurt you so much. To feel hated by the child you love, and want so much to help. Ms. Smith, I think I can help. To summarize what you've told me, you are in a desperate situation with school. You fear that Johnny may not be allowed to continue. That's desperate, but maybe just as painful, you are having difficulty controlling Johnny at home. You are worried about his behaviors toward his sister, and really hurt by the growing distance between him and you.*

**MS. SMITH:** *[Nods to affirm, and sighs deeply, seeming almost in relief as she sinks in her chair.]*

**THERAPIST:** *There are a number of pieces of information that I need to follow up on before we proceed, then I can talk to you about what we ["we" meaning the agency/private practice] can do to help.*

At this point, the therapist follows up on potentially dangerous situations with others (school, sister, mom). The therapist also inquires into Mom's methods of discipline. In each case, he remains genuine and connected to Mom by explaining what he is thinking, at levels she can understand, what he is asking and why. He gathers remaining necessary intake information and obtains Mom's written consent for him to contact Johnny's school: (1) to confirm that Johnny and his mom are receiving agency help, and (2) to get a clearer picture of Johnny's school situation and perhaps offer to consult, if appropriate.

**THERAPIST:** *Now let's talk about what we can do to help. [Remembering to reflect the underlying positive] First of all, I know that you want Johnny to succeed at school. . . .*

**Ms. SMITH:** *Yes. He's really smart, when he's not in so much trouble.*

**THERAPIST:** *. . . And I know you want a loving relationship with him, not this painful, maybe hateful relationship you have now.*

**Ms. SMITH:** *[Nods and smiles, shrugging in relief.]*

**THERAPIST:** *My primary recommendation is for me to work with Johnny individually. I suspect he is hurting, even if he is acting out toward others in that hurt. He seems to be confused and conflicted and moving down paths that, as you know, can predict ever-worsening futures for him. The approach I will take with him is called child-centered play therapy. In that work, he can use his play with me in the specialized playroom as his mode of communication in therapy, much in the same way an adult would communicate with her counselor. [Therapist looks to see that mom seems okay with all of this so far. She does. And as she has vented and been responded to with empathy, she is ready to listen and receive help.] In that work he will be prompted to rethink decisions he is making, especially about who he is and who he wants to be, what kinds of relationships he wants with others [Mom smiles as if to say that would be good]. Look's like that sounds good to you so far.*

**Ms. SMITH:** *[Sounding relieved that someone understands her and seems to know what to do to help] Yes, I want that. But I want to know . . . how long will this take?*

**THERAPIST:** *That will depend on a number of factors. I want us to plan on weekly sessions for Johnny for as much as the next six months [Mom seems to gasp slightly and stiffen some], for Johnny to complete his therapy, but you should see progress well before that. And I want us to meet monthly to discuss his progress. I'll also ask you to rate his behavior for me on a weekly basis.*

**Ms. SMITH:** *[Has gotten more comfortable again and is sitting back comfortably to listen. She also knows that the therapist has said he is willing to contact Johnny's school, both to gather their input firsthand and to seek their continued patience with Johnny if necessary.]*

**THERAPIST:** *. . . A factor that can speed up Johnny's progress is you. There are things you can do. We have an ongoing parent skills group that you can join to work with other parents struggling in similar ways. In that group, you can learn new ways to respond to Johnny and new ways to manage his behavior that will complement what he is learning in his sessions. And another thing,*

> *Ms. Smith, is that I want you to consider working with one of our therapists yourself. You can spend part of the time consulting about your relationship with Johnny, but mostly I want you to focus on yourself. You have been through a lot. If you and Johnny change together at the same time, the two of you can grow to be more harmonious most quickly.*

The therapist and Ms. Smith then discuss the logistics of these options (e.g., the time each takes, the financial costs). In many cases, parents have to prioritize or choose between the options. For example, if they talk further and discern that Ms. Smith seems to know what to do as a parent, but seems to be off-track for personal reasons, individual counseling without parent skills training may be the best of the additional options for her. Or if she seems to be at an acute loss for what to do, parent skills training may be the most imperative intervention in addition to CCPT.

The therapist will also need to address the logistical information for her that parents usually need to know about play therapy (addressed above). The therapist should set at least a few key individualized goals for Johnny with Mom on which she can comment and rate his behavior periodically. If time does not allow for this in a complex situation, a more detailed checklist repeated periodically or a standardized behavior rating scale can be used (see Chapter 12).

## Getting Started With a Parent in a School Setting

In a school, your primary goals in an initial meeting with a parent are exactly the same as in an agency: to make a personal connection through empathy, to hear the problem in the parent or parents' own words, and to convey that you understand the problem—not that you understand every detail of how the problem works or why, but that you get the level of difficulty and the nature of the problems that the parent and her child experience. Secondarily, you will almost always have the same opportunity to provide an initial, small but helpful intervention by addressing the underlying positive message in the parent's description of the problem to you. Once your primary goals are met, you can consider intervention options that seem to make sense, including CCPT, and explain the options to the parent. In the following sections, we walk you through this process as it typically unfolds, but with the variation that is common in school settings in which you or the school initiated the meeting due to a learning or school behavior–related child problem.

Clinicians in schools do not usually refer to or think of the initial parent meeting as an "intake." Rather, that first meeting is seen as an education-related consultation in which ongoing services may or may not be expected. So, as the mental health clinician in the school (whether school counselor, mental health counselor, social worker, or psychologist), you do not have an obligation to informed consent or confidentiality at the parent meeting (although you would still be respectful of the parent's privacy and have obligations to prevent imminent danger and report possible child abuse) and your roles in information gathering and assessing for ongoing treatment options may be less emphasized and less overt vs. agency settings.

In many cases, these initial meetings arise out of teams of educators considering a student's special learning needs or often arise impromptu out of disciplinary, behavioral difficulties. In these cases, you will not likely be the only professional present with the parent.

In our experience in such meetings, when we or our students were working in schools, most of the educators at the meeting assumed only one meeting and assumed or attempted problem-solving roles in the meetings. They tended to ask questions with the assumption that if they uncovered the right parent error, they could give the parent the right guidance to begin turning the situation around. So your role through the primary goals may stand in noticeable and refreshing contrast to the educators' problem-solving focus. Of course, if the problem can be solved with simple guidance, then that is the best course. But in the many situations in which that is not possible, your input from the perspective of a play therapist and a person educated in a mental health discipline is needed (see the example/illustration below).

One recommendation that we find a quite common outcome from the educators' approach is a decision that the parent should follow up with counseling outside of the school for the child. We applaud this idea, but find far too many situations in which this is not likely to happen. There are issues of cost, stigma, transportation, and simply having a parent whose life is too disorganized to follow through on a consistent weekly basis. It is a very difficult, humbling, often humiliating experience for a parent to "admit defeat" or "admit inadequacy" and take her or his child for professional help.

However, you have a number of advantages when working from the school setting:

- You have access through meetings that parents are compelled to attend for educational reasons.
- You can explain your services in terms of educational benefit (increasing readiness to learn, decreasing behavioral and emotional difficulties that interfere with learning).
- You have firsthand access to observe and give and receive feedback into one of the child's major systems—the system of his relationships with teachers, peers, and other school adults (Cochran, 1996).

A mother–child example follows that is very similar to the mother–child example provided for the agency setting. We use the same names and encourage you to picture the same mother and child in the school setting explanation and example. This can allow you to see how the setting contexts are different, while key principles are the same, and to see how mother and child may be quite similar, but present somewhat differently in different contexts.

Also note that while a parent meeting in which you meet your primary goals, address the underlying positive, and proceed to treatment arrangements is the ideal in a school, just as it is the typical practice in an agency for some of the same reasons families sometimes cannot follow up on referrals to agencies, some parents also cannot attend regular school meetings. In these cases, we and many counselors working in schools simply obtain the necessary parental consent and proceed to help the child without the parent contact that we would like. The ability to proceed without parental involvement when absolutely necessary is one of the profoundly beautiful aspects of CCPT in schools—that you can reach and help the child in a significant behavior and life-changing way, even when you cannot reach a parent.

## Primary Goals

In school settings, counselors often establish informed consent by simply stating their role and the purpose of the meeting. You can incorporate this in your warmly stated opening statement, which begins to clarify your primary goal: connecting with the person and understanding her situation. For example, when being seated in a meeting that the parent asked to have with you: "So, I'm glad to meet you, Ms. Smith. I am your child's counselor at Copper Hill Elementary, and I look forward to hearing your concerns for Johnny in the time we have to talk today, and to then consider how I may help you." If you asked for the meeting, you might begin by explaining the difficulties you see: "Thank you for coming, Ms. Smith. The reason I asked you to come is that, as you know, Johnny is experiencing great difficulties in school. He has been in a number of fights, argues with his teacher a lot, and because of these things he's losing a lot of learning time. I am worried for him and want to help. I'd like you to tell me how you understand him and the difficulties he is facing. Then we can talk more about how I can help." If another professional is conducting the meeting and you are sitting in as a staff member, the opening statement may not be yours to make, but your goals should always be to connect and convey empathy and understanding of the situation as much as possible.

In such school meetings, parents often feel intimidated and are defensive. Many parents whose children are having severe and persistent difficulties in schools had poor school experiences themselves, and being called in brings back bad memories. And just as we noted for agency settings, it is very difficult for most parents to admit a need for professional help with the behavioral and emotional development of their child. These reasons underscore the critical importance of your empathy and unconditional positive regard. Your primary goal is to connect with the parent through empathy, to develop your understanding of what she is going through and what she sees that her child is going through. If you see that she has tended to lack the loving care and attentiveness of Johnny or the needed structure for Johnny that you think she should have, you may be able to help her with that after you have connected, but until you have connected with empathy and seen the situation from her perspective, you must put your opinion aside.

Should Ms. Smith deny that Johnny has any difficulties at home, which would be unlikely with the difficulties he has at school, it could be that she is working two jobs and not really aware of him at home (their time together is quite limited), or it could be that he holds it together for her at home and can't continue to contain his emotions at school. It could be that she wants to convince you to see him positively because she fears that the school is angling for some special placement that she thinks will be to his disadvantage. Or it could be that she is simply presenting him to you this way in hopes that you will see him more positively. Whatever the reason, you need to empathically go with her experience and her description. In almost all cases, doing so either helps her be less defensive and more truthful with you or helps you understand her context such that you see that your perspective and hers are both true. Depth and warmth in empathy is needed to get at the complexities of her perceptions.

## Addressing the Underlying Positive

The underlying positive of a parent's admitting the level of difficulty may be less pronounced in schools, especially as the counselor or school may have called for the meeting. However, with sensitive empathic responses, you should be able to uncover the parent's deep unhappiness with her failing child's situation or behavior. This allows a similar reframing of the situation in seeing her dissatisfaction of the current situation as evidence that she wants a better situation for or relationship with him. At some point in your empathic listening, most parents will express their hopes for him to do well, to succeed. This allows you to carefully reflect that and use it as a point of alliance and a point from which to discuss what services you may wish to discuss and the paths you see to continuing to work together.

## Example of Getting Started With a Parent in a School Setting

**PRINCIPAL:** *Thank you for coming in for this emergency situation, Ms. Smith. This is Ms. Morey, a counselor who works with us here at Copper Hill. As you know, it is school policy that after any significant violence at school, the children involved must leave school for the day, and a parent or guardian must pick them up and attend a parent conference before they return. Because we have not been able to get in touch with you so far, we have arranged to all meet with you now to take care of the conference part, to make a plan for how to turn Johnny's behavior around today, so that you don't have to make another trip over.*

**MS. SMITH:** *[Conveys anger, but also seems somewhat shaky, unsure of herself, worried perhaps, as she speaks] Well, thank you. [There might be sarcasm in her voice.] Yes, I did have to take off work to be here. I am not allowed to leave my shift without notice. I may lose my job. Johnny and I will really be in a fix then.*

PRINCIPAL: *We were afraid of that, Ms. Smith. To try to help you, we have kept Johnny in in-school suspension for the afternoon until you could get here, instead of sending him straight home, which is our policy. And we stayed late until you could get here. Most of the teachers and staff have gone home for the day.*

MS. SMITH: *How do you know this isn't somebody else's fault? Johnny is a good boy. He doesn't do stuff like this. . . . [The principal cuts in at this point.]*

PRINCIPAL: *Ms. Smith, Johnny has been in three fights in the three months he's been here. He is in constant conflict with his teacher or others in his class. This has got to change. Now you tell us what is going on so that we can try to help you.*

MS. SMITH: *[Speaking shakily] I get the notes from his teacher. I don't think she likes him very much. [Seeming to find a voice in defiance] He never had trouble like this before. I tell you, he's a good boy.*

PRINCIPAL: *Ms. Smith, I'm sorry, but that's not true. I spoke with Johnny's last principal. I know that they were considering various special services when he left.*

Ms. Smith becomes agitated at this point, shifting in her seat, looking as if she is about to spring out of the room. She responds with a sense of anger and hurt.

MS. SMITH: *Look, what do you want us to do? He's a good boy! He makes mistakes! He's not perfect! [The principal interjects at this point.]*

PRINCIPAL: *[Speaking rapidly, matching Ms. Smith's agitation] Now Ms. Smith, let's keep calm. We are here to help you. I want you to consider counseling for Johnny. I know that there are a number of excellent agencies in the area or . . .*

MS. SMITH: *[Interrupts, beginning to cry as she responds] Look, I want what's best for him. I want help. But I'm working two jobs, and we get threatening calls from collectors all the time. He stays with his grandmother, but she can't drive. You have to leave us alone! [The counselor, who is sitting by Ms. Smith across the desk from the principal, touches her arm to get her to look at her, then interrupts the principal to speak to her.]*

COUNSELOR: *You don't know what you think about all this. You look like you feel trapped and overwhelmed, like you just don't know what to do.*

MS. SMITH: *[Begins to tear up a little and keeps her face toward Ms. Morey, away from the principal] At that other school, they wanted to put him in some kind of special class, but he's smart. He doesn't need that.*

**PRINCIPAL:** *Ms. Smith, you need to understand that special education isn't because a child cannot learn, but because he has needs beyond the regular education resources of the school . . .*

**Ms SMITH:** *[Interrupts, speaking rapidly, very upset] I don't care about that. I know that Johnny can learn and I want him to learn. I don't want him singled out like some kind of . . . I won't allow any sort of [Counselor stops her, gently nudging her arm to draw her attention away again.]*

**COUNSELOR:** *I get the idea that you have big hopes for him and you don't want to see those hopes limited [addressing the underlying positive within a therapeutic reflection]. The thought of any sort of special education for him is very upsetting to you. Will you please take this time to explain how you understand Johnny, whatever difficulties he was having at his last school and how you understand his difficulties here? Then, once we understand him from your perspective, we can talk together about what to do to help him succeed. And also, one of the reasons I came to this meeting is that if you can't take him to counseling at an outside agency, I'll make time to help him here. I know that he is really struggling a lot and that he has great potential.*

**Ms. SMITH:** *[Sighs] I just don't want to see him singled out. The program they wanted at that last school sounded just like jail.*

**COUNSELOR:** *That's important to you, that he not be singled out, especially not in a program that sounds like jail.*

**Ms. SMITH:** *Johnny's father, who I was . . . Johnny's father has been in jail. [Pause] Johnny knows this. We are . . . well, we are not together now. Johnny has seen . . . well, I think Johnny both admires him and hates him for what he saw.*

**COUNSELOR:** *Ms. Smith, it sounds like what you are telling us is very hard for you to say. There is something about what Johnny has seen that upsets you very much.*

**Ms. SMITH:** *[Begins to cry] I don't want you to convict him before he has a chance.*

**COUNSELOR:** *[Speaking to the principal] Mr. Barsalinas, would it be alright if Ms. Smith and I talk alone for about 20 minutes, then get back with you before she leaves?*

The principal agrees and leaves the counselor and Ms. Smith to talk privately.

**COUNSELOR:** *Ms. Smith, I get the idea that you are trying to protect Johnny, maybe at home and at school. I asked for us to speak alone as I thought there were things you want to have understood, but were reluctant to say in front of Mr. Barsalinas. I don't believe Mr. Barsalinas is anywhere near decided, but I think I should admit that, yes, a more restrictive classroom environment is an option that the school might consider. [Ms. Smith starts to interject, but the counselor lifts her hand in a gesture of asking for forbearance.] There are a number of ways that I and others can help here at school to prevent getting to that point. In the 15 minutes or so that we have now, can you help me understand your and Johnny's situation, then I can explain ways that I can help.*

**MS. SMITH:** *[Sighs, then begins] Look, Johnny's father can be violent. I have a restraining order, but I don't trust that. We moved here partly to be further from him. [After a pause] Johnny has seen him, well . . . hit me more than once. I sometimes think Johnny thinks he's supposed to be tough like him . . . like his father. I worry that if we don't do something, he will end up like him.*

**COUNSELOR:** *So that's part of what you mean that he has seen and it seems like a big worry for you.*

**MS. SMITH:** *Yes. He's a very loving boy, but I also know he gets mad easy. He just has to have his way. But, look, he's just confused right now. He'll get through this [raising and calming her tone again with these last two statements].*

**COUNSELOR:** *You know that and you are hanging onto it, but you are also worried.*

**MS. SMITH:** *[Pauses significantly hearing this] Yes. [Tearing a little] I don't want to lose him.*

**COUNSELOR:** *That's a terrible fear for you, that you will lose him. Ms Smith, I think this has been a pattern for Johnny. [Reflecting and moving to assert for treatment] I think you are concerned about his confusion and maybe patterning after his father. I am, too. I want him to have intensive counseling to work out what he has been through and to think through who he wants to be. I can provide that for him here at school. I would suggest that I meet with Johnny twice weekly in the first month and weekly following that. [Counselor sees Ms. Smith tighten in reluctance and responds to this with empathy.] Something that I just said bothers you.*

**MS. SMITH:** *[Responding without being highly defensive, as she has come to confide in and begin to be open with the counselor] Yes it* does. That sounds like therapy. I am his mother. He should work through this with me.

COUNSELOR: So that's a part that bothered you about it, that he should work through his difficulties with you, not a stranger at school.

Ms. SMITH: Well . . . I don't mean this to sound wrong, but we don't know you.

COUNSELOR: That's a big deal in this situation, that you don't know me. [Offering assurance and explanation] Ms. Smith, you will always be important to him. My role is temporary. I think you had noted before that he doesn't have these problems at home. I might guess that that is because he has a sense of what you've been through and how hard all of this is for you. Through my work with you, he will grow in closeness to you that you can keep, as long as you are open to it. Such closeness with a caring, attending mother is what is natural for all children, when it is possible. I think it could be that right now, in his confusion, he wants you to be okay and to know that he is okay, but he's not okay. [Counselor sees that Ms. Smith is beginning to tear again.] This is hard for you to hear.

Ms. SMITH: No. It's okay. I think you are right. He's not okay right now, but he will be.

COUNSELOR: So you are sounding more okay with this.

Ms. SMITH: [Smiling a little for the first time] I am. I don't want to give him up, but I have to help him.

COUNSELOR: You seem a little relieved. [Ms. Smith offers a tearful, small smile of agreement.] And you aren't giving him up. I want to try to set a time when we can meet next week to discuss your goals for him and then to follow-up monthly. I can hopefully find a time to work around your schedule, maybe coming in really early so you can drop him off with the kids who ride the bus, then we can talk briefly before you go to work. If that won't work, we can find a time to talk on the phone. What I want is for us to find a time to talk periodically, for you to let me know how you see his progress, for me to let you know his progress, and for us to talk about other ways you can support his school behavior. I'll explain a little more to you of what our work will be like, then I'll need to explain to Mr. Barsalinas what we are doing and why, and see where he wants to go from here.

You may note that in some schools the counselor would not actually need Ms. Smith's permission, as the counseling is an education-related service. In other schools she might need parental permission for the service. But even when permission is not needed, we would strongly prefer to build a connection with her and to maintain periodic contact with her to support the work of CCPT whenever possible.

Hopefully, the parent and counselor connection is clear in this example, as well as how that empathic connection served to bond the two and shift the qualities of Ms. Smith's interactions with the school. In some cases, when permission is not needed, CCPT can easily proceed without such a counselor and parent connection and with the service being barely noted in the chaotic lives of some families struggling with extreme difficulties. Fortunately for the children of such families, CCPT can still work and be powerfully effective at helping the child gain control over his behavior and mastery over his life within the context that he lives.

## Feedback Sessions With Parents

### General Structure of the Parent Feedback Meeting

We prefer to arrange for feedback meetings with parents after about each fourth or fifth session with their child. We let parents know that they can ask for time to talk more often than that, if needed. Usually, that timing works, but occasionally a parent will have a high need to be heard each week. When that is the case, we set up brief parent meetings following the child's session. Such an arrangement should be rare, as it poses a couple of problems. First, you can't talk about the child in front of the child. Doing so would expose the child to adult decisions, communication, and experience sets that the child cannot and should not understand. Second, doing so may give the child the impression that each week after his session you report his actions to his parent. His believing that would understandably inhibit his self-expression in sessions. If a parent's need to meet frequently with you, to be heard by you and talk to you, is excessive and inhibiting of her child's progress, it may be time to reconsider more appropriate additional services for the parent, such as individual counseling with a colleague where she can address concerns that she finds herself needing to talk about, or parent skills training in individual or group sessions.

Feedback meetings should start with a warm statement of the structure of the meeting: "Hi, Ms. Smith. I'm very glad to see you tonight. I'm very glad to have this time for the two of us to talk. I want to take about half our meeting time to hear how Johnny is doing at home and school. I want to hear if things have improved a little or a lot, or also if any parts of your situation have gotten worse. Whatever it is, I need to hear. After that, I want to talk to you about what I'm seeing in Johnny's progress. We should spend about half our time on each topic." It is important to let a parent know this structure up front because, for example, if the parent doesn't know her time to talk to you is time limited, she may think that when you change the topic it means you were tired of or bothered by what she is saying. Also, the better the parent understands the structure you are working in, the better choices she can make regarding what to say or how quickly to work in her time with you.

## Feedback From the Parent to You

Just as in the intake or initial parent meeting, deep empathy is critical in the first part of the feedback meeting. Your empathy serves to continue your personal connection and alliance, helps her speak freely with you, and helps her get to the core of what she most needs to communicate to you in an efficient amount of time.

You should let the parent speak first because she may be seeing more or less progress than you expected. Each individual child's pace of progress is difficult to predict. It may range from great symptom reduction after one session to only gradual progress after more sessions. When you describe in-session progress, you will speak in terms of stages, but some children make rapid external progress while moving slowly through stages. Others move quickly into stages while making gradual external progress. It might confuse a parent if you begin explaining a child's complex and slow warm-up, when the child was making rapid external progress. Likewise, if you report rapid progress into stages, when the parent is seeing only gradual change outside of the session, this also may be confusing. If you hear from the parent first, you can put what she tells you in context for her when you make your report of her child's progress in CCPT.

## Feedback From You to the Parent

A good way to think of what to say first when providing feedback to the parent is to think of what you imagine the parent's worst fears to be. Those worst fears are usually such things as fearing that you have found that her child is deeply flawed and cannot get better, that you have learned that her child is in great danger, or that her child has "spilled the beans" of some terrible family dysfunction. So, we recommend starting with a statement that allays those fears: "Ms. Smith, I want you to know that Johnny is progressing very well and as expected, given the kinds of problems and oppositional behaviors he has developed. So I see that we are on the right track. I don't see any cause for alarm, and, of course, if I had seen cause for alarm, I would have told you immediately after the session." We find that when therapists begin this way, parents rarely push for details of their child's sessions.

If a parent does voice concerns during this part of the meeting, you should first respond with empathy to the implications of her concern, then explain or answer as honestly and nondefensively as possible. For example, if she asks, "Has he talked to you about what's gone on with his sister?," you may respond, "It sounds like there is something there that concerns you, something you are concerned that I might know or that I don't know. His work in therapeutic play is quite focused on himself, his decisions and choices, which is where his focus needs to be in play therapy. I don't know of any situation with his sister. Is there something that I need to know?"

In this part of the meeting, you can explain that there are typical stages in CCPT (see Chapter 10) and briefly explain what they are. We sometimes rephrase the Aggressive Stage as "Expressive," if we think the parent will be alarmed that her child is being aggressive in sessions. Likewise, we sometimes describe the Regressive Stage without naming it, if we think the parent may be upset by the thought of her child's regressing.

For example, "Johnny is right at the end of his Warm-up Stage and beginning his Expressive Stage, which is about what I would expect at the fourth to fifth session. He has begun to take responsibility for his work in sessions. While he sometimes breaks limits, inadvertently at this point, he is gaining ease in complying with the limits that I have to set. He is learning to tolerate the frustration of limits and to establish self-control so that when a rule is set, he is able to comply, but also able to continue to self-assert and self-express in appropriate and acceptable ways. It is going to take a while for those skills to transfer out to home and school, but he is accomplishing the first step to that. In most cases, those same skills begin to be used at home shortly after they are evident in sessions. So you can look for that progress in gradual ways at home."

You should allow time for parent questions after you talk. Often, parents follow your statements with practical parenting questions, such as how to parent differently to promote the skills at home. This is a natural time for you to begin work on parenting skills, as time allows.

## Working From a Teacher or Principal Referral

Begin with the understanding that you will treat the principal or teacher who is referring a child to you in a school in much the same way as getting started with a parent. Your primary goals are the same. You need to gain an understanding of how the referring person sees the child, the child's context and situation. Because this principal or teacher is responsible and important in this child's life and because she is one of your primary collaborators in helping this child, conveying that you understand the child and his situation in her view and to connect with her experience in the situation remain important primary goals.

You can also often reframe the principal's or teacher's reaction in an accurate reflection by responding to the underlying positive. In most cases, if a principal or teacher is complaining about how bad a child's behavior is, one correct perception of what she is communicating about her experience is that she is very unhappy with his progress and situation at this point and she wants very much to see him change such that he is learning well, behaving in positive and desirable ways, making friends/getting along well socially, and just being enjoyable to be with. We see no purpose in trying to force such a reframe into the conversation if it doesn't really seem true, but we find that it usually is true if we remind ourselves to look for it.

Meetings to receive referrals from principals or teachers are often shorter than similar meetings with parents. For example, you may be meeting with the principal you work with regarding a number of children and school matters, when she says, "Oh, and Demetri Salamone is one of the students I want you to work with. He is really *out of control* (you know she doesn't mean literally out of control). He was in the office for disciplinary reasons three times last week, and it is becoming quite a pattern. I also had an interchange with his mom last week, and I can see where he gets it." So, reflecting by also putting his concerns in context and getting to the business of maintaining alliance, planning for goals and follow-up, you might respond, "So you are worried about him and want me to make working with him a priority. I get the idea you really feel for him after the interchange with his mom. And from how you said it, I get the idea that while his difficulties are a pattern, they are getting worse lately." The principal may then respond by explaining what his pattern has been and how it seems to be changing. She may also explain how she perceived his mom in their interchange: "Yeah, he's always been a handful, but something seems different lately." She briefly explains his pattern of difficulty and recent change.. "And so I got his mom on the phone the other day. While she wasn't able to or wouldn't talk much, she sounded *very stressed* and fed up with him, too—like she's at that point of not even liking him anymore." And you respond, "Okay, I'll check in with Ms. Sanchez (Demetri's primary teacher) for her input and to begin scheduling. It sounds like his primary areas of difficulty are (summarize or categorize from her problem description as you are coming to understand it). I'll also try to connect with his mom."

You may also note that in referral interchanges with most principals, like the one above, the referral interchanges are quite brief. Hopefully, you can also see that empathy is embedded in your understanding conveyed in succinct ways that are made possible through ongoing and well-developed workplace relationships that you have built over time. If you don't have such a relationship yet, you will need to work on it. For the principal to comfortably and effectively refer to you, she needs to know the same five things as parents in turning a child over to your services. She needs to know:

1. That you care for her as a leader and a person with great responsibility for the school and for the student.

2. That you understand the student's and her situation.

3. That you see the underlying positive in who and how she is in describing the problem to you/asking for your help with the problem.

4. That you have a plan for such situations, know what you are doing, and can follow procedures known to work.

5. That follow-up or ongoing communication will be a part of your work.

These should always be at the top of your relational goals with your principal. In the rare, worst-case scenarios where this is not possible, you can still help the children achieve greater school and life success with CCPT and related services, but the work for you and the children will be more difficult.

Table 11.2  **The Five Things Every Teacher Should Know as She Refers Students to You as Counselor**

1. That you care for her and her student.
2. That you understand how she sees her student and her situation with him.
3. That you see the underlying positive of who she is as his teacher.
4. That you have a plan, that you know what you are doing, and can follow procedures known to work.
5. That follow-up or ongoing communication will be a part of your work.

## Getting Started With Teachers

Remember to weave your primary goals into your work with teachers: Listen for her understanding of the child, connect with empathy, convey that you understand the problem and that you are striving to know how this is for her. An example follows.

> **COUNSELOR:** *Thanks for meeting with me, Ms. Sanchez. Principal Howe wants me to work with Demetri Salamone. I want to get your view of him as I plan for how I can help, then schedule his first several meetings with me.*
>
> **Ms. SANCHEZ:** *Oh, he's a handful. He's strange, too, a very unusual child. I think he's always stood out, but this year he's really reached a bad turning point. He's gotten to where the other kids pretty much stay away from him. He's failing most of his subjects. He is constantly arguing. I've got to tell you I've about had it with him. He needs medication and he needs extra help!*
>
> **COUNSELOR:** *[The teacher has an abrasive air in speaking, she really is overwhelmed, and you suspect she is not one of the greatest supporters of your work at the school. You are tempted to say, "I am proposing to provide that extra help!" in a somewhat argumentative way, but you remember your primary goals.] So it sounds like he's been more than a handful for you and he's gotten on your last nerve. You see him as unusually troubled and really want him to improve. [This last phrase was an attempt to address the underlying positive. If it turns out not to be true, you can still make the attempt to address the underlying positive, until proven wrong.] Help me understand his specific behaviors and what seems to be going on with him better so that we can set goals for my work with him that will support his learning and cooperative behavior in the classroom and we can provide each other feedback on his progress.*

From this point, Ms. Sanchez describes Demetri's behavior in specific instances and general qualities. You respond by striving for and conveying understanding. You also continue to respond with empathy to her experience in reaction to him. Following this, the two of you begin to work out goals and observable objectives for his classroom behavior (see Chapter 12). With few exceptions from your work with parents and with principals, the teacher should have an opportunity through your work to come to know:

1. That you care for her and her student.
2. That you understand how she sees her student *and* her situation with him.
3. That you see the underlying positive of who she is as his teacher.
4. That you have a plan, that you know what you are doing and can follow procedures known to work—we find that teachers, in particular, don't need or particularly want to know what you will do with Demetri or why, just to know that you are confident in it as an effective way to help.
5. That follow-up or ongoing communication will be a part of your work.

## Considering a School-Based Array of Services for Child Problems That Employs Effective Use of CCPT

The array of services we would offer in a school setting are centered and grounded in CCPT, as it is effective with a wide, nearly universal array of child problems. (See Chapter 1 for a brief review of the evidence supporting CCPT; Chapter 5 for comments on the range of children that CCPT is appropriate for and also the limitations.) But we still have to decide when a less intrusive intervention will do and what services might be able to help in addition to CCPT. For example, some of our former students, who are excellent play therapists, take a solution-focused or motivational guidance type of approach when the child's problem seems discreet (i.e., singular or autonomous from major underlying factors that may prevent forward progress). For example, if an older child conveys clear goals for a change (not likely in outright statement, but in the counselor's therapeutically listening to his communication and helping him draw out what he wants to be different, seems to really want the change, but still remains hesitant to do different things—perhaps through a somewhat normal and understandable fear of the change), the counselor may be able to help through fairly informal monitoring and encouragement of progress (e.g., upon meeting in the hallway with an opportunity for a semiprivate conversation: "Jason—good to see you! How are you doing with that plan we talked about?" Upon hearing his response, "No, I'm sorry. I still think you can do it. Let's talk about what a doable first step for you might be . . . "). Some of our former students frequently use guidance interventions like this to make simpler, less time-invested interventions when possible.

If you are a school-based counselor, you should be a regular or frequent member of the team that works on behavior management plans and classroom and other school environment modifications to assist with student needs. Especially when the problem is oppositional or conduct-disordered behaviors, it is necessary to provide adult behavior management or modification plans in order to maintain safety and school functioning, and as a bridge to the time that CCPT helps the child build internal motivation to change. At times, these efforts are begun first, and CCPT is an added intervention as your time becomes available or when it becomes obvious that the child is not taking advantage of the behavior change options that school adults are working to provide. Your perspective as a play therapist (i.e., one who studies CCPT and its core change mechanisms and therapeutic qualities; one who studies children and child development, including the role of affect and play) can often be quite helpful to the team's understanding of each child and adult response options.

We also find that skill-teaching options are sometimes helpful in conjunction with CCPT. For example, if a third grader is making good in-session progress in CCPT stages, but not changing his way in the classroom, you might first observe to see if the more positive behaviors are being elicited in the classroom or if the system very strongly, if inadvertently, favors maintaining the old, maladaptive behaviors. If you observe this and find that the teacher is not open to changes the child is trying to make and not receptive to consultation from you regarding classroom changes, you may be able to teach the child a self-monitoring system in which, with your help, he analyzes and gains perspective on what his actions are so that he becomes ideally equipped to make his own self-responsible choices in his actions.

But also remember that CCPT can be a brief intervention for moderate range difficulties. For example, Fall (1999) found CCPT to be effective in six 30-minute sessions for kindergarteners with learning-related self-efficacy difficulties, and we have had success with single-session interventions for children with serious but normal-range separation difficulties at kindergarten. For example, a kindergarten girl was weeping almost all day for her first five days of school. The counselor decided to meet with her for a single CCPT session first thing the next morning, without any suggestion of continuing beyond that meeting in the opening statement (e.g., " . . . This is our special play time *today*. In this time, you can . . . "). In her session, she seemed to work through an initial anxiety paralysis, which the counselor met with warmth and empathy. Then she played with surprising vigor, considering her anxiety and early school behavior, although her play did continue to have a somewhat cautious, warm-up quality, as would be expected. Later that day and for the days following, her teacher reported to the counselor that she had stopped weeping and was interacting as normal with her peers. It could be that she worked through important points of internal confusion in that session, or it could be that she came to see school differently, knowing that she had begun to connect with at least one person, that there was "that guy in the special playroom who really got her and knew she was cool." For whatever reason, she was ready to enter her classroom with only minimal, normal separation difficulties and to engage in the learning tasks at hand.

## Feedback Meetings With Principals and Teachers

Feedback meetings with principals and teachers are usually shorter and less formal than the ones we described with parents earlier in the chapter. Very often, goal-rating sheets with spaces for comments suffice for their feedback to you (see next chapter for examples). Spoken feedback often comes in 5-minute check-in conversations in the empty classroom. Or spoken feedback may come in school-based treatment team meetings.

Regarding your feedback to principal and teacher, often we find that none is expected—that while the principal and teacher care very much about the child's progress at school, they are not that curious about what goes on in session, as long as it seems to be working or as long as they see that you and they are working together as an alliance. When you do need to give feedback to them, it can be in terms of how you see the child or how you see his work in therapy progressing. For example, "I see Johnny as progressing as expected toward more self-responsible and prosocial choices. I hear in some of what you are saying that he seems to in a kind of contemplation stage of this in the classroom. It sounds like he is becoming more aware, but not yet making the choices we want to see." Going a little further to depicting his work in sessions, "One of the things I see him working on, as expected at this stage considering the difficulties he faces, is expressing his angst and anger in appropriate ways and tolerating the frustration of limits when he veers into expressing himself in ways that are inappropriate in sessions. This is an expected first step to his accepting the reasonable limits of the classroom. So, while he's not quite there yet, it is time to watch for and be open to his beginning to make different types of behavioral choices."

## Common Problems in Helping Parents, Teachers, and Principals Support the Child's Work in Play Therapy

### Forgetting to Build a Relationship With Critical, Referring Adults

As you may guess, the number one problem in helping parents, teachers, and principals support the child's work in CCPT is the counselor inadvertently skipping the step of building an empathic relationship and alliance with these key caregivers in the child's world. If this is sometimes done in hurried oversight, slow down—remember the old expression, "Haste makes waste."

Additionally, some counselors and therapists who gravitate to child therapy are more comfortable with children than with adults, and are at times somewhat inhibited with adults. If this is true of you, we encourage you to work through this. You will be greatly limited in your success in helping children if you cannot also connect with the key adults in their lives. Also, it may help to remember and discover through empathy that the adults are just "big grown-up kids"—they need listening, love, and caring just the same as their children or students.

### Trying to Be All Things to All People or Trying to Do Too Much to Please the Adults

There is an important difference between being warm, open to input, and empathic with parents, principals, and teachers and trying to gain their support by pleasing them. For example, if a private practitioner were to offer to lower her fee for a reluctant parent, this may only fan the flames of reluctance. First, that reluctance is being rewarded, which is not the same as being attended to. Second, trying too hard to draw in and keep a reluctant parent can also prompt her defenses. High-pressure sales tactics often motivate people to a purchase in a given moment, but if the choice to purchase has to be sustained, as it does in receiving counseling services, the same sales tactic will not promote a sustained choice. And most people resent high-pressure sales tactics when no longer in the presence of the salesperson.

We find it much more effective to listen well and connect with deep empathy, to convey understanding and competence, and to speak with the confidence of one who knows that what she offers works. Assess the situation and connect while you are assessing. Convey that you understand and see that you can help. Stand ready to listen as the referring caregiver reacts and help her process her reaction.

## Difficulty Taking Parents' and Teachers' Perspectives or Thinking You Understand When You Don't

It can be difficult to take the perspective of a parent or teacher. This can come from a lack of experience, if you have not been a parent or teacher. However, this is not usually the reason. Empathy is quite powerful. Through empathy, you do not have to have had the same experience as another person in order to understand the experience of the other person. This is very important. For example, even if you have parented six children to adulthood with various childhood difficulties, you still may not know what it's like to have had a childhood of painful abuse and insecurity that is now rekindled as a young parent. Or you might not know what it's like to try parenting from a position of poverty. Or you might not know what it is like to have experienced domestic violence or a spouse who developed or turned out to have a severe and persistent mental illness. Or you may have had some of these experiences and incorrectly assume that this parent or teacher's response to these experiences is the same as yours. In summary, it is not likely that you ever really understand what it is like for the caregiver referring to you. But you can learn to come very close to really understanding through developing your skills for deep empathy.

## Too Much the Child Advocate

Another threat to your ability to connect is being too strong a child advocate. If you weren't a child advocate, you would not likely be drawn to CCPT. But feeling or identifying too much with the child's plight can tempt you to see the parent or teacher as the problem vs. part of the solution. In truth, the parent or teacher could be a large part of the problem, but even if so: (1) you just about always have to have their support to avoid what can become crippling sabotage; and (2) with your empathic connection and help, even the most struggling parent or teacher can become part of the solution for her child or student.

## Setting Goals, Evaluating Progress, and Explaining Counseling

It is critical to learn to set goals and objectives and evaluate progress well with parents and teachers. See Chapter 12 for these skill sets.

We also see developing skills at explaining what CCPT is and why it works as an important skill for child-centered play therapists. It is very helpful to be able to explain what you do and why to an interested parent, principal, or teacher. Being able to explain CCPT and its applications for different children is an excellent way to expand and clarify your understandings of CCPT. You probably need to explain how you tend to help and why to your employer, so that she can have a basic understanding of your work. For some parents, an explanation customized to their child can be quite helpful in helping them support their child's work in CCPT.

But while explaining how play therapy works for specific children is important, you also need not get too caught up in this as a primary task. If you develop a strong relationship with each parent and teacher or principal, and you convey the five things that every parent/teacher/principal should know in getting started with CCPT, most don't require extensive explanations of how and why CCPT works. Often, the explanations are mostly helpful to you in an "inside baseball" sort of way.

The most common explanation is that CCPT allows the child to substitute play, which is children's natural mode of deep communication, for our adult mode of communication—talk. The following are examples of customized explanations:

- For a child who is highly oppositional, and often rule breaking, an explanation could be: "In his counseling, Johnny will naturally want to express his angst or anger. He will come to express the worst of himself or what he thinks is the "darkest side" of himself. In doing so, he will encounter the limits of child-centered play therapy sessions. But play therapy will help him experience limits differently. He will be naturally motivated to self-express, which is emphasized in CCPT, yet practical limits will be firm. For this reason some sessions may end early. In this process, he will learn to tolerate limits at home and school, just as in sessions, and learn to find alternative ways to express himself and get his needs met. This will help him develop a new and more cooperative way with you and a more cooperative attitude in life."

- For a child who is highly anxious and restrictive, perhaps experiencing somatic difficulties: "Susie seems to be keeping a lot of emotion bottled up inside. These seem to be emotions that she is afraid to begin to express and that she cannot yet express in words. This therapy can provide an initial place for her to feel safe to begin to let it out. What we are working toward is her ability to express herself to you [parent], to share her emotions or thoughts with you. This therapy will serve as a temporary bridge to her improved relationship with you.

- For a child who is known to have undergone great trauma or abuse: "Some of Tara's behaviors seem due to fear and confusion. She has to integrate into her belief system about life, herself, and her relationships with others that which she cannot easily express or even possibly understand. Play therapy will give her an opportunity to contemplate what she is going through internally, as she has the control to bring to the surface that which she is capable of handling in a nonthreatening manner. She may need to play and replay certain themes or actions. This is much in the way an adult might say aloud internal fears and mixed-up thoughts as a way to sort them out, or as an adult who has been through a recent trauma tends to tell and retell the trauma as she sorts out what she has been through, and what it means to her.

Of course, the explanations you use and how far you go in explaining depend on the unique circumstances and on whom you are talking to. These are a few examples to spur your thinking. The possibilities of how CCPT works to help individual children are as varied as each child is unique. There are many examples available in the works of Virginia Axline and the body of literature from CCPT. We offer a number of recent case studies (see J. L. Cochran, N. H. Cochran, Fuss, & Nordling, in press; J. L. Cochran, N. H. Cochran, Nordling, McAdam, & Miller, in press).

## Activities and Resources for Further Study

- *Activity A:* Review the Primary Skill Objectives to see that they make sense to you now and that you can explain each in your own words.

- *Activity B:* We encourage you to revisit the Application Focus Issues now that you have read and considered the key principles and best practices in helping parents, teachers, and principals support a child's work in CCPT. Work individually or with a group to (1) discern what the errors or omissions were for the therapists or counselors in Application Focus Issues, and (2) what the counselor or therapist may do in order to move forward from the impasses described. You can find our "answers" to this within Skill Support Resources Section F at the end of this book.

- *Activity C:* Work with partners or on your own to develop scenarios that you think of as typical and others that you think of as particularly problematic in working with parents, teachers, and principals when meeting to possibly initiate CCPT services. Employ the primary goals and key principles of this chapter in working through the difficulties in mock sessions. If possible, record your mock sessions in order to discuss or review your errors and celebrate your success. If you can make the time to try three or more mock sessions, you should be able to see patterns in your errors and begin to discern your personality characteristics that seem to be prompting repeated areas of error.

- *Activity D:* Discuss and consider what you think your weaknesses will be in working with parents and teachers. Plan for how you will overcome these weaknesses.

- *Activity E:* Seek peer or professional supervision review and guidance for your work with parents and teachers. We find this work to be among the most subtle of the skill sets you should master as a child-centered play therapist, and ironically sometimes one of the least attended to skill areas. Again, videotaping parent and teacher consultations for review with a supervisor can be very helpful.

- *Activity F:* Create case examples and practice customizing explanations of how that child may benefit from CCPT.

# Goals, Treatment Planning, Reporting, and Evaluating Progress

*I have perhaps been slow in coming to realize that the facts are always friendly. Every bit of evidence one can acquire, in any area, leads one that much closer to what is true. And being closer to the truth can never be a harmful or dangerous or unsatisfying thing.*

—*Carl Rogers*

## Application Focus Activity

By this point you may have decided that the deeply respectful, child-centered approach to therapy resonates strongly with you. You may have seen child-centered play therapy (CCPT) work well in your practice or may have come to experience some of the child and human nature concepts from which it grows at work in children, families, and yourself. You are excited about using CCPT, but then a pang of apprehension hits, as it has for many, and you think, "I can't do child-centered work in a managed care setting (or hurried school environment, outcome-focused agency, or private practice that needs to satisfy parents . . . ). It all sounds great—valuing child expression, each child's unique path to self-worth and self-responsible behavior—but I'll never be able to convince my (employer/parents/teachers) that this will work. I believe in and want to work from this theoretical base, but I'll never be able to do it!"

This chapter is here to assure you, "Yes, you can." In this chapter we will walk you through methods for setting goals and objectives, projecting treatment plans, reporting, and evaluating progress in the powerfully effective child-centered approach. We provide a method that will help you to ensure that the child has made sufficient progress internally (according to and within self) and externally (according to measures and evaluation of others) to start a "countdown of CCPT sessions, and provide a caring and effective ending phase of CCPT sessions for the child. CCPT is rapidly effective in accomplishing *clear, measurable* external behavior change, while remaining maximally empowering for each child and accomplishing *deep and lasting* internal change that is child-led, and that fits and feels right within each unique child's path of self-actualization.

## Primary Skill Objectives

The following Primary Skill Objectives for this chapter are provided to guide you through the chapter and for reflection and review after completing the chapter reading and exercises. By reading and working through the chapter exercises, you will be better able to:

1. Describe a few good reasons to set clear goals with measurable objectives, to establish baselines, and measure progress.

2. Describe the principles of wise goals and generate examples of wise and poor goals, explaining what is wise or poor about each.

3. Explain how individualized goals can be developed in collaboration with parents or teachers and give examples of simple goal-rating systems.

4. Explain the steps to collaboratively setting goals, including the kinds of tasks within and rationales for each.

5. Explain internal-to-the-child and external-to-the-child methods of evaluating progress and why a combination of external and internal measures is best.

6. Describe the six principles of case notes (per-session record keeping) related to CCPT.

7. Describe common problems in establishing goals and objectives and evaluating progress.

8. Describe the criteria to be met in order to end CCPT sessions for a child based on internal-to-the-child and external-to-the-child measures (the child reaching the Mastery Stage), and parent and teacher reports of progress and therapeutic goals met.

# Introduction

We encourage you to set clear goals with measurable objectives and to collect data verifying your objectives. It is a temptation of many therapists and counselors to skip this step. After all, it is the time helping children and families that counselors and therapists enjoy and love. It is the skills of the therapy that you want to master and perfect. But without measured outcomes, your work can lack for the credibility to grow your practice as well as your confidence to do the work that you love. Parents, teachers, and employers are in danger of not seeing progress that is there and could have been clearly measurable. And if you work with very high-risk clients with quite difficult lives, for whom progress will not come easy, you risk burning out and losing steam for your valuable work in helping children and families.

Because CCPT works to reestablish and reinvigorate children's unique paths of self-actualization, you can set goals that would be reasonably expected within that child's normal development, but which seem delayed due to some sort of trauma or inhibiting life situation. And as with the goals of any intervention, you can establish measurable objectives as markers toward accomplishing that goal. As the child uses his process in CCPT to regain full steam to self-actualization (which, when not diverted by trauma and mistaken development (see Chapter 2), will always equal ever "maturing" and prosocial development), he will soar past your goals and objectives on his way to becoming the very best adult he can be.

## CCPT and Levels of Progress Analysis

One can think of goals for counseling services at four levels.

1. **Symptom reduction**—meaning the problem occurs less. This is the lowest common denominator of therapeutic intervention goals. It would be the simplest to measure and may be what most people think of and what therapy managers care most about regarding analysis of progress.

2. **Developing desirable human capacities**—meaning the child develops self-responsibility, self-control, the capacity to love and relate well to others, self-esteem, a desire to learn, and so on. This is what most parents and teachers want for children in therapy, at least once they have moved beyond a feeling of desperation for symptom

reduction, when the referral is made from a desperate situation. At this level, you will usually need to think through what behavioral evidence for the desirable capacity for that child will look like and measure those behaviors, but sometimes you can simply rate the capacity or use a rating system that can do that for you.

3. **Personality change or wellness**—a level of change at which a parent or teacher might happily say, "He's just not the same kid anymore!" When succeeding at this level, symptom reduction will have been accomplished along with numerous human capacities, some having been planned and some pleasant surprises. Consider that most adults come to counseling for symptom reduction. But if deep change was needed and therapy is successful, what they gain is personality change, wellness, and a more integrated or solid personality, with symptom reduction accomplished along the way.

4. **Flourishing**—we often think of this level of change with filial therapy (see Chapter 13 on filial therapy), where, for example, not only have the parent and child come to stop fighting or get along, work well together or live harmoniously, they have become a very well working family where each person naturally works to further the other's development. A metaphor for flourishing can be a special houseplant for which you have tried providing different nutrients, different light conditions, different methods of pruning—and it has lived well enough along the way—until finally you find just the right set of internal and external conditions and it begins to flourish. It takes on its best color ever, grows rapidly, and blooms in ways that it never has before. This is the ideal for therapy, where the outcome is not just "good" or "better," but is optimal and very long lasting.

In CCPT, progress will be discernable at all levels of analysis. Symptom reduction will be accomplished while your client is succeeding through greater human capacities and overall wellness. You don't have to choose one level over the other. Provide excellent child-centered play therapy, measure progress well, and you will see your clients grow at all levels.

## Overview and Initial Guidance in Choosing Measures

In this chapter, we guide you through goal basics and principles, measurable objectives, steps to setting goals, and external- and internal-to-the-child measures of progress. You will find different methods of evaluating progress more important at different times. For example, you may regularly evaluate stages as it is no extra work for you and provides input on the child's process that can be invaluable beyond measuring progress. And you should always employ some methods of evaluating external progress. But you may only use standardized measures when you need more sensitive and unbiased assessments. At other times, you may decide that easier, simpler, individualized rating systems will suffice. The ideal would be to employ each type of measure each time. However, we also realize that you will often select only parts of an ideal evaluation process. The key concept that we want to convey is that you can and should evaluate progress by children in CCPT.

## Goal Basics: "Wise" and "Poor" Goals

The key question to consider with each goal and objective for CCPT, as with any therapeutic intervention, is: Is it a reasonable goal? Is it a reasonable expectation for that child's development? Examples of poor goals and wise goals follow. We recommend selecting goals in consultation with key adults in the child's life, usually parents and teachers. This selection normally requires a conversation in which you ask the parent's or teacher's main areas of concern, turn the concern around to be worded as a positive area of growth, and give input to help the parent or teacher select wise goals.

Our principles of wisely selected goals are that the goal should be (1) within the range of normal development for most children, with consideration of the abilities and context of the particular child (this principle can often mean that the goal would be relevant for similar peers in similar context); (2) stated for positive expectations; (3) specific vs. global; (4) in keeping with accepted thought regarding children's mental health; and (5) achievable from the therapy you provide with minimal additional interventions. Watch for these principles as you consider the five examples below. We discuss measurable objectives for each example in the following section.

## Example 1

### *Poorly Selected Goal: "Stay Seated and Quiet"*
While this may be the wish of many a caring parent or teacher of a child whose behavior has worn her nerves thin, it is an unreasonable wish. In many cases such expectations are impossible for the child to meet and

set the child and parent/teacher up for failure. If you hear it implied in a parent or teacher meeting, we suggest that you warmly reflect the parent's or teacher's feeling toward the child and then assert for more useful goals: "Ms. Beyers, I get that you are quite exasperated with Joseph. You see that he is not learning and you worry that he is falling behind. So you are frustrated with his disruptions. A part of what I want us to do in our time today is to develop three or four goals over which we can measure his progress. Tell me your thoughts on a few specific areas of improvement for Joseph. . . . "

*Wisely Selected Alternative: "Be on Task Comparably to Peers"*
This is a more reasonable version of the preceding poorly selected goal. It takes into account what is probably normal for children in the context for which the behavior will be measured.

## Example 2

*Poorly Selected Goal: "Stop All Arguing and Fighting!"*
You may have learned that this child's parent views him as arguing about almost everything, and that she, as his mother, is frustrated, "at her wit's end." Also, this child is described as constantly fighting with his sister, and the parent is worried for his sister's safety. The base desire behind these wishes probably can be accomplished, but these goals are stated in negative and absolute terms. It is better to state goals in positive and relative terms. Also, there seem to be two separate issues here that should be stated separately.

*Wisely Selected Alternatives*
You may generally describe what this parent wants as, "a more harmonious home life." A reasonable goal from this description may be *"follows most instructions."* We leave the word *most* in because we believe that no one follows all instructions and that in life some instructions should be questioned, unless the instructor is remarkably omniscient. Should there be important problems in the ways that Mom gives instructions, this will often naturally correct as their system of interactions change with his changes through therapy—this is the principle of "it takes two to fight." In a situation where Mom inadvertently keeps a fight going, perhaps giving unreasonable instructions and maintaining impossible expectations for compliance, you can help her adjust her ways once he has made significant internal progress in play therapy. At that time, small changes from her will be immediately rewarded, as he will have become receptive to her.

Regarding part 2 of the poorly selected goal above, a reasonable and positive restatement can be *"responds to his sister in kind and respectful ways most of the time."* Such would seem to be within the range of most sibling relationships, given normal rivalry. As with the alternative to part 1, if the family context does not support this change, you can help the family make adjustments in how conflicts are resolved with parent skill training that will be readily received and easily successful, once your client is well begun in his internal progress.

## Example 3

*Poorly Stated Goal (for a Child with Abnormally Aggressive Behavior): "Be Less Aggressive"*
Two problems here: This goal is stated in the negative, and it is nonspecific. You would need to help the parent or teacher develop a description of specifically what the problem is and what a more positive way of being would look like.

A wisely stated alternative can be: *"Plays/works cooperatively with peers most of the time."*

## Examples 4 and 5

*Poorly Stated Goal: "All A's"*
It might well be within most children's range of possibilities to earn some A's at school. When normal self-actualization is not inhibited, children want to learn and most are motivated by grades. But "all A's" should not be within most children's ability, and if a parent is striving for this, the outcome may be perfectionism or discouragement vs. optimal learning success and mental health.

*Poorly Stated Goal: "Learn to Read at Grade Level"*
The problem with this goal is that it requires at least two other elements, which are beyond the therapy you will provide. Reading at grade level is dependent on a child's intellectual abilities. And recovering skills that are within a child's abilities, but were perhaps delayed by emotional distress, requires time in a nurturing learning environment.

*Wisely Stated Alternative: "Demonstrates Motivation and Effort in Learning"*
Different from poorly selected goals 4 and 5, which are more dependent on environmental context and ability, this goal addresses motivation and effort, which is normal for all children regardless of ability level.

## Measurable Objectives

The following examples of objectives stem from the preceding goals. Our purpose is to demonstrate simple versions of the kinds of objectives that can be measured from CCPT. Such simple parent/teacher observations for individualized goals are very helpful in establishing alliances with key adults in the child's life and in creating an atmosphere of positive, practical expectations. For accurate and complete evaluation of progress, we recommend combining such measures with standardized behavior ratings, open-ended parent/teacher reports, and internal-to-the-child measures. We discuss these tools in later sections.

## Goal Example 1: "Be on Task about the Same Percentage of Time as Peers"

In a conversation with a teacher, you could discern the meaning of "on task" to her (e.g., members of the class are each mostly engaged, focused in the learning task at hand, with acceptable amounts of daydreaming, wiggling, and other lapses in focus). You should write down the meaning of such a key term for guiding ongoing ratings. Also, discern the approximate range of percentages of time that most are on task in the classroom (e.g., 75%–90%—this is never 100%). Then, on a chart of 1%–100% that reminds her of her definition of "on task," she can mark her perception of his on-task behavior at predecided days or weeks and immediately following one or more predecided key periods of learning. An outside observer could make more accurate assessments of on-task behavior, but this is beyond the needed or available resources in most situations. The long-term objective is for your client to be on task within the percentage range of most of his peers. If his baseline for on-task during key learning periods is 25%, you may anticipate monthly increases of 10%–15%.

Because grades and achievement scores should naturally improve with increases in on-task behavior, you could also set goals and objectives around these. For example, if your client has particularly poor grades, assumed to be below his intellectual abilities, you might anticipate increases of one letter grade in five of the seven grade areas within the first full grading period following the start of CCPT.

## Goal Example 2: "Follows Instructions"

Assuming a baseline points to arguing with or ignoring instructions a lot of the time (80%), the long-term objective could be to reverse that to *"follow instructions 80% of the time."* You might ask the parent to observe, reflect, and discern a percentage, plus write a brief comment on this goal in daily preselected moments (i.e., not right after a struggle over bedtime, but in a quiet moment).

## Example 3: "Plays/Works Cooperatively with Peers"

Improved conduct grades can be one area for objective measure. Having one or two good friendships, in which he and friends enjoy playing cooperatively together, can be another, assuming the child is of an age for cooperative play. Observation-rating systems can be set up as with Examples 1 and 2 as well.

## Examples 4 and 5: "Demonstrates Motivation for and Effort in Learning"

Observer rating systems can be established for this one in the same way as Examples 1 and 2. Also, Fall and McLeod's (2001) Self-Efficacy Scale for children is an easy to use, nine-item rating from teachers or parents that has good validity and reliability in estimating teacher or parent perceptions of children's self-efficacy, especially related to learning tasks, when taken in context with other measures.

## Steps to Setting Goals

### Hearing the Presenting Problem

The first step in initiating therapy for a child in need is sensitively listening and connecting to the referring parent or teacher. The first step in setting goals is also listening to the referring parent or teacher. We often find that very good therapeutic listening helps the parent or teacher express the problem understandings you need, but we also follow up with questions as needed. Our goal in listening as a first step to goal setting is to gain as clear an understanding of the problem and context as possible. For an example of the kinds of things we would be listening for or asking, consider the following areas of interest related to a situation of frequent tantrums or behavioral emotional outbursts. While listening for these items, you would also be thinking of possible comparisons to these starting points as the child improves.

- How frequent are the tantrums (e.g., daily, multiple times of day, weekly)?
- How long do the tantrums last? What happens? How do they end?
- How severe are the tantrums? We often ask for a rating on a scale of 1 to 10 and ask for an explanation of the rating, if the parent/teacher doesn't naturally offer comments.
- What happens surrounding the tantrums, just before, right after?
- What do the tantrums seem to be about, related to?

You may note that with the items listed, we are not fishing for a simple solution to the problem. If a simple solution were possible, it would have already been done. We would want to know what the tantrums seem to be about, not to suggest some simple change in parenting or classroom management, but because early signs of change may be related to the contexts and "content" of tantrums, as well as to frequency and duration.

## Your Input Toward Goal Formation

As you may note from our examples of wise and poorly stated goals above, most referring parents and teachers do not happen to state goals well. In most cases, the parent or teacher is struggling emotionally or he would not be making a referral to you. That struggle will likely make it difficult for him to suggest wise goals without your help.

Help the parent or teacher shape goals to achieve the principles of wisely selected goals. Following from those principles:

1. Give your input to help the parent or teacher think through what is within the range of normal development for the child.
2. Help the parent or teacher restate each goal for positive expectations—what the child can be doing that is the opposite of or will preclude the negative behavior.
3. Help the parent or teacher be specific and clear in what he wants and will monitor.
4. Help the parent or teacher understand what wishes or preferences are within reasonable expectations for children's mental health and optimal development and which are not.

5. Listen for and focus your planning, at this time, on goals that are achievable from the therapy you will provide (i.e., not dependent on resources that are not at your disposal, such as special reading teacher time—you should also be your client's advocate, but that is separate from the goals you set for counseling/therapy.

The process often goes something like: First, hear the problem. State that this is a problem that can be addressed in the counseling/therapy you provide, if indeed it is (the range for CCPT is huge). Then ask the parent or teacher to help you set a few goals so that you and he can know the directions you both want to go and so that you both can know when you are making progress. Ask him to describe for you what it would look like when his child's/students' behavior is as he would like it to be: "How will it look when he is doing much better?" Apply the five principles above in conversation with the parent on your way to selecting wise goals. Suggest measurable objectives that occur to you and accept parent/teacher input on this.

## A Standardized Measure

Along with establishing goals in conversation with the referring parent or teacher, we recommend using standardized measures, such as the Child Behavior Checklist (CBCL, Achenbach & Rescorla, 2001) or Conners Rating Scales (Conners, 1997). Such standardized measures can be much more sensitive to behavior change and less sensitive to parent and teacher affect in response to children. These measures can often (1) give additional insight into the nature of the child's problems and can help you better help parents or teachers understand the child's difficulties, (2) formulate more inclusive and sensitive goals, and (3) more clearly recognize progress. Watch for these elements in the following research-based examples.

In two recent case studies from our recent research (J. L. Cochran, N. H. Cochran, Nordling, McAdam, & Miller, 2009), 6-year-old boys were referred for very severe and persistent attention and aggression difficulties for which other interventions for behavior change had been ineffective across more than one school year. Based on referring teacher descriptions of problem areas alone, there would have been no reason to select goals in areas other than attention and aggression and important progress may have gone unrecognized. Consider the role of the standardized measure in the brief summaries below. The boys' names are fictitious.

### Anton: Anxiety Underlying Misbehavior

While his referring teacher had not noticed high anxiety levels, his CBCL scores (confirmed by the therapist's impressions in early sessions) did. The research team later conceptualized his behavioral difficulties as stemming from hypervigilance, worry, and stress. Following treatment, his scores improved overall, but his greatest improvements were within the Internalizing Composite rather than the Externalizing Composite. His decreasing anxiety seemed to lead to his behavioral improvements. Anticipating this in advance for a child like Anton would not change the treatment, but could help his teacher have a better understanding of him and help his therapist and teacher set more inclusive and more sensitive goals and objectives. More sensitive goals and objectives for a child like Anton can help therapists and other caring adults avoid missing this first encouraging and important progress.

### Berto: Depression Underlying Misbehavior

Like Anton, his referring teacher had not suggested depression as a reason for referral, but his CBCL scores (confirmed by his counselor's impressions in early sessions) showed depression as his most severe problem area. Following treatment, his CBCL scores improved overall, including areas most associated with the reasons for his referral, but as with Anton, having the more sensitive understanding early in treatment could help a counselor and teacher better avoid missing important and encouraging early signs of progress.

Additionally, in open-ended reports (e.g., in response to "How is Anton doing in your class?"), his teacher did not describe much progress. But in the much more sensitive and less affected standardized measure scores, her ratings indicated very significant progress. In open comments, many caring teachers only admit progress even when behavior ratings indicate progress that is highly significant. We see this to be because what she wants is to know he is going to be okay, perhaps live "happily ever after." With that as her internal goal for him, anything less than that may not register as progress.

## The Question of Predicting Duration

The length of time needed for each child's work in CCPT is different for each child. A normal or "rule of thumb" time expectation for a child to reach mastery stage is 15–20 sessions. If you need to give a parent an indication of how long therapy will be needed (i.e., for the parent to plan for payment), after emphasizing that the length of time varies for each child and that consistency of sessions and that parental support toward goals will increase efficiency, it is also reasonable to project about six months to completion, with measurable progress realized along the way. Most parents and teachers see progress relatively early in that time, and thus their commitment to allowing the work to continue grows. Some counselors in fee-for-payment practices project the dollar costs for parents in order to allow them to make a fully informed commitment to the service for their child. We find the keys to parental commitment to be your empathic connection, your confident judgment that what you offer is highly effective and will work, and forming an alliance around goals and objectives.

Regarding duration, we should also note that CCPT can be quite brief. When applied to more normally occurring concerns, progress can be much quicker. For example, we have effectively applied CCPT in single-session assistance to kindergarteners experiencing separation difficulties, and Fall (1999) has demonstrated its application to children's nonclinical learning-related self-efficacy difficulties in a brief format (six 30-minute sessions).

## Evaluating Progress

Children's internal and external paths to progress are not always clearly matched. For example, a highly anxious child may do tremendously important work in simply becoming comfortable with you and the playroom and beginning to play freely. This may result in very early, significant external change at a time when she is only beginning to fully engage her internal work. For a child with hard-learned negative beliefs about himself and others, resulting in long-learned habits of misbehavior, you may see important internal progress before his changes result in significant external behavior change. Therefore, we urge you

**Table 12.1** **Two Types of Measures Indicate Progress**

| External-to-the-Child Measures | Internal-to-the-Child Measures |
|---|---|
| • Parent or teacher report in feedback meetings | • Your observation of the child's process and progress through typical stages of CCPT |
| • Weekly ratings and comments on goal-related qualities or behavior areas | • Your observation of individual child qualities or themes in play therapy |
| • Standardized measures | |

to develop your skills in gauging both internal and external measures of change and in discussing those measures of change with the referring parents or teachers in your clients' lives.

## External-to-the-Child Measures of Progress

### The Parent's or Teacher's Report in Feedback Sessions

In your feedback sessions with parents or teachers (usually occurring every fourth to fifth session; introduced in Chapter 11), listen to the parent's/teacher's report of the child's progress. Listen for obvious statements of progress and anecdotes that exemplify progress. Listen for changes in the qualities of how the parent or teacher describes her child/student. For example, has a mom seemed to shift from tearfully telling of a son's difficulties to describing similar difficulties with less affect? Perhaps she uses similar words to describe behavior but is less affected. If you reflect this change in her, it may lead to awareness of progress or to a better understanding of their relational context. Or if you notice words of positive affection creeping into a teacher's description of still troubled behavior, you may reflect and gain aware-ness of early progress or relational shifts. If descriptors shift from "out of control" to "a high-energy handful who is still one of my biggest problems," that is probably not your end goal, but probably is a good sign of early progress.

### Objectives Ratings in Weekly Feedback

If you have collaborated with the parent or teacher in discerning individualized goals and measures for which a parent observation rating and comment is utilized, which we recommend when possible, you may want to collect these ratings and comments weekly. This can serve several purposes:

1. Weekly collection can help you *track* changes. Such ratings can be highly variable, affected by particularly good or bad incidents. They are better indicators of trends through time than in any single day or week.

2. Collecting them with this frequency helps the parent or teacher know you are regularly listening for her input.

3. They help prevent the parent or teacher from trying to give a report or complaint at the beginning of the child's session. In most situations you cannot listen to the caregiver's comments at that

time, as it would require having an adult conversation about adult matters regarding the child in front of the child and because it would interfere with the child's hour. You can discuss the trends and important seeming moments in these more frequent ratings in feedback sessions.

### Standardized Measures

If you are collecting standardized behavior ratings, it may be helpful to collect those ratings the session before the feedback meeting to give yourself time to score the measures and prepare to discuss the implications of the scores with the parent or teacher.

## Internal-to-the-Child Measures of Progress

### Stages

Learning to discern the typical stages of CCPT (see Chapter 10) is a critically important tool in the evaluation of progress. It takes practice. Qualified supervision in this work is very helpful. Once you can assess the stage of a child's work in play therapy accurately, you gain:

- Confirmation that the mode of treatment is working
- A tool for communicating the child's progress in appropriate ways with parents and teachers
- A clear and confident confirmation of a child's readiness to begin a countdown to termination

### Individual Child Qualities in Therapy

In our practice, supervision, and research so far, we have found the stages to be almost always present in children's work in play therapy. But there are always exceptions to any rule. In rare situations, children do not move through the typical stages, or do so in ways that are so unusual or overlapping as to be nearly impossible to categorize. In those cases, your observations of changes in the child's behavior and *ways of being* in the playroom become important measures of progress in themselves. For example, if a child who is very slow to warm up, who had worked to keep his play "hidden" from you and had seemed remarkably restricted in his play, begins to indicate that he wants you to see what he is doing and begins to play more freely, this may be a sign of progress. If a child who had been reluctant to separate in the waiting room each week becomes easily able to separate, that may be a sign of progress. If a child who had seemed fixated on "torturing and punishing" a baby doll for several sessions shifts to soothing and feeding the baby, that can be a sign of progress.

# The Course of Progress and Examples of Progress Charting

Some agencies with which we have worked require progress projections in treatment planning. When this is needed, you can set benchmarks within objectives at regular intervals. On average, your clients will meet the benchmarks. An example is provided in Skill Support Resource Guide at the end of the book.

However, you should not expect an individual's progress to be incremental. Growth of most living things is not incremental, even though it can appear to be when the growth of many in the same category is averaged. Children's physical growth or learning can be seen as coming in spurts vs. increasing in the same amounts each week and month. As you are tapping into naturally occurring, internal-to-the-child developmental processes with CCPT, your individual client's progress will likely be in spurts. A client may take weeks in CCPT readying himself to take on more self-responsible ways of being outside of therapy, experiment with or sort of test out new behaviors in a given week, then suddenly display a whole new skill set the next week, and perhaps regress back into old ways on occasion, while settling into a consistent and positive new way of being.

## Case Notes

We offer the following per-session record-keeping guidelines with respect to CCPT. Specific record-keeping requirements will vary between settings.

## Write "Just Enough"

Describe themes and patterns in play just enough to spur your memory while avoiding recording any more details than necessary. If you are seeing many clients each week, it is helpful to review a child's play from recent sessions before beginning a new session in order to help you more quickly engage in that child's unique themes and play patterns. Additionally, reviewing themes and patterns periodically can help you be aware of how a child's play is evolving and aid your evaluation of his progress. At times, play therapists have concern that a child is stuck in repetitive play. In our moments of such doubt, our notes have been enough to spur our awareness that the client's play is evolving forward. The notes have reassured us of the purposeful nature of his play and encouraged us to keep faith in and let him work his process in his pace.

But while notes of play themes and patterns are helpful, you should avoid noting aspects of play that you may be uncomfortable explaining later. Remember that you can never have complete control over who reads your notes—the family's confidentiality and the child's privacy can be breached.

## Don't Speculate

Avoid speculating on the meaning of specific actions in play. Even clinicians who do play-based child assessments, which is not your role in CCPT, only speculate on repeated themes and patterns in combination with other aspects of evaluation, never on specific single actions in play alone.

## Note Imminent Danger

If you have to handle reasonable suspicion of abuse or other imminent danger following a session (see Chapter 16), note this carefully, addressing what you suspected, based on what (this should almost always be a child's statement, but could also include explicit actions in play), and what you did to ensure the safety of your client or other vulnerable persons.

## Note Well-Being

You can generally note a child's well-being in play therapy, as you would in talk therapy for an adult. For example: "Jamar separated easily from his mom in the waiting room and readily engaged in CCPT. He appeared well kempt, healthy, and vigorous."

If you note a significant concern in the child's well-being, note how you will address it. For example: "Jamar is becoming more comfortable with CCPT, asking fewer questions, and requesting less direction. However, he also has seemed lethargic, perhaps overly tired in the last two sessions. Will discuss this in upcoming parent conference on June 2."

You should note parent conferences/feedback sessions in detail following the same principles of any adult client consultation meeting, including topics you raised as well as parent concerns and any treatment decisions.

## Note Indications of Progress

If a parent or teacher is giving you weekly ratings with comments on individualized goals, file this with case notes. You may also note observed progress. For example, from a child whose relationship with father had been distant: "Jamar was eager to greet his father following the session. There seemed things he could hardly wait to tell him on the way out. James [Jamar's father] responded with calm interest." For a child who has struggled with ending sessions, note how many minutes it took for her to end the session when you first realized the problem: "Rachel expressed disgruntlement over ending sessions. She repeatedly refused to leave, first asking to 'just let her finish her artwork,' then asserting with mild anger that the end time was not fair. It took her about nine minutes to accept that her session was over for today." As she expresses what she needs and you respond with empathy and consistent structure, you can note the lessening minutes that this process takes her over the next few sessions.

## The Case Note Advantage of the Comprehensive CCPT Model

Because CCPT is a comprehensive individual therapy model, you do not need to take much time in your notes describing your actions. Therapists who take eclectic approaches in individual counseling need to

## Table 12.2   Case Note Reminders

- Write "just enough"
- Don't speculate
- Note imminent danger
- Note well-being
- Note indications of progress

*Consider the advantages of the CCPT model for note taking.

spend much more time explaining what they do and why in individual sessions as their actions may vary greatly from week to week and would thus need to be carefully explained and justified with each shift.

## Common Problems

### Not Setting Goals and Establishing Measures

Striving for the accountability to support your work well can be an extra step that is very tempting to skip. A recent intern arranged to provide CCPT in a highly troubled school. Near the end of her internship, she was frustrated with reluctance of teachers to help her schedule her sessions and of parents to meet with her. While she had permissions to provide counseling, of course, she had ignored advice to establish collaborative goals and at least simple outcome measures. She had done good work with her clients, but individual child progress may not stand out in a context with many, many seriously troubled children. While her offer of help was warmly received early in her work, support for it waned as the school year wore on and she prepared to end her work. We believe that collaboratively formed goals and systematic feedback from key adults regarding child progress on goals would have helped the adults see progress more clearly and support her work more consistently.

### Not Establishing a Baseline

Please pardon our possibly obvious advice, but don't forget to establish some sort of at least minimal baselines to measure progress against. This may be as minimal as helping a parent articulate clear and specific problem descriptions, or it can include much more. But if you forge ahead with treatment and skip this step, it is very difficult to go back and establish this point of reference later. And, over time, the credibility of your work can suffer without clear points of reference from which to measure progress.

### Collecting Only Minimal Feedback/Lacking Multiple Measures

Whenever possible, we encourage you to use the most complete measures of progress possible. As with Berto, mentioned earlier in this chapter, his counselor was collecting minimal feedback of periodic teacher meetings for anecdotal reports. When describing his progress to the researcher, the counselor explained that she saw great progress, but that the teacher would not say he had gotten better. Much to the pleasure of the researcher and counselor, the researcher was able to respond, "Actually, she did." Her ratings in standardized measures indicated highly significant progress.

It can also be important to overlap progress. As a minimum, this should almost always be done by comparing a child's internal progress, discerned through the counselor's observations of the child's stage in CCPT as well as individual child qualities in therapy indicating possible progress, with external measures, at least parent or teacher anecdotal reports.

But the more progress data you can overlap, the better. In some cases, we have found that parent ratings are much more sensitive than teacher ratings for a child—assumedly because the teacher has many more children to observe. In other cases, we have found teacher ratings to be much more sensitive; assumedly in those cases the teacher's ratings were less affected by personal reactions, as it is a part of her profession to be a keen observer of children.

## Concluding Thoughts

We know that multiple measures are not always practical, and we encourage you to seek as many measures of progress as you can make practical in your work. Never shy away or simply avoid measuring the effectiveness of your work. Your work in CCPT can be powerful and efficient. We want you to have full credit for that. The more credit for good work you earn, the more good work you will have the opportunity to do. And that equals more help to children and families in need.

## For Further Learning

### Mock Parent Sessions

- *Activity A:* Review the Primary Skill Objectives to see that you have accomplished each. If not, review chapter sections to mastery of each.

- *Activity B:* Practice, practice, practice. Many great therapists serving children are actually quite shy around parents and teachers and avoid collecting data. One way to master this is to work with a group of peers, in supervision, or in your individual reflection to:

1. Speculate problems that you expect to encounter in establishing goals and objectives and evaluating progress (remember, this work is not easy and not the favorite part for many counselors and therapists). Plan for how you will overcome your weak areas and strengthen and grow in your work.
2. Plan for the measures that you may use in the settings/populations where you will serve. Identify a few standardized measures that you think will be particularly applicable in your work. Describe the role that these measures will have in the goals you establish and the progress you measure. Apply your thoughts to real or hypothetical case examples.
3. Anticipate sets of problem descriptions for case examples and describe likely progress and measures of progress. Generate examples of goals and objectives. Describe which measure and methods of evaluation you choose, which you may omit, and why.
4. Do mock parent and/or teacher session segments in which you work to discern individualized goals and observation/rating plans for those goals.
5. Troubleshoot possible problems with the observation plans and goals.
6. Generate examples of case notes that meet the principles as related to CCPT.

- *Activity C:* Practice taking the perspective of parents and teachers can be critically important in your development. There are three parent or teacher scenarios provided below. Work individually or in groups to discern what you think the parent or teacher is feeling in each and why. Describe aspects of your life, times you may have had similar feelings, that help you identify with the feelings of the parent or teacher in each scenario.
  1. Eight-year-old Lizbeth begins the morning with her mother first coaxing, then pleading, and then physically pulling her out of bed. She slumps over her breakfast, refusing to eat, and then fusses for 20 minutes over what to wear. Her jeans are "too tight" and her sweater is "too itchy." After a shouting match with her little brother, she is finally rushed out the door to catch the bus. By the time she reaches school, she cannot seem to begin even the simplest of tasks without her teacher's one-on-one

assistance. After some free time to work a puzzle, when Lizbeth is asked by her teacher to return to her desk, she refuses and appears to completely "fall apart." She scatters the puzzle pieces and begins to cry.

2. Four-year-old Deanero clings to his mother's skirt at the doorway to his preschool classroom. When the teacher approaches to welcome him, he quickly buries his head and will not look up. The teacher invites Deanero's mother to come in and stay for a while, but after 15 minutes, little Deanero still sits in his mother's lap—holding on tight. Deanero's mother doesn't want to leave, but she must go to work, so she allows the preschool teacher to physically pick up and hold on to her son—who is screaming and crying now—and has to be physically held by the teacher and an assistant. This is how this mother's workday has begun for the past week. She begins to cry as she walks down the long hallway.

3. Ten-year-old Kurtis has always been "happy-go-lucky"—a "straight-A student" and never a behavior problem in school. In the past few weeks his parents have noticed, with increasing concern, notes sent home from his fifth-grade classroom teacher for "inattentiveness and clowning around." At home, he constantly sulks, and if questioned about his mood, he becomes angry and withdraws to his room to work on his computer. Today, his parents have received a phone call from the school principal. Kurtis has been kept after school for "cursing, showing disrespect, and talking back." Both parents are shocked and confused. They anxiously wait in the office for a meeting with the teacher, school counselor, and principal.

- *Activity D:* The skill of discerning stages becomes simple and somewhat obvious, once you have mastered it. However, the stages can be subtle. So, mastering this skill is not as easy as it may sound. Practice this skill as much as possible. Discuss your clients' work in play therapy with colleagues in terms of stages (in settings that fall within your confidentiality commitments, which usually include supervision and consults within agency—with child privacy protected and respected, of course). If possible, work with a group of colleagues who can knowledgeably discuss your classification of a child's stage in play therapy.

# Filial Therapy: Involving Parents and Caregivers in Child-Centered Play Sessions With Their Children

## 13
### Chapter

*To each child, let us convey the uniqueness of our relationship, not its fairness or sameness. When we spend a few moments or a few hours with one of our children, let us be with him fully. For that period, let the boy feel that he is our only son, and let the girl feel that she is our only daughter. For the moment to be memorable our attention must be undivided.*
*—Haim G. Ginott*

*I wish we could stay in special play time all week!*
*—Quote from a child in filial therapy*

*I didn't know Dad could play—he's really good at it!*
*—Quote from child in filial therapy*

*Our whole family feels better!*
*—Quote from a parent in filial therapy*

## Application Focus Scenario 1

James (age 7) and Alecia (age 5) have made very good progress in child-centered play therapy (CCPT). The background of their situation is that Alecia was found to have suffered sexual abuse by her father during shared custody. Both children had symptoms of severe depression and anxiety from the trauma of their situation. Now that the divorce is final and their mom, Jenny, has stabilized their new home and gotten her life more organized, including progress in her individual counseling and with substance abuse issues now under control, she has expressed her concerns to James and Alecia's counselor that she just doesn't know how to relate to them anymore. She feels terribly guilty and is wracked with self-blame.

James and Alecia are, of course, still bothered by the situation. They seem to know that they love their father, even though they know he has done wrong and can never be alone with them (at this time they have very limited visits supervised by a social worker). Jenny explains that when they are upset, she just tries to distract them. Upon reflection, she realizes that they have to be able to feel and be upset, but she feels like she "just can't stand it." She knows that they are doing quite well now, but she also sees that they seem increasingly distant from her.

Their counselor, Susan, has discerned that Jenny is ready and able to commit to filial work, and the agency's treatment team has discussed and supported the possibility of filial therapy—a process where Jenny will learn to have filial sessions or "special playtime" (SPT) with her children. Susan explains the benefits of filial therapy. She explains that the work will help Jenny reestablish connections with her children; that it will help her establish a new, balanced, and consistent level of closeness with her children. It will help them express what they need with her as they continue to adjust, and it will help her listen, accept, and structure their communications and connection accordingly. She explained that it can facilitate their ongoing growth and healing through an ongoing therapeutic relationship with her as their mother and now sole caretaker. It will allow her to better meet their ongoing emotional needs.

She explained the commitment needed for this work, commitment to the training and to consistent SPT. She also explained the support and supervision that she would provide. Jenny was excited to hear about this opportunity, eager to get started, and so this new phase of their work was begun.

## Application Focus Scenario 2

Helen is a therapist working in a residential treatment center that serves children who have been removed from their homes and placed in residential care for three to six months. The children are transitioned back to their homes as soon as their behavior has stabilized and they have begun to meet their treatment goals (those who do not have homes to return to are transitioned to foster or other longer term placements). Filial therapy is a normal part of the transition back to parents' homes and sometimes to foster homes. Parents are taught the skills of SPT in groups. They begin to practice SPT under observation in visits to the center. They progress to videotaping the practice in home visits. By the time their child is released, parents are ready to continue SPT on their own at home. The center follows up in weekly, then monthly, then quarterly meetings with parents after the child is released. In these meetings, the issues of the transition, home adjustment, and ongoing SPT are discussed.

## Application Focus Scenario 3

Tom is a social worker who manages many foster placements. For placements with no signs of ongoing or significant trauma, he provides filial therapy training, support, and supervision to groups of foster parents. The agency has found that this addition to their support services has made a profound difference in the success of their placements.

## Chapter Overview and Summary

Filial therapy (FT) is an approach for training parents (as well as grandparents, foster parents, and other long-term committed caregivers) to conduct filial sessions or "special playtime" (SPT) with their own children. The method has been used to train parents in a variety of therapeutic formats, including moderate-length groups, short-term groups, and individual parent or single couple sessions.

Although a number of teaching/training approaches have been used, in general, the FT process includes the following components: initial skill training with the parent(s) or caregiver(s), advanced skill refinement and training through supervision of parent–child play sessions, assisting the parents to successfully transition to conducting filial sessions at home, and termination. In FT, the role of the therapist differs significantly from traditional child interventions in that the therapist is initially an educator–teacher–trainer for the parent, and later, when SPT has begun, a supervisor. Other therapist skills such as exploring the parent's life history or current life experiences (and examining group process in the case of group FT) are only emphasized when such things are interfering with the parent's ability to acquire and utilize the play therapy skills that they are being taught. Effective filial therapists are able to implement clear, systematic, but flexible teaching strategies and methods; adapt such methods to the needs of a given parent, couple, or group of parents; consistently use empathy, positive constructive feedback, and modeling; and know how to keep the learning process a positive experience for parents.

FT can sometimes be a free-standing intervention (i.e., with no other therapy required first or in conjunction), but is often provided as an addition to CCPT, capitalizing on gains the child has made in CCPT, especially in the readiness for closer and more balanced relationships with parents or significant others that children often gain in CCPT. At times there are other pre-requirements, such as individual counseling or case management to help a parent become stable enough to engage filial sessions and the required training over a significant period of time.

## Primary Skill Objectives

The following Primary Skill Objectives are provided to guide you through the chapter, and for reflection and review after the completion of the chapter. By studying this chapter, you will:

1. Develop a knowledge of the historical roots of FT.
2. Identify the goals and outcomes of FT.
3. Be introduced to the outcome literature on the effectiveness of FT.
4. Identify criteria for determining when FT may be appropriate.
5. Be able to identify the major stages of the FT training process and the tasks associated with each stage.

## The Historical Roots of Filial Therapy

FT is a family-based therapeutic approach in which parents or significant caregivers are taught how to conduct filial play sessions on a one-to-one basis with their own children. The filial methodology was developed by Bernard Guerney, Jr., in the early 1960s (Guerney, 1964). Significant further development and refinements to, and the tireless promotion of, the method were contributed by Louise Guerney (1976, 1980a, 1983a, 1997, 2000, 2008; Guerney & Ryan, in progress) from the days of its early development to date. The development of FT was influenced by a number of dramatic changes in the mental health field at that time. First, the field was moving away from the exclusive

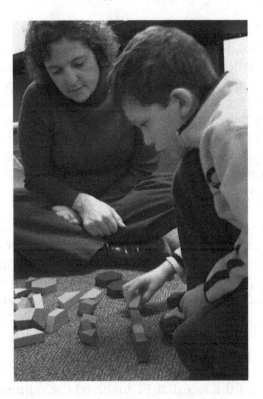

Figure 13.1

use of individual therapy to address human problems, and it was the dawn of the development of marriage and family therapy models. Second, new "skills training" approaches to counseling and psychotherapy were being developed (e.g., Ellis's Rational Emotive Behavioral Therapy). Third, the community psychology movement was trumpeting the need to more effectively "give psychology away" through the use of psychoeducational programs and through the training of paraprofessionals to conduct such programs. The community psychology movement also advocated the use of group-level interventions, since they posited that there would never be enough mental health professionals available to meet existing needs if all therapy were conducted in individual format. These developments in the field deeply affected the thinking of the Guerneys.

Additionally, the Guerneys strongly disagreed with the traditional thinking in the field that parents should be viewed primarily as the source of children's psychopathology, and thus the therapist should engage the child in individual therapy and generally exclude parents from the treatment process. The Guerneys viewed this type of thinking as extreme and shortsighted in that even in cases where this might be true, nonetheless, the parent–child relationship is virtually always the most central relationship in the child's life, so that there was great potential for training the parents to become therapeutic agents of change and healing for the child's current problems, and to prevent future problems developing within the family. The Guerneys were also deeply influenced by the work of Virginia Axline to extend client-centered therapy to work with children—child-centered play therapy. They were optimistic that parents could learn the skill sets necessary for conducting and approximation of the core principles of CCPT with their own children.

At the time of its development, FT was remarkably innovative in its own right in that it did not simply emerge years after these new ways of thinking had entered the mental health field and been instantiated in a variety of therapeutic models. Instead, FT became an early exemplar not only of each of these advances, but also of these advances collectively. Thus, FT became a psychoeducational, skills training–based, child-centered-focused, group-delivered, family therapy that engaged parents and the parent–child relationship as therapeutic agents for the children and the family system. Even more innovative, and highly controversial, was the fact that FT involved the training of parents to function in a role that was previously thought of as only for therapists or counselors—the conduct of therapeutic play sessions with children. In FT, parents were not only no longer viewed as the source of children's problems and extraneous to therapeutic healing, they were viewed as intrinsic to therapy and capable of becoming the primary therapeutic agent. The role of the therapist was radically transformed from that of the wise expert who engaged in therapy with children to save them from the effects of dysfunctional parents, to the skillful educator/trainer/supervisor who transfers knowledge and skills to parents so they can effectively promote healing and growth in their children and function more effectively in the future as parents. Again, in its early days, FT was not only remarkably innovative and controversial, it was viewed as heretical by some within the mental health field. In personal conversations with the authors, Bernard Guerney recounted times in the early days when presenting at professional conferences he was "booed" by professionals in the audience. Today, almost 50 years after its development, and with numerous outcome studies supporting its effectiveness, FT is still innovative in that it remains one of the few family therapies for children, which trains parents to provide therapeutic interventions for their own children.

Table 13.1  **Therapeutic Goals for Filial Therapy**

1. Symptom reduction in child
2. Personality growth in child
3. Improved parent–child relationship
4. Improved parenting skills
5. Personality growth for parent
6. Improvement in functioning of family system (especially when all children of play therapy age are included)

## Goals and Outcomes of Filial Therapy

FT shares two of its seven major goals and outcomes with CCPT, namely, (1) symptom reduction and (2) growth and maturation in basic human capacities of the person that are integrated into the personality structure of the child. Areas of growth include the development of emotional intelligence, capacity for self-expression, increased frustration tolerance and impulse control, self-mastery, self-responsibility, positive realistic views of others and self, and the ability to develop and maintain relationships with others. In addition to these two goals shared with CCPT, FT also has three additional goals and outcomes of (3) directly improving the relationship between parent and child; (4) teaching parents skills that can be generalized beyond the context of filial play sessions and integrated within their everyday parenting; and (5) fostering positive personality changes of the parents themselves, especially those that have significant deficiencies.

This fifth goal of positive personality changes in the parents is not a goal that is generally targeted or shared with parents, but it is a real outcome and valuable growth experience that naturally occurs as parents learn the skills and attitudes entailed in conducting filial sessions with their children. Although many parents have solid parenting skills, capacities, and philosophies, the FT training process is especially helpful in fostering new capacities for parents who find it difficult to set firm limits, tend to be overcontrolling and set too many limits, or find it difficult to be receptive to the emotional lives of their children.

The sixth and seventh goals of FT are also shared with CCPT: (6) the ability to provide a supportive environment for sustaining therapeutic change, and (7) the ability to foster flourishing beyond just symptom reduction. Unfortunately, it is not always possible for a therapist to continue to work with a child once the child has experienced a reduction of symptoms and the personality structure of the child is within "normal" limits. In the case of FT, however, once a parent is trained to an acceptable level of competence in conducting filial sessions with his children and has demonstrated success doing so in home sessions, the parent can continue to provide filial sessions for his children for purposes of both support and continued growth. One additional benefit of FT is that once parents have mastered the filial session skills, they can use it with each of their children not only if problems develop, but proactively for promoting their growth and strengthening relationships with them.

## Filial Therapy Formats

Given the context of its origins, FT was originally conceived of as a group-level intervention. Although fathers and mothers were both included in the training, initially they were trained in separate filial parent groups to eliminate the possibility that couple dynamics would interfere with the training process. After the initial outcome study of the effectiveness of FT supported that parents could successfully be trained to implement filial sessions with their own children and that the children benefited therapeutically (Guerney & Stover, 1971; Stover & Guerney, 1967), subsequent groups incorporated the training of both parents together in the same group. The early FT groups were of moderate length and involved approximately 24 sessions over a period of six months. Over the past 5 decades, additional contributions to the development and promotion of the method have been made by the many colleagues trained by the Guerneys, including Rise VanFleet (2005), Barry Ginsberg (1997), Michael Andronico (1983), William Nordling (Ryan & Nordling, 2003), and Virginia Ryan (2007; Guerney & Ryan, in progress), who have trained professionals to use the filial methodology with individual families and groups.

In 1991, Garry Landreth, PhD, developed a 10-session short-term filial group model called Child–Parent Relationship Therapy (CPRT), which he has continued to refine and research with his colleagues (Landreth, 1991; Landreth & Bratton, 2006; Bratton, Landreth, Kellam, & Blackard, 2006); a summary of the history of the development of the CPRT model and the significant research on the model can be found in Landreth and Bratton (2006). More recently, Wendy Caplin and Karen Pernet have also developed a short-term filial group format adapted from the Guerney model called the Caplin–Pernet Filial Group Program (Caplin, Pernet, & VanFleet, in progress).

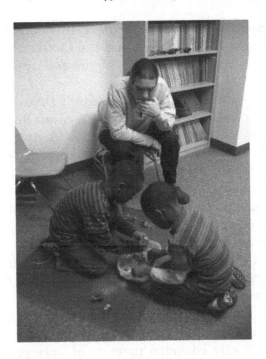

Figure 13.2

## Outcome Research on Filial Therapy

Empirical support for the effectiveness of FT comes from four areas of the psychotherapy outcome research literature: (1) support for the effectiveness of CCPT, which is the foundation for FT; (2) general outcome studies on the various formats of FT; (3) outcome studies on its effectiveness with a diverse group of parents; and (4) outcome studies demonstrating the effectiveness of FT across cultures. A meta-analytic study of play therapy by Bratton, Ray, Rhine, and Jones (2005) found play therapy to be effective with an effect size of 0.80. Humanistic/CCPT play therapies were found to have higher effect size than other models, with the exception of FT, which had the highest effect size of 1.08. The reader is referred to Bratton and Ray (2000) and Ray, Bratton, Rhine, and Jones (2001) for literature reviews and examination of studies that were included in the meta-analytic study and to Bratton and Ray (2002) for a more focused review of the outcome literature on the CCPT model. Like the therapy outcome literature in general, research studies on play therapy, and more specifically on CCPT, vary in terms of the quality of experimental design. A number of recent outcome studies of CCPT have utilized a randomized experimental design and are therefore especially note-worthy include: Ray, Schottelkorb, and Tsai (2007); Danger and Land-reth (2005); Garza and Bratton (2005); Jones and Landreth (2002); and Shen (2002).

There is a significant body of research that demonstrates the effectiveness of the Guerneys' original FT group format (Dematatis, 1981; Guerney & Stover, 1971; Oxman, 1972; Sensue, 1981; Stover & Guerney, 1967; Sywulak, 1977). There is very sizable and growing literature that supports the effectiveness of Landreth's 10-session short-term FT group model (Bratton & Landreth, 1995; Chau & Landreth, 1997; Costas & Landreth, 1999; Glass, 1986; Glazer-Waldman, Zimmer-man, Landreth, & Norton, 1992; Glover & Landreth, 2000; Harris, 1995; Kale & Landreth 1999; Landreth & Lobaugh, 1998; Tew, Landreth, Joiner, & Solt, 1997; Yeun, Landreth, & Baggerly, 2002).

Because FT involves the training of parents or caregivers to conduct filial sessions with their own children, one measure of the usefulness of such an approach is the potential to train a wide variety of types of parents. For example, if the method could be successfully taught only to highly educated parents, or only parents with high socioeconomic status were able to successfully implement FT in the home environment, then FT would be effective for only a small percentage of the families that come for treatment. Fortunately, evi-dence exists that FT can be utilized with a variety of families. The initial filial groups conducted by the Guerneys on which the first outcome  studies were based included a sizable proportion of parents from lower socioeconomic groups from rural settings. Other outcome studies have demonstrated the effectiveness of FT with challenging family situations, including single parents (Bratton & Landreth, 1995), divorced parents (Bratton, 1998), custodial grandparents (Bratton, Ray, & Moffit, 1998), teen mothers in foster care (Celaya, 2002), non-offending parents of sexually abused children (Costas & Landreth, 1999), incarcerated mothers (Harris & Landreth, 1997), incarcerated fathers (Landreth & Lobaugh, 1998), parents court-referred for child maltreatment (Walker, 2008), and parents of chronically ill children (Tew, Landreth, Joiner, & Solt, 2002; VanFleet, 1992).

Another measure of the usefulness of a methodology is whether it is adaptable and effective for a wide variety of cultural groups. Filial therapy has proven useful with a variety of cultural groups, including African-American parents (Sheely, 2008; Solis, Meyers, & Varjas, 2004), Chinese parents (Chau & Landreth, 1997; Guo, 2005; Yuen, Landreth, & Baggerly, 2002), German mothers (Grskovic & Gotetze, 2008),

Hispanic/Latino parents (Ceballos, 2008), Israeli parents (Kidron, 2004), Jamaican mothers (Edwards, Ladner, & White, 2007), Korean parents (Jang, 2000; Lee & Landreth, 2003), and Native American parents (Glover & Landreth, 2000).

In summary, the play therapy outcome literature provides substantial support for the effectiveness of FT in a variety of formats and with a wide variety of children's problems. In addition, FT has emerged as a practical and useful approach with a variety of challenging parents and diverse cultural groups.

## For What Parents and What Children Is FT Appropriate?

Filial therapists normally encourage parents to include not only the child that is experiencing a problem (e.g., the "identified" client), but all children in the family between the ages of 3 and 12. For these "nonproblem" children, the play sessions will serve as opportunities for individual growth and relationship building with parents. Including all children in FT allows for the parents to get additional practice in the method, minimizes the possible stigma that the "bad" child has to go for treatment, and that the "good" children are being punished by being excluded from what quickly becomes evident is a very enjoyable one-on-one time with a parent. Filial therapists may choose to exclude the "nonproblem" children from the FT process if it would be overwhelming for a given parent(s) to have to schedule numerous play sessions per week once sessions begin at home.

Although many parents can be appropriate for FT, some are not. The major reason that some parents are not appropriate would be if they cannot reliably attend training sessions or be expected to *consistently* provide filial sessions for their children. Although FT is flexible, and many logistical issues related to training parents can be overcome, nonetheless, if parent(s) cannot attend training sessions regularly, then the process will result in frustration for all. Additionally, if a parent were to begin filial sessions with a son or daughter who has abandonment or attachment issues, then ends sessions abruptly, that child could perceive the abrupt ending as an additional and quite personal parental abandonment. Filial therapists must monitor very carefully for such risks and should not engage parents who cannot complete significant training and commit to consistent filial sessions.

Another reason to exclude a parent from FT is if a parent is jaded, full of rage, and unwilling (or unable) to expend emotional energy and time on behalf of their child. Although it is not uncommon for many parents to be frustrated and angry with their child, most still possess enough concern about the child's future, basic love, and a willingness to help their child. When these are not present to some extent, perhaps due to pathology or a personality disorder, it will be difficult for the parent to commit to the filial training and to learn skills such as empathic responding and limit setting, as well as to find the time to implement play sessions at home. In such cases, it is generally wise for the child to be seen individually and then possibly as things get better for the child, over time the parent will become more workable and be able to learn how to conduct filial sessions once work with the therapist is complete.

A third criterion for excluding a parent from FT is if they are severely depressed and do not have the energy, attention, focus, or motivation for learning the filial skills. However, this criterion is rarely the reason parents are excluded, since, although many parents needing help may be anxious and depressed, they are not depressed or anxious to the extent that their ability to learn the skills and follow through is compromised. Also, renewing connections with one's child can give many a parent a new reason for self-improvement—so for many moderately depressed or anxious parents, making and being helped to keep the commitment is a part of their recovery.

Finally, on very rare occasions, the filial therapist may believe that the fit between the child's problem and probable behaviors in the play sessions may be too much for a given parent. For example, the filial therapist may believe that a very anxious and passive parent may be emotionally overwhelmed by the behaviors of her sexually abused son who is acting out sexually at home and may very well do so in the playroom. In such cases, the filial therapist may opt to provide CCPT and, once that treatment is successful, then involve the parent in filial sessions.

## The Filial Therapy Process

Regardless of whether FT is conducted in an individual format with a single family or in a group format, there are common phases in the process. These include training in skills approximating CCPT, building and refining skills through supervision of parents as they engage in play sessions with their children, preparing and supporting parents in initiating play sessions at home, and the process of termination of formal meetings with parents while preparing them to maintain on-going sessions at home. In order to be successful in these tasks, filial therapists must possess certain qualities. We will outline these qualities and overview the phases of the FT process.

## Filial Therapist Qualities

A filial therapist is first and foremost an educator, skills trainer, and supervisor. Certainly, a filial therapist needs to be experienced and highly proficient in CCPT. It would be difficult to teach a parent to use skills that approximate CCPT with his own children if you were not proficient with the skills and had not done enough of that work to encounter many of the pitfalls and difficulties that a parent hoping to approximate the work may encounter.

As an educator, a filial therapist must go into each session with a clear lesson plan that indicates the content (e.g., material to be covered and skills to be taught) and learning objectives. This lesson plan may not necessarily be written down, but she is responsible for giving structure and direction to the learning process. Without at least a "mental" lesson plan in place, there is a risk that parents will instead use the time for other admirable, but nonetheless off-task activities, such as talking about the child's behavior in school today, asking for parenting advice, or turning the meeting into their own individual/group therapy session. The plan need not be overly detailed. For example, the plan for an early session might include: give summary of what meeting will cover today, review parents' home assignment, introduce rationale for empathic responding skill, demonstrate skill, parent practice, feedback to parents, parent questions, and parent home assignment.

With this said, a filial therapist must be flexible enough to know when to slow down and when to adjust teaching methods to meet the learning styles and needs of parents (Ryan & Nordling, 2003). Although a filial therapist must be careful to avoid turning the session into individual or group therapy, she should nonetheless be willing and able to use her therapy skills to help parents work through feelings and beliefs that interfere with their learning of the filial skills. For example, if a parent finds it difficult to set limits because he feels guilty about allowing his child to be physically abused, the filial therapist may need to spend some time responding empathically before explaining how setting limits in the filial/child-centered model will help his child develop self-control and ultimately be much happier. This balance of the "didactic" and "dynamic" elements of FT is explored in a classic article by Adronico, Fidler, Guerney, and Guerney (1969).

A filial therapist must also be patient, positive, and encouraging with parents. An essential goal is that parents must never feel like they are failing. A filial therapist must be prepared to break larger skills down into steps or smaller skills so that parents can succeed. In giving feedback, she should start with positive praise for things the parent has done right before giving constructive feedback. In addition, she should limit feedback to one or two things to work on, reserving further learning for later sessions rather than overwhelming parents. Finally, she should be proactive in preparing the parent to be successful for any task that they are asked to do within session or at home.

## Training Parents in the Skills for Special Play Time

As indicated earlier, the first major task of a filial therapist is to teach the skills of structuring, tracking, empathic responding, limit setting, responding to questions, and role-play to parents and caregivers. In general, she should teach these skills systematically one at a time via a process of giving a rationale for the skill and linking it to how it fits with the overarching child-centered philosophy, demonstrating the skill, and then giving parents the opportunity to practice the skills and receive feedback.

There are many methods for teaching skills and allowing parents to practice. For example, in practicing empathic responding, one filial therapist may act out a scene (e.g., of a little boy who is frustrated that his drawing is not turning out like expected) and have a parent or group members respond empathically to what the child is experiencing. Another filial therapist may choose to engage in free play with toys, as if he were a child, and have parent(s) spontaneously make empathic responses. Other learning tools utilized to demonstrate skills may include the use of actual play therapy sessions between a therapist and child (this assumes appropriate permission for use has been obtained), or short demonstrations with the parents' own child(ren). Although some of the filial skills can be taught in isolation, often a filial therapist will help parents to begin to use all the skills together. Before parents are asked to do even short play sessions with their own children, they will have an opportunity to do "mock" play sessions in the playroom with the therapist, who will be in the role of a child whose actions require the parent to demonstrate all of the play therapy skills they have learned. Once a filial therapist is confident that the

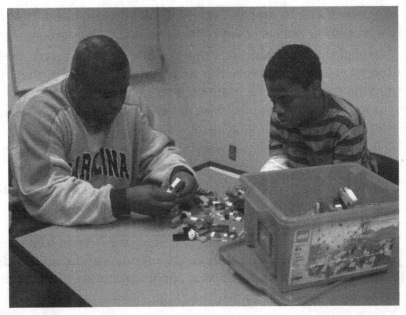

Figure 13.3

parent has reached a reasonable level of proficiency, the next stage is having parents begin play sessions with their own children.

## Parent Play Sessions With Their Own Children

Once a filial therapist is confident that parents have reached a proficiency in the skill set, parents are asked to conduct short "demonstration play sessions" of 10–15 minutes with their own children in order to refine the parents' skills prior to the parents' beginning full length sessions. Filial sessions are dyadic intervention, meaning one parent or caregiver plays with one of the family's children. If there are multiple children of appropriate age in the family, and both parents are participating in the training, then parents may alternate demonstration sessions with different children so that each child gets a turn. Demonstration sessions are generally conducted at the therapist's office while the therapist observes (although in some group filial models parents may be asked to tape the demonstration sessions at home and bring them in for supervision). Following the demonstration sessions, a filial therapist gives the parent feedback. A general feedback process includes:

1. The filial therapist (and group members when applicable) gives a parent positive feedback on one or more things that the parent did well.

2. The filial therapist asks the parent to identify any areas in which she would like help or believed that she had trouble applying skills.

3. The filial therapist addresses the parent's area of concern and, if necessary, also identifies the area judged by to be the most important skill needing improvement.

4. The filial therapist demonstrates through role-play with the parent (or other group leader if available) how to utilize the skill seen as deficient; the parent (and possible other group members) gets a chance to practice the skill.

5. The filial therapist ends the feedback with additional positive praise for other areas of the demonstration that went well.

The total time for a specific parent demonstration and feedback to the parent would generally be about 25 minutes, and thus multiple demonstration sessions and feedback opportunities are available in a given individual or group format meeting.

## Preparing and Supporting Parents in Home Sessions

When the filial therapist has had to observe the parent's demonstration play sessions and assesses that the parents are likely to experience success at home, part of a parent meeting is used to prepare parents to begin home sessions. Such preparation generally includes identifying an appropriate place to hold sessions, a good day and time for parents to have their individual weekly play session with each participating child, and troubleshooting around child-care arrangements for other children (if any) so that interruptions of filial sessions do not occur. In cases where a family has a number of children, it may be necessary for a parent to divide children up (e.g., in a family with four children of reasonable age, each parent may have individual filial sessions with two children in a given week and then switch children the next week). A filial therapist also gives guidelines and assists the parents in identifying appropriate toys to acquire for their playroom at home. However, often this step in home preparation may occur earlier in the therapy process, since it may take some time for the parents to gather the play materials.

Once filial sessions have begun at home, a filial therapist will continue to monitor how the parents are doing through discussions with parent in regular meetings. Even after the parents begin home sessions, they may be asked to continue to bring their children to the meetings so that continued demonstration sessions and feedback can continue in order to refine skills (or, alternatively, some filial group sessions may focus on feedback given to videotaped sessions of parents' home sessions).

## Preparation of Parents for Ending Meetings With the Therapist

One of the strengths of FT is that parents can be adequately trained to conduct play sessions with their own children in a relatively brief period of time. Some time-limited filial group formats specifically are scheduled to meet for only 10 sessions of 90–120 minutes in length. Individual parent/family formats tend to tailor the therapy to the needs of a given family, and may not set a specific number of meetings, but generally are completed within 8–12 meetings of 50 minutes in length. The goal of FT training is for parents to have basic competence in the skill sets (not perfection) and for the parents and filial therapist to have confidence that the filial sessions can continue at home without additional regular ongoing support and feedback. Parents are generally asked to continue to conduct regular individual weekly play sessions with their children for approximately six months following termination. Although formal regular weekly meetings with parents may stop, it is a best practice to schedule a follow-up meeting with parents by phone or in person one month, three months, and six months following termination. In addition, parents are encouraged to call the filial therapist and/or to come in for a formal consultation meeting if they have questions or if problems arise. However, it should be noted that in most of the cases that parents do call to schedule additional consultation meetings, as well as in the majority of normally required follow-up meetings, very positive or uneventful reports of success and progress are the norm.

## Concluding Thoughts

FT is an innovative, powerfully effective family therapy model that is a complement to and extension of CCPT. The focus on training parents to be therapeutic agents with their own children brings with it the possibility of therapeutic outcomes, which are often more difficult to obtain (e.g., parent–child relationship improvement or parenting skills improvement or personality growth in the parent) using CCPT alone. The outcome research supports the usefulness of FT for a wide variety of

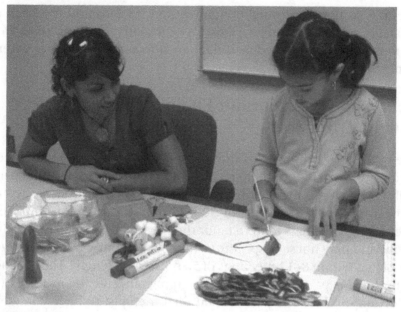

Figure 13.4

problems and in a variety of formats (e.g., individual parent/family and group), and across a variety of cultures. A successful filial therapist must be willing to embrace the transition from therapist/expert to educator/ skills trainer/supervisor and the associated qualities with these new roles as they train the parents in the filial skill sets, supervise them in filial sessions with their children, and prepare them to conduct sessions at home and to continue the sessions after the training has ended. The incredible transformations seen in many families who complete FT make it well worth the effort to master this innovative model.

## Activities and Resources for Further Study

The following activities provide opportunities for contemplation and academic practice of critical key concepts. They can be completed alone, with a partner, or in a small group or classroom.

- *Activity A:* Re-read the "Historical Roots of Filial Therapy" and "Goals and Outcomes of Filial Therapy" sections of this chapter and identify the philosophy, values, and goals that underlie filial therapy. Then think about how closely these values and goals match your own as a therapist.

- *Activity B:* Conducting filial therapy involves a significant change in your professional role—from providing therapy yourself to becoming a teacher/trainer/supervisor of parents. Think about experiences you have had in the past as a teacher, trainer, or supervisor and consider the following questions:
  - What did I like most about being in the role of teacher, trainer, or supervisor? What opportunities would becoming a filial therapist provide me for enjoying such roles again?
  - In terms of skill sets, what are my strengths as a teacher, trainer, or supervisor? What new skill sets do I think I would need to learn or improve upon in order to be an effective filial therapist?
- *Activity C:* Filial therapy has been utilized successfully with a wide variety of cultural groups. Read one of the following articles (see References) and discuss how filial therapy was successfully utilized with this cultural group: African American parents (Sheely, 2008; Solis, Meyers, & Varjas, 2004), Chinese parents (Chau & Landreth, 1997; Guo, 2005; Yuen, Landreth, & Baggerly, 2002), Hispanic/Latino parents (Ceballos, 2008), (Edwards, Ladner, & White, 2007), Korean parents (Jang, 2000; Lee & Landreth, 2003), Native American parents (Glover & Landreth, 2000).

# Helping Children Capitalize on Gains Made in CCPT

## 14
### Chapter

*From the outset the therapist has no desire other than to use his relationship to assist the child to be free finally of the need for his specialized help. The child's feelings are at the center of the experience, and the therapist is in a position to encourage the child to use him in whatever ways he can to grow toward a clearer awareness and acceptance of his own child's self with all that is involved in living with parents, siblings, and companions.*

—*Frederick Allen*

## Application Focus Scenario 1

Imagine that you are a school counselor serving in an elementary school. You know that one of your clients—a young girl who had begun the year with one emotional outburst after another, and had struggled to remain in class long enough to learn—has made very good progress in CCPT. She no longer misses class and is not sent to the office for discipline. She is now able to attend and learn in class. Still, her teacher is not completely satisfied with this progress. You may find, as we often do, that when using a standardized measure that helps the teacher be specific about frequencies or levels of behaviors, even though the child has made very good progress, the teacher does not *see* the change. It may be that the child's misbehavior has reduced from high in the clinical range to a borderline range between what would be expected of a child referred for significant counseling intervention and "normal." Yet her teacher wants the child to be better still. She wants her to have no misbehaviors that stand out as more than her peers.

A probable reason for this teacher's ongoing concerns may be that she and this child have fallen into a system of negative interactions. It may be that inadvertently the teacher is not expecting or asking for better behavior. The child is now healthier and more capable of relating in a better manner, but doesn't perceive that her teacher wants something different from her than in previous interactions, and thus both are left dissatisfied and at odds with one another.

Yet another possible reason for ongoing concerns may be that systems of interaction patterns with peers are shaping this child's behavior to be at least somewhat like it used to be before her work in child-centered play therapy (CCPT). It may be that her new outlook, choices, and decisions from CCPT are pushing her in one behavioral direction, but her social systems are pushing her in the other. These competing forces may allow her to make some progress—progress that you could build on now, but progress that is not yet what you and her other caregivers will be satisfied with.

In the first part of this chapter, we introduce options for multi-faceted, multisystemic interventions that can be used to capitalize on progress made in CCPT. The possibilities for this are limitless. We review a set of interventions that show excellent promise for helping therapeutic gains made in the playroom to transfer to home and school.

## Application Focus Scenario 2

Imagine that you are a therapist in an agency or private practice setting. You have been providing CCPT to a young boy who presented with highly defiant and aggressive behaviors at home and school. You know that his mom, whom you have had regular contact with, who brings him to sessions, and provides you with regular feedback, is satisfied with her son's progress in many areas, but still she wants more from him.

For example, perhaps his interactions with his mother have changed, but she sees that he and his sister still fight and would like to know how to help them get along better. Or perhaps she sees that while her son has made good progress at school and overall, he and his father are still not close, and that without meaning to, they tend to antagonize each other. Or perhaps she sees that he has made progress, but laments that he and she do not have the closeness that she would like.

In the latter part of this chapter, we introduce options for additional interventions within the family system, one of which could certainly be filial therapy (Chapter 13), but we introduce a number of other options that include utilizations, alternatives, or additional interventions that we have found helpful when the child has ended CCPT sessions and is ready to capitalize on gains made in therapy.

## Chapter Overview

CCPT is a powerful and highly effective intervention in and of itself. But no counseling or psychotherapeutic intervention should have to stand alone at all times. Changes made in CCPT are often sufficient in significantly changing the course and direction for a child who previously was blocked in development from his full potential. Time and again we have seen the deep, internal change of a child in CCPT become the change that causes the entire system to change. However, humans live in complex systems, and a single therapeutic intervention will not always foster all the growth needed. Sometimes change for a system can be threatening, so there have been times that we have seen the pressure of a system limit a child's progress. Most interventions for serious psychological difficulties should be multifaceted and multisystemic. Whenever possible, we want to intervene to help a child overcome systemic barriers to external change, in addition to helping the child accomplish deep internal change in CCPT. In the early sections of this chapter, we introduce additional interventions that are particularly relevant to school settings to help children and systems capitalize on progress made by children in CCPT. In the latter sections, we introduce similar additional interventions that are particularly relevant to agency and private practice settings that work with parents to help encourage the child's progress at home.

## Primary Skill Objectives

The following Primary Skill Objectives for this chapter are provided to guide you through the chapter and for reflection and review after completing the chapter reading and exercises. By reading and working through the chapter exercises, you will be better able to:

1. Describe the implementation of CCPT in a multifaceted, multisystemic set of services.
2. Describe the implementation of multiple additional intervention strategy options to follow or accompany CCPT in school settings.

*Table 14.1*  **Sample Multifaceted, Multisystemic Skill Set for a School Setting**

- Child-Centered Play Therapy
- Teacher Consultation
- Parent Consultation and Parent Skills Training
- Peer-to-Peer Conflict Resolution
- Opportunities for Group CCPT or Other Group Counseling
- Mental Health Skill Teaching in Classrooms

3. Describe the implementation of multiple additional intervention strategy options to follow or accompany CCPT in agency or private practice settings.

4. Be aware of the empathic communication for conflict resolution among children model (ECCR), and the extension of the model known as STRETCH, and how it can work to support progress made in CCPT by changing peer-to-peer interactions or teacher–child interactions in schools.

5. Understand group counseling as an option to help individual clients capitalize on progress made in CCPT.

6. Describe how parents may utilize aspects of CCPT to help children capitalize on gains made in CCPT.

# Multifaceted, Multisystemic Interventions to Follow or Accompany CCPT in School Settings

## Teacher Consultation Strategies

It is always advisable, when ending with a client in CCPT, to help make the transition a smooth one by letting others know that the child will be ending sessions and, when possible, setting up a meeting with the teacher for a consultation about this transition. If the teacher is still seeing the child struggle in interactions with her in the classroom, this meeting takes on added importance. Some goals for this meeting would include:

1. Listening to the teacher to let her voice any concerns, or ask questions about what to expect during the transition

2. Helping the teacher see the child's readiness for new ways of interacting with her

3. Teaching empathic attending, especially around structuring and limit setting as a way for the teacher to build her relationship with her student child (this can be done in earlier consultations as well)

4. Helping the teacher think through other ways of building her new relationship with the child

5. Helping to address how current behavior management plans in the classroom can be enhanced through empathic listening possibilities in interaction with all children in the classroom

6. When necessary, arranging a teacher–student meeting to encourage a "fresh start." This is especially beneficial for those children who seem to have fallen into a negative pattern of interactions with their teacher. This meeting gives you a chance, with the child present, to model empathic listening and responding during interaction.

For more on effective teacher consultation, review Chapter 11.

## Parent Consultation or Parent Skills Training

Parallel to teacher consultation, parent consultation is often also possible in school settings. In agency settings, the parent usually must bring the child to counseling. So the opportunity to also work with parents seems obvious. But we urge those of you in school settings not to neglect this important option.

The opportunity for parent consultation often arises when a child is in a school-related crisis (see Chapter 11 for an example). But offering a parent support and education program, such as the Parent Skills Training (Guerney, 1995), in a school is also an excellent method for community outreach. Whether consulting with individual parents related to specific situational needs and parenting skills or providing parent support and training in a group, working to enhance a parent's relationships with her children can be a key multisystemic intervention to accompany your work in CCPT.

## The Conjunction of Behavior Modification Programs and CCPT

A good behavior management plan can work hand-in-hand with CCPT. While one approach changes behavior from the outside in, the other changes behavior from the inside out. A weakness or very difficult hurdle in behavior management plans is the problem of making the transfer from externally rewarded behavior to behavior that is intrinsically motivated and thus self-sustaining. A problem with CCPT alone is that in some situations seriously disruptive or dangerous misbehavior must be managed in the short run in order to (1) give CCPT time to work—no matter how efficient CCPT can be in generating positive change early in the child's process, it rarely produces immediate change; and (2) give the adults responsible for the care and safety of a troubled child a goal, focus, and guide for their immediate interactions with the child in their care.

Behavior management plans used in conjunction with CCPT do not need to be different from those commonly known to be effective. Such behavior management systems can range from immediate and tangible reward systems for young children to points systems earning highly rewarding privileges and/or school to home contingency plans for older children. However, as a child-centered play therapist and an advocate for a child-centered approach, you may be able to help the team members implanting the plan to think in terms of what each aspect of the plan says about their relationship to the child. A few examples follow:

- Does the plan attend more to what the team would like to see vs. what they would not like to see? Does the plan itself suggest a negative behavior or mistake focus vs. presenting an expectation of growth and progress?

- If a form of "time-out" is used, does its use seem to be a punishment, like jail for being bad, or as a time for the child to take a break when he appears headed for a big mistake, which makes explicit a way that well-functioning adults normally use to avoid letting stress overloads erupt into behavioral errors?

- Do the words the team uses suggest *conditions* for positive regard, like "when you are being good/bad . . . " vs. choice-based wording, such as "when you are making wise choices/poor choices . . . " Such minor seeming wording changes can prompt perspective changes in the team and imply a lot to the child about how the team sees him. Do they see him as valuable and lovable, whether he is succeeding or failing with new behaviors in a given moment? To do so can be much more easily said than done.

- How and when can expressions of empathy be integrated within the plan and its procedures?

# Empathic Communication for Conflict Resolution (ECCR)

ECCR (Cochran, Cochran, & Hatch, 2002) assists children with inter- and intrapersonal skills in interactions with peers by guiding them through a practiced form of interaction when in conflict that features empathic listening and responding. Many times, your child clients from CCPT will quite naturally have already become quickly proficient in these skills due to their work in CCPT. But still they may benefit from additional intervention in the form of guidance that reshapes their interactions with peers. ECCR can be provided to enhance relationships among children and empower them to reach out to others with empathy and their expressive and listening skills to peacefully resolve conflicts. It is loosely based on the model of couples counseling known as relationship enhancement (Scuka, 2005).

An additional benefit of ECCR is that it can be taught to school teachers as a way to change the system of peer interactions in the classroom. A variety of the ECCR approach has been developed by our colleagues, Barb Higgins and Dawn Breitung, and is known as STRETCH: Student–Teacher Relationship Enhancement Toward Classroom Harmony. This model offers teacher and support staff of preschool through second graders training in the ECCR approach. This training can usually take place during three 2-hour morning sessions. Teacher and staff training allows the intervention to take place more immediately and directly (in the classroom) and provides added assistance to the teachers and staff working with grades preschool through second grade—the all-important early intervention grades. All too often, children with difficult behaviors are placed in classrooms with teachers who are just starting out.

If your child client who has made gains in CCPT is still having classroom struggles, one-on-one consultation with the teacher is not always time efficient for either of you. Offering a group of teachers STRETCH is a way to provide added assistance, especially to teachers and staff working hard to provide a harmonious classroom environment.

If you are working in schools, especially if you are a traveling play therapist or itinerant counselor, offering such trainings is an excellent way to build solid relationships with the teachers and staff you work with, and to reach out in the community you serve. (For more on the importance and benefits of this, see Chapter 15.) Teacher training sessions in ECCR can include time for sharing with peers, snacks, in-depth training to include mock role-plays, and useful handouts that will prepare teachers to more effectively respond with empathy and consistent limits to classroom disruptions and to supportively resolve peer conflicts by helping children learn to listen to and respond empathically to each other when in conflict, and generally in the classroom environment as well.

## Opportunities for Group CCPT or Other Group Counseling Interventions

We see excellent opportunities for group counseling in schools. For a child who is highly inhibited from successful relationships with peers, individually applied CCPT can serve as an initial intervention to get the child ready to succeed in group work. The child who has become ready for group work through CCPT can then use the group to capitalize on his readiness for new, healthy relationships with peers. School settings offer the opportunity to provide stratified, heterogeneous groups (meaning that not all the students in a group need to have terrible acting-out behavior—that would be a gang—or need to be all depressed, all anxious, all truant, etc.). Homogenous groups cause a number of complications, while heterogeneous groups, with similar but stratified difficulty levels, would seem to offer greater opportunities for success through functions such as group members modeling and supporting each other's development. In our view, the groups can range from CCPT in a group format, which would feature group process over instruction, to more directly psychoeducational groups, with wise counselors selecting formats based on contexts.

## Mental Health Skill Teaching in Classrooms

And, of course, we see the mental health skill teaching in classrooms, often called classroom guidance, which is normally provided by school counselors, as an excellent context addition to CCPT. Children in the normal range of development and beyond often benefit from skills learned in classroom guidance. Failing to learn skills that peers are actively coming to use and master is one good sign that therapy or a significant counseling intervention is needed. We have known of many children in CCPT who referenced things they learned in classroom guidance lessons. We remember one who referred to his "mud mind," meaning muddled, angry, or confused thinking, which we later learned he had picked up from a classroom guidance lesson. We remember another relating back to his realization of universality

Table 14.2 **Sample Multifaceted, Multisystemic Skill Set for an Agency Setting**

- Child-Centered Play Therapy
- Filial Therapy
- Parent Skills Training/Parent Consultation
- Individual Counseling for Parent(s)
- Couples Counseling for Parents

and normalization as he realized that everyone has emotional difficulties at times, that everyone "has a heart." It seemed clear to us that they were using their session time to contemplate the meaning of guidance lessons for themselves. Additionally, as with readiness for group counseling, many children become ready to incorporate lessons in classroom guidance, some of the same lessons that they would have turned a deaf ear to in the past, through their work in CCPT.

# Multifaceted, Multisystemic Interventions to Follow or Accompany CCPT in Agency Settings

## Filial Therapy

Counseling agencies provide the most common setting opportunities to provide filial therapy (FT). As it is usually a parent who will bring the child to counseling, it can be assumed that many parents in agency settings are both motivated for help and past the point of realizing the need for help. Once an agency counselor is confident of a parent's readiness (motivation, stability, ability to commit) and openness to filial therapy, filial training could begin. A parent could begin the required training in FT, while her child is making progress in CCPT and thus, in a way, getting ready to work with her in FT.

Large agencies can provide the added benefit of enough parents ready and open to FT to form filial groups. In this way, parents can support and challenge each other as they develop their "special play time" skills together.

## Parent Skills Training

Short of FT, perhaps for a parent who cannot yet make the time commitment needed for FT, agencies often provide parents other skill support. This can be simply providing the one-on-one counselor time to help a struggling parent think through behavior management or strategies to support her children's success at school. But as with FT groups, for some large agencies, this service can also include ongoing parent support and training groups, in which parents come to acquire skills themselves as well as to help others.

## Marriage and Family Counseling

Agencies can also often provide marriage and family counseling in addition to CCPT. If there are two parents present, but they are in constant discord, the parents can inadvertently prolong their child's difficulties when in fact she was long ago ready to be different with them.

## Individual Counseling for Parents

You will, of course, encounter parents who are struggling with such significant mental health difficulties themselves that they are unable to grow or improve as parents, not ready to learn FT, and even are poor candidates for marriage and family counseling. In such cases, it often works well for the agency to provide one counselor for the parent, while another works with the child. This helps the child's counselor avoid such dilemmas as that of being the child's counselor and therefore advocate, while also being heavily emotionally involved and invested in the parent's individual difficulties and development. In many cases, the parent's sessions can be scheduled in the same time blocks as the child's, as long as the parent and his counselor understand that their session may be interrupted if the child's session needs to be ended early.

## Finding Additional Resources for the Children You Serve in the Community

Children normally develop a readiness to self-express, receive nurturing, and reach out to others through their work in CCPT. Counselors in both school and agency settings can often serve children and families by helping connect children with new opportunities to relate and connect. We've often known principals or mentors who had long been trying to reach out to a troubled child suddenly find success following the child's work in CCPT. Other opportunities that counselors might help with can include community art or music programs, sports, or well-administered mentoring programs such as Big Brothers Big Sisters of America (bbbsa. org). When the child's drive to self-actualize has been reawakened and has found its rightful direction through CCPT, the opportunities to build on success are unlimited!

## Activities for Further Learning

- *Activity A:* Imagine a context in which you work. "Brainstorm" the set of services that you may provide in addition to CCPT in that setting. Discuss likely benefits and possible difficulties for each. Remember to think in terms of intervening in multiple relational systems at once (i.e., peers, family, teachers, mentors). Share your thoughts with peers or classmates.

- *Activity B:* Working alone or with a partner/small group, imagine a setting, and outline and detail how you can apply the ECCR model to engage peer interactions that help capitalize on gains made in CCPT. Include descriptions of which clients/type of clients you see the application benefiting, specific setting contexts, and strategies for overcoming difficulties that you can anticipate encountering.

- *Activity C:* Describe at least four additional services that you may provide along with CCPT in your school or agency setting. Give rationales for each.

- *Activity D:* Work alone or with a partner/group of peers to outline and detail group interventions to capitalize on progress made in individual CCPT. Include CCPT as well as psycho-educational group ideas. Decide which clients or which types of clients you will include and why. Describe your steps to client selection, screening, and group planning. Describe your setting/anticipated setting, including its advantages and disadvantages for this intervention. Include descriptions of how you may overcome difficulties that you can anticipate encountering.

- *Activity E:* Describe at least a few strategies or approaches in working with parents that can help parents capitalize on progress their child has made in CCPT. Use a real situation(s), with identifying information protected or hypothetical situations in order to help you be specific and anticipate potential problems in application and ways to overcome them.

- *Activity F:* Plan a Parent Skills Training group in your school or agency setting. Be as specific as possible, including such things as who you hope to have in the group, how many, how you will reach them, when and where you will meet, how you can encourage attendance, and how you will overcome barriers to progress that you can anticipate in this intervention.

- *Activity G:* Plan a specific strategy for a parent to implement skills that accompany work their child has done in CCPT, but that are less than the requirements of FT, when FT does not seem applicable. Include specific context, including problems that may be encountered and how you may help the parent overcome them in the application you envision.

- *Activity H:* Investigate and report on any of the variety of additional services that we have mentioned and only briefly commented on in the context of this chapter. Share your findings with peers.

- *Activity I:* Revisit the Primary Skill Objectives for this chapter and see if you have mastered them to your satisfaction at this time. If not, seek additional readings, practices, and discussions for clarification, and in order to master them to your satisfaction.

# Reaching Diverse Clients With the Child-Centered Approach

*The freedom to have ideas, values, and beliefs—the permission to be oneself—the right to be different—exist in a counseling climate that is marked by a deep respect for the individuality and uniqueness of the child. In the final analysis, each individual must discover personal uniqueness. It is in an atmosphere where uniqueness is fostered and difference is valued that the full discovery of self can be achieved.*

*—Angelo Boy and Gerald Pine*

*The child-centered approach is uniquely suited for working with children from different socioeconomic strata and ethnic backgrounds since these facts do not change the therapist's beliefs, philosophy, theory, or approach to the child. Empathy, acceptance, understanding, and genuineness on the part of the therapist are provided to children equally, irrespective of their color, condition, circumstance, concern or complaint.*

*—Garry Landreth and Daniel Sweeney*

*If we are to achieve a richer culture, rich in contrasting values, we must recognize the whole gamut of human potentialities and so weave a less arbitrary social fabric, one in which each diverse human gift will find a place.*

*—Margaret Mead*

## Application Focus Scenarios

### Scenario 1: "Ibrahim"

Ten-year-old Ibrahim has been in the U.S. school system for most of a year. He is part of a refugee family outreach program. He speaks just enough English to get around school and get his needs met. He requires an interpreter in class for his studies, and though he is learning English, he still relies heavily on his own variety of "sign language" and a few words and short expressions. This is very frustrating and often causes him to explode in anger at his teachers and peers, or withdraw unexpectedly from activities at his school. The school counselor has had short exchanges with Ibrahim, and believes that with the help of his interpreter for the first few sessions, he can help him through providing child-centered play therapy (CCPT). On the day of his first scheduled session, his counselor says "hello" to welcome him. Ibrahim quickly extends his hand for a stiff handshake, but then tucks his head and will not look up. With the help of the interpreter, the counselor invites Ibrahim into the play therapy room. He follows slowly in and then stands in the middle of the room, seemingly baffled and taken aback by the setting. The counselor and interpreter convey the opening message and Ibrahim begins to loosen up. He smiles and shakes his finger at his counselor, teasingly, as if scolding him, "Toys in the school . . . toys are not for school . . . this is not good, Mister!"

## Scenario 2: "Gavin"

Three-year-old Gavin has been "suspended" from preschool due to "inability to follow instructions and communicate with others" and aggressive behavior that his teachers "cannot control safely." He has seen a clinical psychologist and has been diagnosed with Asperger's syndrome. This psychologist refers Gavin for CCPT with a therapist in his agency. During the first 10 minutes of his first play therapy session, Gavin has not acknowledged or made eye contact with his therapist, and has spent most of the time with his back to her—digging his hands into the sand. As he digs and sifts the sand repeatedly, he carries on a running monologue about insects. Occasionally, he jumps up and rocks excitedly back and forth—before retuning to the sand tray and his "running monologue."

> **GAVIN:** *The exoskeleton of the insect molts, and the stages between are known as instars! Before the new hard exoskeleton develops, the insect is very vulnerable to predators. . . .*
> **THERAPIST:** *You are letting me know about . . .*
> **GAVIN:** *[Quickly interrupting and talking over the therapist] The insect's body wall is sclerotized. Insects don't have bones . . . insects don't have bones. . . .*
> **THERAPIST:** *Insects don't have bones. . . .*

**GAVIN:** *[Briefly directs his gaze at the therapist with a stern glare.] Stop . . . you're not supposed to say that!*

**THERAPIST:** *You don't like it when I say that . . . you want me to stop . . . to be quiet!*

**GAVIN:** *[For the first time makes sustained eye contact and smiles with seeming satisfaction in reaction to the therapist's remark.] That's right!*

## Scenario 3: "Destiny"

Nine-year-old Destiny lives part-time with her maternal grandparents, her "Mama Lynn" and "Papa James," who are Caucasian, and part-time with her paternal grandmother, "Grandma Lilly," who is African American. Her mother and father were young teens when Destiny was born and are not married to each other. Her mother has remarried, lives in another state, and has a baby girl 4 months old. Her father is attending a community college in a nearby town and is considering joining the military. Though she sees them occasionally and during holidays, her relationship with both of them has always been similar to that of a younger sibling. The joint custody arrangement between Destiny's grandparents has been very friendly and worked well, and up until recently Destiny has seemed to thrive at school and in both home settings. She has always been a "straight-A student" and never a behavior problem in school. She has always been "full of smiles," according to her Papa James, and "a happy little drama queen—a dancer and a singer—willing to try anything," according to her Mama Lynn. Her Grandma Lilly agrees, saying, "She's always been a quick learner and never been one to shy away from a challenge." At the beginning of her fourth-grade school year, however, Destiny's grandparents have noticed that she seems to have "lost her sparkle." They report a noticeable change in her mood, and that she watches too much TV and overeats. She complains of stomachaches and frequently wants to stay at home from school. When Destiny begins secretly rubbing raw marks on her arm with a pencil eraser, the three grandparents are distraught and at a loss as to how to help her. All three decide to make an appointment to consult a highly recommended play therapist at a private practice in their town.

Scenarios such as these are common to school counselors, private practitioners, and agency therapists. Children in need of counseling come from a variety of socioeconomic and cultural backgrounds, and enter counseling with a variety of symptoms, conditions, and diagnoses. It is therefore essential that the counselor be self-aware in regards to her own feelings about working with children who are from different cultures, lifestyles, circumstances, and/or who have mental health diagnoses. In attempts to help children, we all too often fall into the trap of becoming overinvolved in assumptions, stereotypes, or expectations based on cultural differences, prior diagnoses, and other background information about the child before we begin to provide therapy. It is often helpful to remember that CCPT is by design an open and particularly freeing therapy for the individual child—no matter what the "presenting problem" may be, or the background situation or scenario. By providing the core conditions of empathy, genuineness, and unconditional positive regard, the therapist provides an atmosphere where the individual child is allowed to set his own pace, and use the language of movement, play, art, music—and even the language of shared silence—for self-exploration, self-expression, and growth.

Preparing you in gaining self-awareness and knowledge around issues of diversity in relation to CCPT, and for assisting each child you counsel as she shares her "pure voice" or "diverse human gift" is the goal of this chapter.

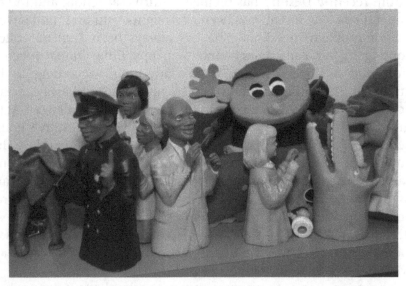

Figure 15.1

## Chapter Summary and Overview

The concept of human diversity is both complicated by, and over-simplified by the many attempts to define and understand it. We, as counselors, often narrow the concept of diversity to include only those persons of a different ethnicity, gender, and geography from our own. This chapter will encourage play therapists to think broadly about the concept of diversity and apply this thinking to how counselors can best provide a therapeutic atmosphere and relationship that ensures that each client's natural and unique language is present, and accepted, and understood.

Vignettes (and scenarios) of children who all experience significant barriers to communication—including cultural differences, behavioral and emotional disabilities, gender identity issues, posttraumatic stress, and/or a combination of these experiences—are presented to highlight how the language of play, art, and, perhaps more importantly, the opportunity to freely express, can lead to optimum healing and a sense of enhanced human connectedness between counselor and client.

## Primary Skill Objectives

The following Primary Skill Objectives for this chapter are provided to guide you through the chapter and for reflection and review after completing the chapter reading and exercises. By reading and working through the chapter exercises, you will be better able to:

1. Explain and generate illustrations for four ways that CCPT addresses and encompasses issues of diversity.
2. Explain and describe the importance of and ways to overcome four "pitfalls" related to cultural assumptions and ethnocentricity that should be important to play therapists.
3. Explain and describe how to avoid four common problems of novice play therapists related to cultural differences.
4. Describe difficulties that *you* expect to need to overcome related to providing CCPT across cultures, including your "buttons" that you think some children's behavior, temperament, or style of self-expression may push.

# How CCPT Encompasses and Addresses Issues of Diversity

## The Culture Within

Glauser and Bozarth (2001) described the person-centered approach as addressing "the culture within" (p. 142). They review research evidence and provide illustrations to counter the "specificity myth" (p. 142), that is, that particular techniques can be matched to particular persons based on the populations and categories that the client is assumed to represent. We use their phrase "the culture within" to introduce our view that (1) each person is of, from, and a part of the sets of cultural groups that make up her context; (2) each person makes individual meanings of all life experience, including cultural context; and thus (3) each person's culture is a combination of her context and the meanings she makes of her context, especially her culture most relevant to her counseling experience, is her "culture within."

We assert from the notion of "the culture within" that it makes more sense to address the cultural within through a therapeutic relationship that helps the person realize her culture and the meanings she has made of it, relevant to her current situation vs. trying to match techniques to counselor assumptions about her external culture. Glauser and Bozarth also address the body of counseling and psycho-therapy meta-analytic research indicating that the therapeutic rela-tionship explains the largest part of counseling outcome, with specific techniques accounting for a much smaller portion of change, a portion of change matching that accounted for by the placebo effect.

CCPT boldly and profoundly addresses each child's culture within. It is distinctively culturally sensitive as it is, by design, especially responsive to each individual child as a unique and "unrepeatable" human being. It is focused in the therapeutic relationship as a means to facilitate each child's unique need for and forms of self-expression, each child's unique path to greater self-direction and ever maturing behavior.

## The Child Has a Right to Be Different

The child-centered approach also embraces the notion introduced by Boy and Pine (1995) that each child has "a right to be different." A child-centered counselor accepts each child as he is in each moment of his development. We have often known parents to bring their child to

## Table 15.1  Addressing Diversity Through CCPT—Remember to:

- Respond to "the culture within" as well as the child's external culture
- Respect each child's right to be different
- Relate to each child as an individual first and foremost
- Connect across cultures with empathy, genuineness, and unconditional positive regard

therapy having internalized messages from society (schools, extended family, medical doctors or other experts)—messages that tell them that because their child stands out as different, there is something wrong that must be fixed, medicated, or rehabilitated. In consultations, parents often realize and are much relieved to hear that their son's therapist sees their child as unique and as an individual with a right to be him- or her*self*. Behaviors and emotional difficulties are signs that their child is struggling, but this does not mean that something is "broken" or in need of fixing. Learning this attitude from the therapist, many parents learn to model the child-centered approach of addressing difficulties, which includes structuring and limiting behavior as needed, but above all accepting and prizing their child for the unique (i.e., different) person that he is. When coming to this realization, one father of a boy we knew who could be described as fitting Asperger's syndrome (American Psychiatric Association [APA], 1994) went to his coworkers, who tended to be bright engineering and computer science professionals, and he described his worries about his son and the Asperger's diagnosis that had been given to his son by previous clinicians. They decided that while they shared his concerns for what his son was going through, they also could accept his son's right to be different. They concluded, after talking about their own childhood experiences, that they would all fit the description of being "Asperger's children!"

On a related note, we don't want to suggest that diagnoses are not made by counselors and therapists who work in the child-centered approach. Diagnoses of children are often required for necessary services, and can be additionally helpful in understanding children and families. When needed or helpful, child-centered play therapists utilize diagnoses to justify reimbursement or understand children's or families' difficulties in functioning in the same ways as counselors or therapists who work in other approaches. For instance, "wrap-around" services for children with diagnoses to include school and medical interventions; occupational, speech, and physical therapies; social skills education; and parent education are often the very positive results of accurate diagnosis, and are highly valued services for children with special needs. For a child who additionally has emotional and behavioral difficulties, CCPT is often the intervention that "pulls it all together" and enhances these other services by helping the child to fully utilize and benefit from all services offered.

## Relating to the Child as Individual First and Foremost

Each child who comes into CCPT is given the opportunity to begin *where he is* as opposed to where others assume *he should be*. Each child who comes into CCPT receives the opportunity to share with a unique "voice" of her own *what it is she needs to express*, as opposed to *what it is others feel she should express*. Because CCPT allows the child to lead and provides a time for freedom of expression within a safe structure, the individual—the whole self—is accepted and allowed to fully be. This notion is a part of the unconditional positive regard facilitated by limits when needed that CCPT embodies. This way of relating empowers children through their play to accomplish the abstract, existential tasks of an adult in counseling—tasks of seeing oneself as one really is, and thus choosing to change, or seeing oneself clearly and fully and realizing that oneself is largely acceptable, not flawed, and unlovable as previously feared.

## Connecting With Deep Empathy, Genuineness, and Unconditional Positive Regard

Each child who comes into CCPT experiences the empathy, genuineness, and unconditional positive regard of a therapist who is steady and consistent in providing these core conditions. Empathy means that the counselor will try to come as close as possible to what the child is experiencing in the moment to include his unique set of cultural experiences. Genuineness means that the therapist brings an honest self into the counseling relationship and does not make changes in relating or the therapy hour based on the child's background, gender, or culture. Unconditional positive regard means that the therapist accepts and prizes the whole child—his culture, temperament, and expressive style. It is through this deep acceptance of the child, and genuine valuing of her uniqueness that the true sensitivity to her culture can occur.

# Avoiding the Pitfalls of Cultural Assumptions and Ethnocentricity

The image of "pitfalls" may be a helpful image for understanding the topics of this section. Our guidance here is meant to help you avoid unexpected problems in your work—to help you avoid a situation where you are steadily working along, aiming to provide good CCPT services, when, without noticing, you stumble into a hole. It's difficult to discern how you have missed this hidden gap in the road, but now you must work your way out and continue on toward helping the children and families you serve. The four areas of guidance at the bottom of the page will hopefully help you avoid most unseen "pitfalls" by preparing ahead, and having an awareness of potential problems and what the causes of these are.

## Client Expression That Is Difficult for You to Accept—The Need to Develop Your Self-Awareness and to Expand Acceptance

It is inevitable that you will encounter client expressions that are hard for you to accept. If you strive to practice in open ways, your chance experiences will include clients who "push your buttons." It is important to develop self-awareness of your own attitudes. Developing your awareness and expanding your range for acceptance can come from introspection and reflection on your feelings about issues of diversity, including gender, religion, race, and socioeconomic status. When you find that you have assumptions, explore the legitimacy of each, and if found to be based in ethnocentricity or misinformation, learn from this.

## Table 15.2

| Danger Areas | | Prevention Tasks |
| --- | --- | --- |
| Encountering client expressions that are hard for you to accept | → | Continually develop your self-awareness and expand your ability to accept |
| Connecting with children without connecting with their communities | → | Make yourself known and reach out to your clients' communities |
| Inhibited parent connections | → | Strive to love, respect, and welcome each parent just as you would each child |
| An inadvertently insensitive setting | → | Take care to provide a diverse playroom that is user friendly to your diversity of clients |

Identify your internal cultural values, your unspoken beliefs that affect your acceptance. Consider the following example that was challenging to the counselor involved.

### Example: Brandon's Intense and Graphic Aggressive Stage Play

Coming out of his warm-up stage, Brandon has begun to fiercely "attack" the baby doll in his play. He pretends to beat it, to bite it, to torture it. He ties one foot to a chair and keeps a plate of food just out of reach. He yells at the doll, "Don't try to move," and whips it fiercely with a rope. Every now and then he begins to comfort it from crying, but then he begins whipping and kicking it again. This Aggressive Stage action is all pretend play, but it is still gut wrenching for his counselor to watch and experience with him. Perhaps understandably, she responds with tracking and empathy that is noticeably less than, and that does not match, Brandon's experience in play. In some of the worst moments, she winces. She is watching but distracted by being bothered by his play, and she is therefore only partly connected with him through his play.

Brandon brings the play closer and closer to her view, as she holds back. He seems to try to invite her to take part, giving her a role as baby-sitter, with initial instructions that suggest to her that he is going to have her whip the baby in the same way he did. But when he sees her less than enthusiastic reaction and starts to suspect her revulsion, he goes back to the work on his own.

While this example is an unusually graphic aggressive play scenario, it is true that some children, for various reasons, including anger release and shared reality, need to go far into bizarre and disturbing themes in aggressive play. It seemed in supervision that this counselor's inability to go to some of the dark, aggressive places that Brandon needed to go prolonged and intensified his aggressive work. It was as if he were saying through his behavior, "This is something I need to share with you, this is something I need you to hear. Oh, you didn't hear me? Well, you must need me to repeat it for you, or play it again louder for you."

His counselor took appropriate steps to prevent potential danger or risk. She had frequent contact with his mother and new stepfather. They understood that based on circumstances that he has likely experienced as rejection, he probably has a well of anger and resentment. They carefully monitored around areas of potential danger to others (e.g., younger children or animals) or himself. They helped her monitor his behavior outside of counseling and confirmed that while he was highly oppositional with them—so much that they were unsure if they could parent him—he was not self-injurious or aggressive toward other children.

But still this counselor remained revolted by his play. His play struck chords of sensitivity in her that made his play—this part of him— almost impossible for her to accept. It helped her (outside of sessions) to analytically speculate what the play might mean—perhaps seeing parts of himself as unacceptable and deserving of torture, perhaps the vulnerable, needy parts of himself (his opposition to his parents was as if he was all grown up, showing them up, showing that he doesn't need them). But it was more important for her to work through her sensitive spots that his play was reaching, those "buttons" that triggered her recoil. She discovered that she had some difficult-to-face sensitivities around violence, especially to the unprotected. This same caring that drove her to work very hard for children now kept her from connecting well with a child who so needed her acceptance and unconditional positive regard. Realizing her vulnerability in this way helped her see Brandon for Brandon, for the unique individual that he was, who happened to *need* to express harsh things in that moment. This thought process did not completely change her reaction, but it helped. In subsequent sessions, her faith in the child-centered process strengthened as she was with him as he moved forward in play to Regressive themes, Mastery play, and well-being in life. This experience helped her grow, and she was better prepared for the next time.

Whatever the reasons for our unique, individual "buttons" that can be pushed, we all have them. To become excellent and efficient therapists, we must continue to work through them, to make our vulnerabilities less by knowing and accepting them. It is also important to realize that this work is never finished. Our vulnerabilities, our "buttons," are never fully gone, and in the infinity of human conditions and children's play, there is always a child to find a new one for you! We find this to be not a burden, but a constructive aspect of the work of an excelling play therapist. It keeps your self-actualization process working particularly well and consistently, so long as you are careful to attend to it.

## Connecting With Children without Connecting with Their Community—The Need for Community Outreach

While your play therapy room is a separate, safe place for each child, and it may be the center of your work, it should not be an isolated workspace for you. Whenever possible, you should reach out and go out into the communities you serve. This provides an exceptional way to better understand and reach out across cultures.

### Outreach to Community Schools

If you work at a community agency or private practice that gets a number or referrals from a particular school or schools, you will be more helpful to the children and families you serve, as well as earn more referrals, if you also are at least an occasional presence at the school. With appropriate permissions that allow you to consult, you could offer to provide your understandings of particular children, in person or in writing, in school-based meetings regarding how the school can best educate individuals that are your clients. Adding your perspective to the outlook and work of the school-based professionals can be a very significant addition to how you help your clients. Remember that your child clients spend nearly as much—or, in some situations, more—time at school than with their parents. If your understandings of clients can help the school provide better educational services, this is a significant advocacy intervention for your clients. And also remember that professionals at the school, who may know your clients very well, can certainly improve your understandings of your clients and their families. Before this consultation, your knowledge of your clients' school experiences was filtered and altered through the perceptions of at least a couple of individuals before received by you.

You might initiate school contact at the request of a parent who is concerned about her son's situation at school, perhaps a child who has had a problem with fighting or aggressive behavior and now is facing possible expulsion or referral to a "last resort" external program for children with extremely difficult behavior. Even if the parent was late in seeking assistance that you can provide, and the school is understandably frustrated and needing to protect the education and safety of his peers, you may be able to share your hope of turning the situation around, as you explain what you will be doing in his therapy, how it will work, what to expect in change, and in what time frame.

Your offer to work with the school should be made in unassuming ways. Note that we did not say your offer to *help*, but your offer to *work with*. Schools often do the most important work for children and receive the least appreciation. Perhaps for this reason, school professionals may be sensitive to offers of *help* that may come across as condescension. If your first few offers to work with a school regarding clients you are serving are not accepted, your next one may be. Every situation is different. And if your humble offers to work with the school are not accepted, but you get "credit" for willingness and possibly thus more referrals (if not officially from the school, but from school staff members in community contexts), then that is a good thing, too.

Once a relationship is established, you may be able to offer an in-service workshop for teachers on understandings of particular child problems from your perspective, or skills that you learn from your work with children that you think could also help children in the classroom. Perhaps with a working relationship established, you can also offer contributions for the school newsletter that includes helpful insight or guidance for parents. These kinds of ideas are important outreach client services. Secondarily, they could expand your practice, a positive by-product if it occurs, more than a goal of your outreach, but good all the same!

### Outreach to Community Groups

Regardless of the school or agency base for your services, it will be to your and your clients' advantage to reach out to the community groups of your service area. You may be able to reach out to area churches to let them know what you do in the community, to help them understand some of your passion to serve and the services you provide. In doing so, you may learn more about what they do, why and how, and their passions to serve.

If you are culturally different from many of your clients, the community may be understandably reluctant to accept the very effective services you would provide. Remember that when persons in the community come to you for help, they are in a vulnerable state. If you work through your own initial discomfort, and make yourself at least a little vulnerable in reaching out to the families in the community you wish to serve, you make those families' access of you less worrisome and uncomfortable, and so more possible and likely.

## Inhibited Parent Connections—The Challenge of Consistently Loving, Respecting, and Welcoming Each Parent

While therapists and counselors focused on serving troubled children commonly say they want to serve and connect with the parents and families of troubled children, too, this is often not quite true. At times this inhibition is based in a lack of personal confidence, perhaps from a worry that sounds something like, "The parents would not take me seriously. I can provide this therapy for the child, but I won't have all the answers to what this parent should do in the complexity of his situation. And what will I do then?"

Whatever the reasons, we often see the evidence of such inhibition. In schools, we have often seen the relief, thinly masked as exasperation or disappointment, when a counselor or teacher reports: "Mr. or Mrs. _____ failed to show up for a meeting again!" We have also seen meetings with parents who were expected to be difficult or contentious jam-packed with enough school personnel and officials to surely subdue these parents with ease, and whether intended or not, to very effectively intimidate them.

Whatever the reasons for possible inhibitions, you must find the capacity to care for, respectfully communicate and welcome each parent, just as you do each child. These connections are sometimes sought by asking for meetings that don't seem to be desired at all by some parents. This may be with parents who are reluctant to access services, or with parents who through their own inhibitions coupled with high need are willing to turn their child over for help, or are willing to leave the school with the sole responsibility for, and thus control over, the education of their children. These connections can be sought through listening well with deep empathy and reaching for unconditional positive regard and deep connection with each parent in meetings. And these connections can be sought through the community outreach advocated above.

## An Insensitive Setting—The Necessity to Provide a Diverse, User-Friendly Playroom

Your setting and space must be open to widely divergent modes of play and expression. There should be opportunities for various forms of visual art, drama, music, and other play that may interest your clients. If you see a number of children with special physical or occupational needs, certain adjustments and accommodations can be made (see Activity G: Activities for Further Study). You should have toys that allow for various forms of Aggressive Stage play and Regressive Stage play. You must take care to have a balance of toys that you would expect to appeal to different ages, and to boys and to girls. And, of course, you must have toys that are culturally sensitive. For example, among your dolls or other human figures, you should have dolls that represent all the ethnic groups you serve, including enough to put together family sets of dolls from the various ethnic groups as well as mixed sets. The acceptance and accessibility of your toys and playroom speak for your acceptance and accessibility across cultures.

# Common Problems of Beginning Counselors in Providing CCPT across Cultures and in Unfamiliar Territory

## Prejudgment of What Is Best for the Child

Some beginning counselors struggle with assumptions based on "too much information" in the reason for referral of the child (background information combining cultural and context information with problematic symptoms, circumstances, concerns, or diagnoses). Indeed, some helpers become so caught up in this predicament that the therapy hour for the child can soon become the missing component in the overall treatment plan. Unfortunately, when this happens the child as an individual gets "lost in the mix," and we miss the opportunity to allow the child's unique being—the self—to grow and carry with him internal change, and a sense of self-efficacy and internal locus of control. While it may seem obvious in reading now, it may also be important throughout your career to remember that your aim is always to help an individual child and family vs. to help a member of a particular cultural group, context, or diagnosis.

## Overrating the Importance of Language

There is a limitation in assuming that children who will not speak (those with selective mutism, some forms of autistic spectrum disorders) or children who do not speak the same native language as the therapist cannot—due to problems with spoken or heard language—fully benefit from CCPT. One of the great advantages of CCPT is that it offers the therapist and child an opportunity to relate without relying heavily on words. This way of relating through being with, through tracking and empathic responding that is sensitive *first* to the feelings of the child, in a sense is the initial and most important "gap" across cultures that is bridged—that between adult and child.

Because a counselor who is skilled in CCPT responds with empathy and unconditional positive regard in her being, this is felt by the child. It is seen by the child whenever he looks up from his play to her face. Her face in those moments becomes a significant reconfirmation of who he is, and her empathy and acceptance is heard in the tone of voice she uses while tracking his actions and moment-to-moment experiences. Indeed, so much is communicated in facial expressions and tone of voice that it becomes less important whether the child understands every word of his therapist's responses or not.

## Paying Too Much Attention to Differences

At times, beginning counselors or therapists may try too hard to understand the meanings of a child's cultural, ethnic, and socioeconomic background. For some, this can cause anxiety. For others, it can prompt subtle but important misunderstandings of an individual child's experience in the moment. It can cause unnecessary and inefficient inhibitions in connecting.

Remember that in CCPT the first connect is through tracking and empathy to feelings expressed in the here-and-now. When you as counselor begin here—attempting through your way of being to reach out, human to human—then it becomes easier to truly understand the whole child, inclusive of all he is. The child's background can be very important to your case management functions in addition to CCPT or in wrap-around services, but in CCPT sessions, background is never as important as the here-and-now.

## Difficulties Accepting Unusual Modes of Play Due to Temperament

Some beginning play therapists have difficulties with long silences, children who play quietly and off to themselves, or difficulties with loud, high-energy, constantly engaging play. If you find this true in you, strive to remember that because CCPT allows the child to freely choose self-generated activity to self-express, the child's predominant temperament and personality are present and acknowledged, accepted, and prized in CCPT. While most children will play in a variety of styles, and engage in a variety of play activities at differing energy levels throughout the CCPT process, it is necessary to realize that by nature some children are shy and reserved, and others are boisterous and talkative. For one child, painting with watercolors while quietly humming to herself for 20 minutes is a Mastery expression of herself. For another child, joyfully jumping rope 100 times in a minute is a Mastery expression of himself. Having tolerance for differences includes that the child's individual temperament and way of being is prized and accepted by the therapist.

## Difficulties With Acceptance Due to Personal Judgments in Regards to Gender Identity

Some beginning play therapists have difficulties putting aside personal judgments in regards to a child with significant gender identity issues, or have difficulties when a child in CCPT overtly and consistently plays out roles and themes that indicate obvious distress over biological gender. Because the child in CCPT is given the opportunity for a safe, confidential time *to be and feel fully accepted and prized*, and because empathy, unconditional positive regard, and genuineness are the core conditions in CCPT, it is important that you reflect on personal feelings concerning children and gender identity, and that you seek supervision and guidance if children with gender identity issues pose difficulties or personal challenges for you in regards to your full acceptance and unconditional positive regard.

## Return to Scenarios From Opening of Chapter

We suggest you return to the Application Focus Scenarios now that you have read and contemplated the guidance of the chapter. Think about how you might view them differently. In Activity A of Activities for Further Study, we suggest that you work with peers or alone to consider the problems, pitfalls, inhibitions, or thought errors that you or a novice therapist may encounter. Then please see our concluding thoughts on the Application Focus Scenarios in Skill Support Resource H.

## Concluding Thoughts

Silently finger-painting on a canvas . . . actively role-playing out scenes of horrific death and destruction . . . twirling, dancing, and singing joyfully and without inhibition . . . pounding, smashing, flattening clay . . . silently sifting sand through tiny fingers . . . there are a myriad of expressions in play. Play will differ depending on early life experiences from infancy to toddlerhood, as well as cultural background and ethnicity, the child's temperament, and the child's lifestyle and unique "way of being."

How a child uses his time in CCPT will be different from child to child, and from session to session. Knowing this, the skilled child-centered therapist is careful not to place judgment on the child's play, and to remain steady and consistent in providing the core conditions of empathy, genuineness, and unconditional positive regard. She uses what she knows about counseling to connect with each child she serves as an individual first and foremost, and thereby reaches—one by one—a diverse group of amazing, courageous children.

## Activities for Further Study

The following activities provide opportunities for contemplation and academic practice of critical key concepts. They can be completed alone, with a partner, or in a small group or classroom.

- *Activity A:* Reread the Application Focus Scenarios. Journal alone or discuss with a group of peers the difficulties that you think you might encounter as the play therapist in this scenario. Consider the pitfalls thinking about treatment errors that some novice play therapists might fall into. Then see our thoughts on this in Skill Support Resource H.

- *Activity B:* Discern and describe the difficulties that you expect to need to overcome related to providing CCPT across cultures, including your "buttons" that you think some children's behavior may push. This activity is particularly helpful to discuss with peers, if possible.

- *Activity C:* To further develop your understanding of diversity as it applies to a child-centered approach to counseling, we suggest that you read, consider, and discuss with others "Person-Centered Counseling: The Culture Within" (Glauser & Bozarth, 2001).

- *Activity D:* We also recommend for reading, consideration, and group discussion, two articles by C. H. Patterson: "Multicultural Counseling: From Diversity to Universality" (1996) and "Do We Need Multicultural Counseling Competencies?" (2004).

- *Activity E:* Immerse yourself in the study of cultures, and experiences in communities, churches, and school systems *other than those that feel common and familiar to you.* Discuss with others your feelings after taking part in a religious service in a church (or place of worship) or visiting a school system or community that is culturally unusual or not familiar to you.

- *Activity F:* Read articles and books by those counselors, play therapists, and teachers who have worked with and have extensive experience with children in cultures different from their own. A suggested book chapter is Geri Glover's (2001) "Cultural Considerations in Play Therapy," found in Landreth (2001).

- *Activity G:* If you plan to work predominantly with children with special needs, three excellent resources to review are Karla Carmichael's (1994) article, "Play Therapy for Children with Physical Disabilities," "Play Therapy with Learning Disabled Children" by Louise Guerney (1979), and "Using a Person-Centered Approach with Children Who Have Disability" by W. C. Williams and George S. Lair (1991).

- *Activity H:* Educate yourself! Search, find, and review journal articles for further education to include play therapy work with children with autism spectrum disorders, homelessness, physical disabilities, learning and developmental disabilities, medical conditions, and/or other differences and special situations that you expect to encounter in your work.

- *Activity I:* Discuss the broader concept of diversity to incorporate the following statements from Boy and Pine (1995): "The Child Has a Right to Be Different" (p. 210) and "The counselor accepts differences in the child because the counselor knows that where differences cannot be accepted, individuals cannot be" (p. 211), as well as "The Rights of Children in Counseling" (pp. 206–214). If you have access to Boy and Pine, you can see that we highly recommend their perspective. If not, work alone or with peers to discern the meanings you make/your views related to the topic titles in the quotes above following your study of this chapter.

- *Activity J:* Work alone or with a partner/small group to generate as many examples of potential significant cultural differences, and differences in value sets that you may encounter (or have already encountered) in your counseling work in communities. Include descriptions of different communities, client populations, and specific setting contexts (schools, agencies, shelters, residential care settings). Share your personal reactions and self-reflections for overcoming difficulties that you anticipate encountering in reaching out across cultural differences and differences in value sets to reach all children in need of counseling.

- *Activity K:* Learn more about cultural and religious differences through the reading of more general sources on culture and psychotherapy such as the classic text, *Ethnicity and Family Therapy* (McGoldrick, Giordano, & Garcia-Preto, 2005).
- *Activity L:* Revisit the Primary Skill Objectives for this chapter and see if you have mastered them to your satisfaction at this time. If not, seek additional readings, practices, and discussions for clarification, and in order to master them to your satisfaction.

# Legal and Ethical Issues From a Child-Centered Perspective

|  |
| --- |
| *16* |
| Chapter |

*The issues are: (1) accountability, (2) evaluating counseling, (3) the rights of children in counseling, (4) the rights of the counselor, (5) the use of information in counseling, (6) cognitive therapies, (7) counseling and testing, and (8) psychodiagnosis. They are issues of justice, fairness, objectivity, judgment, equal treatment, and respect for the person, especially the child with problems. . . . To child-centered counselors, counseling's response to these issues represents the future of the profession.*
—*Angelo Boy and Gerald Pine*

## Application Focus Issues

In the intake, Ms. McAdams anxiously describes the opposition that her son Seth shows toward both her at home and teachers in school. She is at a loss to explain what is the source of his misbehavior and expresses some concern that nothing will help him. Ms. McAdams agrees to bring Seth for play therapy sessions, but asks, "Will you tell me what he does in each session so I can understand what is going on with him and can I watch some of the sessions?" The therapist responds empathically to Ms. McAdams' concerns for her son and desire to know what is underlying his behavior. Following this, the therapist explains that although Ms. McAdams has a right to know the details of such sessions, that her agreeing to grant her son privacy with regard to what is expressed in sessions is likely to be important for progress to occur. The therapist assures Ms. McAdams that she will be notified immediately if anything disclosed in sessions results in concern by the therapist for the safety of her child or others, and commits to meeting with her regularly to share information with each other about progress being made at home, school, and in therapy sessions. Ms. McAdams seems satisfied and agrees to this arrangement.

After completing an initial intake session with Mr. and Ms. Collins, a professional counselor assesses that filial therapy (FT) would be a really good fit for treating the Collins family. The counselor has recently taken a two-day training in FT, but has not had any practical experience with the method. The counselor decides to contact a local therapist she knows who has practiced the approach for a number of years in order to get supervision with what will be her first case providing FT.

Dr. Ranasinghe has mostly utilized cognitive behavioral strategies in a practice consisting of mostly older children. He has recently completed an extensive training program in child-centered play therapy and wishes to begin working with younger children with the method. He has worked with about a dozen children under the supervision of a Registered Play Therapist-Supervisor (RPT-S) who specializes in CCPT, so he believes that he has basic competence with the method. However, he has never worked with children who have experienced physical or sexual abuse, and he expects that as he begins to take more play therapy referrals he will inevitably begin to work with such children. He decides to take some additional workshop training pertaining to play therapy with abused children. In addition, he arranges to consult with his previous CCPT supervisor in the event that he needs help in determining whether a given child's play suggests that abuse has occurred.

Ms. Uru has recently taken a job as an elementary school counselor. She is working with a child who frequently throws temper tantrums and shows signs of being angry and depressed. The working policy of the school is to place all such children on behavioral plans as the exclusive treatment. Trained as a child-centered play therapist, Ms. Uru is concerned that although utilizing a behavioral program may address the child's behavior, it may not address the underlying emotional distress of the child that is the foundation of the tantrums. She approaches the school principal, explains her concerns, and gains permission to utilize CCPT in addition to the implementation of the behavioral plan.

## Chapter Overview and Summary

Both laws and ethical principles guide child-centered play therapists in their efforts to provide the highest quality services to children. Play therapists are governed not only by laws established by state licensing boards and ethical guidelines developed by national-level professional associations for therapists in general, but also by more specific laws and guidelines related to the provision of services to children, specialty guidelines related to play therapy in general, and the values underlying the therapeutic approaches which therapists choose to utilize. Ultimately, it is the therapist's own personal moral code integrated with such laws and ethical guidelines that ensure children and parents receive the best care, rather than the "minimum" necessary to meet professional obligations.

This chapter examines the major legal and ethical issues governing the child-centered play therapist including informed consent, confidentiality, mandated reporting of child abuse and neglect, note taking and maintenance of records, and ensuring professional competence. This chapter is not meant to serve as a comprehensive introduction to ethical and legal issues facing therapists in general, or even child/play therapists more specifically, but should serve to sensitize the reader to how a child-centered play therapist approaches and integrates ethical principles and legal guidelines for these areas into their work with children.

## Primary Skill Objectives

The following Primary Skill Objectives for this chapter are provided to guide you through the chapter and for reflection and review after completing the chapter reading. By reading and reflecting on chapter information, you will:

1. Develop an understanding of the various levels of ethical principles governing the practice of child-centered play therapy including: state laws, national organizations, specific ethical principles applying to work with children, specialty guidelines related to play therapy, acting consistently with regard to principles underlying the child-centered play therapy methodology, and honoring and acting in accord with one's own personal moral code and values.

2. Be able to understand the importance of the informed consent process and to identify the components of the informed consent process.

3. Be able to distinguish between confidentiality as a right of the parent and privacy granted to the child as a necessary condition for effective therapy.

4. Become aware of legal and ethical responsibilities related to the mandated reporting of child abuse and neglect.

5. Develop a basic understanding of what makes a competent child-centered play therapist and why ongoing supervision is important.

6. Develop an awareness of how the values underlying CCPT impact the way that the therapist meets legal and ethical responsibilities.

# The Importance of Ethical Principles and Legal Guidelines

Ethical principles and legal guidelines preserve the rights of those receiving therapeutic services and encourage play therapists to provide high standards of care consistent with best practices in the field. Legal guidelines are generally promulgated through state laws governing the practice of a given profession (e.g., psychologist, clinical social worker, and professional counselor), but recently federal laws have also begun to influence mental health practice (e.g., Health Insurance Portability and Accountability Act of 1996 [HIPAA]). Compliance with such state and federal laws is enforced with the full force of law.

Play therapists are also bound by codes of conduct, ethical principles and guidelines of national professional associations that they voluntarily join, such as the American Psychological Association (2002), National Association of Social Workers (2008), American Counseling Association (2005), and American Association of Marriage and Family Therapists (2001). In addition, specialty practice professional associations such as the Association for Play Therapy offer more play therapy-specific ethical guidance for play therapists (e.g., "APT Play Therapy Best Practices" [2009a], "APT Paper on Touch" [2009b]). Such guidelines established by national and state level professional associations often influence what are considered the minimal "customary standards of care" and the exemplary "best practices and standards," as well as influencing state and federal laws. Therefore, ignoring such professional association guidelines may ultimately result in either legal consequences or civil lawsuits.

Ethical principles, codes of conducts, and state and federal laws are all generally founded on a set of values regarding what is due the client. These values include beneficence and nonmalfeasance (i.e. "do good and do no harm"), fidelity and responsibility, integrity, justice, and respect for people's rights and dignity (APA, 2002). These basic values underlie the aspirations of each of the mental health professions, all therapeutic formats (i.e., individual, marital, family, group therapies), and specific therapeutic methodologies (e.g., play therapy). However, the practice of each therapist is also governed by *her own set of personal values and ethical principles*, as well as the ethical principles specific to the therapeutic methods that she chooses to use with clients. Indeed, often therapists choose a particular approach, like CCPT, because it is congruent with their own personal ethical code.

## Specific Values of the Child-Centered Play Therapy Method

Child-centered play therapists and counselors share with all mental health professionals the values of "do good and do no harm," fidelity and responsibility, integrity, justice, and respect for people's dignity, and these values guide their practice. In addition to these shared values, a central value of CCPT is the view of the child as a person with profound capacity for change and growth, and as such emphasizes fostering the development of foundational human capacities such as self-awareness and self-expression, coping skills, self-control, developing positive views of self and others, perception of self-efficacy/competence, ability to value and develop secure relationships with others, and to freely make choices and decisions that are prosocial.

CCPT also adopts a holistic view of the person. As such, CCPT certainly appreciates that certain childhood (and adult) problems are strongly influenced by biological factors and may require medication. In addition, given its emphasis on the potential for growth and development, CCPT sees value in therapeutic approaches which utilize skills training perspectives such as parent skills training which enhances parent's human capacities and cognitive behavioral therapies with older children that enhance children's cognitive strategies for coping. However, child-centered play therapists and counselors are concerned that such interventions are often used in a reductionistic manner simply to control behavior or reduce symptoms. Often, treatment is discontinued once symptoms are relieved, but before positive personality growth is experienced, thus the more foundational capacities of the child or parent and capacity for growth and development are neglected. Therefore, the CCPT approach may include in the treatment plan a referral for medication, parent education, or the teaching of social skills, but these will be seen as *augmenting* the use of CCPT or FT aimed at fostering personality growth.

In interactions with parents and children, CCPT strongly values the use of relationship to foster growth and change. The therapeutic relationship is not simply a foundation for doing therapy, it is part of the therapy. The therapeutic relationship is not primarily one of doctor to patient, or expert advisor, or teacher, but is a relationship that allows the parent or child to shape the direction of therapy.

These values of the CCPT shape all aspects of the therapeutic relationship. They shape the intake interview, treatment planning, and implementation. They also are integrated with and color the way in which the CCPT views and implements ethical principles in the areas of informed consent, confidentiality and privacy, mandated reporting of suspected child abuse, note taking and record maintenance, and ensuring professional competency.

## Informed Consent

Informed consent is a process by which a mental health professional provides the client with information relevant to making a free and informed choice whether or not to enter into a therapeutic relationship with the therapist. The informed consent process generally begins with a discussion of the limits of confidentiality that is held prior to any self-disclosure by the client so that the client realizes possible repercussions of sharing certain types of information. The process continues throughout the initial intake interview and includes providing the client with information about the therapist's qualifications for providing services, fees and agency/setting policies, treatment recommendations and possible alternative treatments, possible risks and anticipated benefits of treatment, and expected duration of treatment. Informed consent is not a one-time event. The therapist and client give and receive feedback throughout the therapeutic process and discuss whether to continue or modify the initial treatment plan, and ultimately decide when to end the therapeutic relationship.

Because the ability to fully understand and freely consent to treatment requires developmental capacities not generally possessed by children, ethical guidelines and state/federal laws delegate to parents the responsibility for making decisions about participation in treatment. Given their deep respect for the child and her developing capacities, the play therapist attempts to involve the child in the informed consent process in a manner appropriate to the child's developmental level. Given the core values underlying CCPT and those who practice it, and the emphasis of CCPT on fostering freedom and self-determination, it should be noted that the play therapist does not treat the informed consent process as a mere formality and does not allow a lax casualness to creep into the process. Because CCPT values hold equally in interactions with both children and adults, the play therapist sees the informed consent process as something owed to both the parent and child as persons with dignity.

## Respecting the Confidentiality Rights of the Parent and the Privacy of the Child

Privacy is a constitutional right of an individual to decide for himself whether or not and what private information he wishes to reveal to others. In the mental health field, respect for client's privacy has been mandated through state and federal laws and ethical guidelines of professional associations by means of the client's right to confidentiality. With few exceptions such laws and guidelines forbid mental health professionals from releasing client records, videotaping sessions, or discussing information about the client unless prior permission has been obtained from the client. Laws governing confidentiality vary from state to state, but, in general, exceptions are made for the mandated reporting of child abuse and neglect and for taking action when there are threats to the safety/life of the client (e.g., imminent threat of suicide), and often when the client is threatening the life of others.

In most cases, states view the parent or the child's legal guardian—not the child—as the holder of the right to confidentiality. For the mental health professional this means that the parent has a right to know what goes on in the child's therapy session and to access the child's clinical case record. Although the child-centered play therapist has deep respect for the parent's concern for their children and their desire to be kept informed of the therapeutic progress and/or be involved in the treatment of their children, the therapist is also aware that the creation of the very conditions that make therapeutic change possible—unconditional acceptance, not feeling judged, no threat of shame, freedom to express difficult things, ability to make decisions and test or break limits, and feeling free to engage in fantasy play with both Aggressive and Regressive themes—may be difficult or impossible to accomplish if children do not feel the basic content of sessions will be kept private.

It is important for the therapist to have an open discussion at the intake, as part of the informed consent process, about the reasoning for why there is a need for the child's sessions to be kept private. In most cases, if the therapist assures the parents that they will be kept informed of general therapeutic progress and that the parent will be notified immediately if the therapist concerns about the safety and welfare of their child arise, then parents will be willing to grant privacy for the child's sessions. The therapist should note the parents' agreement to allowing privacy for the child in their clinical case note.

In cases where the parent will not agree to grant privacy, then the therapist may decide that in some cases it would not be clinically sound (and possibly also against the therapist's own value system) to commit to seeing the child individually in CCPT. However, in such cases, if the parent is willing to be involved in the treatment of the child, then the therapist may recommend filial therapy, parent skills training, or some other form of family therapy, assuming that the therapist assesses that such treatments would be appropriate for the parent/family.

## Mandated Reporting of Suspected Child Abuse and Neglect

All states have laws governing the mandated reporting of child abuse and neglect by mental health professionals. However, states vary in terms of the criteria for when reports must be made as well as the procedures for reporting. Therefore, it is very important for play therapists to know their state laws. Although state laws vary in their criteria for mandated reporting, many states require mental health professional to contact Child Protective Services (CPS) departments whenever there is "reasonable suspicion" of child abuse (physical or sexual) or neglect. Once the criterion of "reasonable suspicion" is reached, in general the responsibility of the play therapist is to file a report with CPS which then takes over the investigation, rather than the mental health professional engaging in an investigation which if done incorrectly could jeopardize the criminal case against the abuser.

Because the determination of "reasonable suspicion" resides with the mental health professional, and the negative consequences for either failing to report when abuse is occurring or for reporting when no abuse has occurred is great, it is important that mental health professionals responsibly seek out education in the area of child abuse and neglect as well as mandated reporting of sexual abuse (Kalichman, 1999; Lau, Kraus, & Morse, 2008). Given that CCPT and many other play therapies involve children's expression through symbolic play, and since not all symbolic play containing themes of violence toward the child or sexual themes is indicative of physical abuse or sexual abuse of the child, it is important for play therapists to seek education through reading and attendance at workshops pertaining to how physical and sexual abuse appear in play sessions. When in doubt, it is always wise for the play therapist, whether highly experienced or new to play therapy, to consult with a trusted colleague to ensure that the best decision is made.

In keeping with child-centered values (and more broadly person-centered values), when the criterion for mandated threshold has been reached and reporting is required, the play therapist may decide to involve the parent(s) along with the therapist in making the call to CPS (especially if the parent(s) is not likely the source of the abuse), unless doing so may place the child in danger. This process can allow the parent to take an active role in the protection of their child.

## Ethical Issues Regarding Case Notes and Record Maintenance

A common concern of mental health professionals of all experience levels is the determination of what to put in one's clinical notes. This issue is made even more complex when documenting CCPT sessions in which much of the content of sessions is symbolic expression through play by the child rather than direct verbalizations by the client or directive actions taken by the therapist, as would be the case in adult therapies or structured child therapies. However, CCPT shares the same purposes for documenting therapy sessions as therapists working with adults or using different child therapy methods:

1. To record therapeutic progress for one's own use
2. To record the therapeutic progress in a form that can be understandable to other mental health professions who currently or will in the future work with the child
3. To document decision making and actions taken by the therapist on behalf of the client to plan and implement treatment, comply

with state laws and ethical principles, assess and ameliorate risk to the client or others, and terminate treatment

4. To adhere to good risk management strategies

Since the play therapist is governed by the principle of "do no harm" and because the clinical case record may be read by other therapists, parents, and even lawyers, the play therapist must compose case notes in a manner which is both understandable and not likely to be misinterpreted, cause unnecessary concern, or be misused (e.g., legal proceedings). In general, this means that the CCPT must not record the "raw" data of the sessions, which may be provocative and would likely be provocative for parents, misinterpreted by other mental health professionals not familiar with CCPT, and misused in legal proceedings; instead, the case notes should include the therapist's understanding of what themes or therapeutic issues are represented by the symbolic play. Although the CCPT therapist is ultimately interested in the personality growth of the child, it is both wise and collegial for the therapist to also link such themes to therapeutic goals that are shared in common with other therapists (e.g., concrete behavioral goals). The therapist should also avoid using terms that would be understandable to other child-centered play therapists, but not parents or other professionals (e.g. "the child is in the Aggressive stage") unless such terms are given context.

### *Example of a problematic case note entry:*

Johnny engaged in a role-play in which he was the student and the therapist was the teacher. When told he had to do a class assignment, he told the teacher to "shut up." He instructed the therapist (as teacher) to continue to demand that the student do the class assignment and then he took a dart gun out and pretended to shoot the teacher while saying "die!" He repeated this scene numerous times. Toward the end of the session, he varied the scene and instead of pretending to shoot the teacher he threw a block at the therapist (in the role of the teacher). When the therapist set a limit against throwing the block at her, Johnny angrily replied, "That rule is stupid and you are stupid," but he did comply and did not throw another block. Johnny is in the Aggressive stage at the present.

Because a parent or even another child therapist who does not understand the child-centered approach might be confused about the freedom granted to the child to verbally insult the therapist and to express aggression in fantasy role-plays, this note is problematic. It would not be helpful in informing a future mental health professional about therapeutic progress and, if read by the parent, might cause embarrassment to the parent and possible repercussions for the child. A better case note entry would be as follows:

Johnny's play included themes of frustration and anger when others ask him to do things he doesn't like to do, and themes of desires to be in control. However, during the session, when the therapist set a limit, although Johnny did verbally express his frustration with the limit, he did comply, rather than continuing to test and/or break the limit, as in other sessions. This suggests that Johnny is beginning to develop the capacity for verbal self-expression as an alternative to reactively acting out. This is a movement in the direction of self-control, and when generalized to home would be expected to decrease the frequency of noncompliance to parental requests and tantrums. The themes in today's session are ones typically seen in the second (of the four) stages of the child-centered play therapy process in which issues of control and self-control are worked through.

In addition to questions concerning what to put in the clinical case note is how long one needs to store a clinical record once the child stops treatment. Each state has its own requirement regarding both the length of time records must remain accessible to the client or client's guardian. Some states set a specific number of years past the date the case is closed as the dates when records can be destroyed. Other states allow records to be destroyed some period after the child reaches majority. In addition, the federal HIPAA guidelines, which govern many mental health professionals, establish not only requirements for length of time but also the manner in which records are stored, and mandate that mental health professionals comply with the most stringent of the requirements when state and federal requirements differ. In short, it is important that you be familiar with both your state laws and federal HIPAA guidelines (web site: www.hhs.gov/ocr/hipaa/).

## Becoming a Competent Child-Centered Play Therapist

Child-centered play therapists as mental health professionals are required to be competent in the knowledge and skill areas required to provide high-quality services that meet the needs of children and families. These areas of competence include assessment and diagnosis, treatment planning, play therapy skills, and the skills to work cooperatively with parents and other professionals who impact children's lives and/or are part of an overall treatment plan. Child-centered play therapists must possess knowledge and skills of their broader mental health profession, *and* must also possess the general knowledge and skills necessary for working with children and families, as well as CCPT methods.

## Competence in Assessment and Diagnosis

Given the child-centered play therapist's deep respect for the uniqueness of each child and the inherent potential to grow and develop, there is a natural reluctance to use diagnostic labels, which imply that the child can be identified as simply an exemplar of a specific childhood disorder. Diagnostic labels also have a tendency to be casually and sometimes even disrespectfully used to describe human beings, and once diagnostic labels are given, they can often "stick" with the child even though the child experiences considerable growth and change. Nonetheless, it would be inaccurate to say that the therapist is not obligated to become an expert at utilizing standardized assessment instruments and using diagnostic criteria such as the DSM-IV-TR (APA, 2000) in order to understand childhood problems. Knowledge of both normal child development and child psychopathology enables the therapist to determine whether play therapy is appropriate as a primary or adjunctive treatment methodology, and when play therapy is the primary treatment, it allows the therapist to formulate a comprehensive treatment plan. However, in the play therapy sessions themselves, such diagnostic labels must not influence the therapist's perception of and respect for the uniqueness of each child, nor be allowed to impact the therapist's hopeful and positive anticipation of growth in the child.

## Competence in Treatment Planning

Although the child-centered play therapist will often choose CCPT, or its family level version, FT, as the primary treatment method, the competent child-centered play therapist understands the necessity of viewing childhood problems from a comprehensive and systemic perspective. Many childhood problems require other interventions with parents and teachers in addition to play therapy. Some childhood problems will require school interventions, some a focus on relationship between parents (e.g., couples therapy or parent counseling), and some may require medical interventions (e.g., prescription of medication by a psychiatrist). In some cases, a referral for extensive psychological and/or neuropsychological testing may need to be made in order to gather more information about the strength and deficit areas for the child, and to better understand the emotional functioning of the child so that all the needs of the child are addressed. The therapist must avoid professional "laziness" by assuming that CCPT or FT will always be the only intervention needed. In order to practice in an ethically competent manner, this means that the therapist must know when to refer to other professionals and must develop cooperative relationships with such referral sources.

## Competence in CCPT Skills

The three hallmarks of developing competency include education, training, and supervision in a method. Reading the current text is a good example of education. However, to be competent in CCPT requires that a therapist seek out additional education, training, and supervision opportunities. Given that CCPT is one of the most widely utilized play therapy methodologies, postgraduate continuing education workshops are offered by professional organizations, freestanding play therapy training institutes, and university-based play therapy centers. The web site of the Association for Play Therapy (APT; www.a4pt.org) maintains a fairly comprehensive listing of play therapy training opportunities both in terms of graduate-level course instruction and post-graduate continuing education; however, since this organization promotes all play therapy, it is important to verify which sites offer training specifically in CCPT.

We want to emphasize the importance of getting supervision as you begin to apply the CCPT method with children. Although CCPT is a very accessible approach in terms of its basic theory and skills, which is why even parents can be trained to use it with their own children in FT, nonetheless, to acquire the level of mastery required for a mental health professional to use it confidently and effectively with children experiencing a wide variety of problems requires a period of supervision to attain. Again, the APT web site has resources for locating a RPT-S, but the reader will need to inquire whether a given supervisor utilizes CCPT and, if desired, more specifically the Guerney variation of CCPT.

Table 16.1 **Keys to Developing Competencies as a Child-Centered Play Therapist**

1. Broad training in a mental health profession (e.g., clinical social worker, professional counselor)
2. Education in the assessment and diagnosis of childhood disorders and problems
3. Competence in treatment planning (i.e., determining the appropriate intervention(s) for a given child)
4. Basic training and education in CCPT (e. g., college courses, workshops, training programs)
5. Supervised practice of CCPT with clients by competent play therapy supervisors
6. Lifelong learning (e.g., ongoing peer and self-supervision, books, continuing education courses)

In addition, there are a number of play therapy training institutes that provide not only basic and advanced training in CCPT, but also intensive supervision in the method. The National Institute for Relationship Enhancement (NIRE) provides excellent basic and advanced CCPT training and supervision, based on the Guerney approach, and closely matched to this book.

## Summary

Mental health professionals enter the field because they want to help their clients. State and federal laws, ethical guidelines formulated by national and state professional associations as well as specialty professional associations, help to form the values underlying various therapeutic methods which help to ensure clients receive the best quality care. Becoming familiar with laws and ethical guidelines in the areas of informed consent; confidentiality; mandated reporting, note taking, and record keeping; and ensuring professional competence are essential to good practice. In addition studying comprehensive texts on both professional ethics (Bersoff, 2008; Koocher & Keith-Spiegel, 2008) and professional risk management (Bennett et al., 2006) can help the therapist develop skills in ethical reasoning and judgment and elevate the quality of one's practice.

However, one's own principles and the values underlying therapeutic methods which you choose to use as a therapist significantly and profoundly influence the nature of the therapist–client relationship, the assessment process, and treatment planning and implementation. Accordingly, choosing to utilize therapeutic methodologies founded on values and understandings of the person consistent and congruent with your own personal values is a powerful combination.

## Activities for Further Study

- *Activity A:* For one or more of the major ethical principles covered in this chapter (e.g., informed consent, professional competency, etc.), read and compare the ethical guidelines of the American Counseling Association, American Psychological Association, American Association of Marriage and Family Therapists, and National Association of Social Workers. Each is accessible online.

- *Activity B:* Reread Chapters 3 and 4. In what ways are the values and theoretic underpinnings of the child-centered approach similar to your own, and in which ways do they differ?

- *Activity C:* Choose one of the major profession's ethical guidelines (e.g., American Psychological Association), choose a section of the guidelines, read it, and then think about how a child-centered play therapist might rewrite the guideline to make it more consistent with CCPT.

# Your Ongoing Development

### 17
#### Chapter

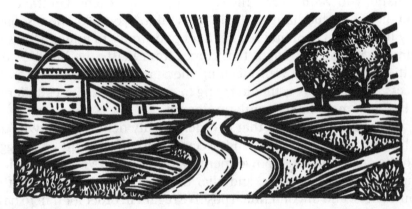

Figure 17.1

> On the way to becoming a play therapist, one must understand oneself,
> one's own beliefs, attitudes, values, the qualities of one's being, the nature
> of one's life, one's internal proclivities, resources, and tendencies, and
> external talents and skills. To know oneself in truth and fully is the direct
> path to being receptive to and knowing others.
>
> —Clark Moustakas

## Application Focus Issue 1

A few years or a few weeks into your use of CCPT, you will meet the
child or family that confounds or discourages you. Variations of people
and predicaments are infinite. So our guidance, no matter how comprehensive, cannot be complete.

And there will also be the times of your own personal struggle—
where you begin to lose heart—and it becomes painfully difficult to

accept the at times tragic circumstances that children you want to help have endured. So how do you continue to adjust, grow, and develop? This chapter provides guidance for self-care and personal development as you face the ongoing challenges of being a child advocate and providing child-centered play therapy (CCPT).

## Application Focus Issue 2

There is a paradox inherent with the child-centered approach. On the one hand, you want to end the suffering of each client. On the other hand, if you try too hard to "fix it" or "end it," you take the responsibility from your client and restrict her opportunity to find the blessing of greater personal strength that comes from mastering her life's difficulties. While many well-meaning therapists attempt to "hurry the process," the paradox is that in trying to end the child client's suffering for her, you may inadvertently prolong it.

A paradox of CCPT is that in order to truly help children who are in distress, you must allow and accept a certain amount of struggle with the angst and disempowerment that the child *feels*. You must join your client in his struggles, and offer the core conditions of empathy, genuineness, and unconditional positive regard in order for him to have the opportunity to tap into internal resources and find his "own way." It is counterintuitive but true.

As a result, there is a risk that you will eventually experience symptoms of counselor burnout, and as frequently happens in this type of burnout, you will try to *do* more to take over your clients' lives—in false expectation of being able to "find a quick fix" or "end the suffering." Your faith in the child's ability to "lead the way" will waver, and you will look for another path—a path you choose for the child.

Addressing your ongoing development consciously and proactively can simultaneously prevent these type errors of counselor burnout and develop you into a maximally effective agent of positive change for children, families, schools, and communities. For this reason, please consider the guidance for ongoing development of this chapter.

## Primary Skill Objectives

- Consider and plan for mastering your CCPT skills, developing your confidence, and satisfaction in your work.

- Consider, value, and plan your strategies for ongoing study, supervision, and support from like-minded colleagues.
- Consider and plan your development of "wrap-around" skills that make sense in your anticipated context.
- Consider your self-care from the perspective of the ways you care for your clients in CCPT, including self-empathy, self-acceptance, using limitations wisely, and the "empathy sandwich."

## Chapter Overview

From our experience, as well as that of our supervisees, peers, and continued learning from our colleagues and the literature of our professions, we see the keys to developing for excellent and sustained work as:

1. Mastering efficient CCPT skills through supervised experience and training

2. Building confidence through experiencing success and measuring outcomes

3. Seeking qualified supervision as well as the collegiality of like-minded peers

4. Developing wrap-around skills, as well as studying in areas that support your work

5. Caring for yourself as you would your clients—through self-empathy and realization of your own limitations

In this chapter, we offer our thoughts and recommendations in these and related areas.

## Mastering CCPT Skills and Developing Confidence and Satisfaction in the Work

Following your study of CCPT with this book, as a qualified mental health professional, you should be ready to begin applying your CCPT skills. But as you can see, the work of a child-centered play therapist is both simple and complex. You don't have the pressure of needing to know little Johnny's way out of his internal predicament because as you facilitate, Johnny "knows the way." Yet, you have many decisions to make in what are often fast paced sessions: which questions to answer and which to let him struggle with, which of his requests or commands will facilitate self-expression if followed, and which may inhibit his self-expression. And you have balances to achieve: how much to track and when, involvement in role-play vs. more observational empathic responding, limits that facilitate self-expression vs. limits that prohibit self-expression. Many days you will leave play therapy feeling calmly meditative, satisfied, and content. But just as your client's important work is not usually easy for him, you may also leave some play therapy sessions physically or emotionally drained and scratching your head, not really sure if you made the best decisions and maintained the best balances.

We found that such feelings of confusion and uncertainty in our work decreased over time, and as we developed as therapists through experience and supervision, our satisfaction increased. But, of course, our greater feelings of satisfaction with our works in play therapy were not accidental. We have continually worked to master our skills to efficiency. Then, seeing our clients succeed, we gained confidence and an ability to stay steady in the work.

> For when I accept what is, and I am not clinging to what used to be or wishing for what might be, I can step into doing what I can for myself and others, which helps bring me peace of mind . . . the antidote to despair.
>
> —*Anonymous*

## Ongoing Study and Self-Care

We have continually studied the child-centered approach, person-centered and related theories, child development, and the nature of play and families. We find that there is *always more to learn* and we constantly find new writing, concepts, or ideas from others that inspire, encourage, or challenge us to think in new ways, or to *be* better.

Every therapist's or counselor's path of ongoing study for self-development should be a unique search for meaning, work, and personal support. For us, our "studies" supporting our work in play therapy and our self-care have included such seemingly unrelated areas as our personal development in meditation, spirituality, time spent outdoors, time spent with loved ones, and even time spent relating to and playing with our dogs! From meditation we have learned that one can find calm, focus, and acceptance in the midst of almost anything. To us, this can also be true from some approaches to spirituality, that by acknowledging a higher power we find strength in accepting what we have no power over, and in simply doing what we can do to make the world a better place. Time spent outdoors often reminds us of the interconnectedness of all things in life and gives us a sense of humility. From our dogs, we receive many lessons in the power of unconditional positive regard, and from our loved ones we learn from many opportunities to give and receive love in relationship. We encourage you to find and develop your personal sources of strength as well.

## Supervision and Support

We readily seek supervision and the support of like-minded colleagues and friends. We found that initial supervision in graduate school was incredibly important. And we've found postgraduate supervision or training toward specific certification additionally important to building efficient skills and depth of understanding. We also think that this process never ends. We stay continually involved in our fields and professional associations and we continue to make new friends who we find to be "further down the path," whatever one's individual path may be unfolding to be, and we find new energy, challenge, and excitement when we meet those new friends.

## The Importance of Measuring Progress and Research

We also encourage you to carefully measure your client's progress. Whenever possible, go even further than the clinical, individual studies required for good work, described in Chapters 11 and 12, to measures of your client's progress that approach empiricism. Research your work and measure the outcomes of your programs. Just like the caregivers in your clients' lives may sometimes, out of caring, see no progress until they can "know with certainty that the child they care deeply for will live happily ever after," you may fall into this same trap of absolute thinking that discards the positive. Out of deep caring, you may also find yourself dissatisfied with your work unless you can know that *all* your clients will "live happily ever after." Many a caring counselor or teacher remembers much more strongly the client or student whose negative environment overwhelmed all attempts at progress, than all the many students or clients who progressed to well-being and mastered self-control in "out-of-control" environments. Strong research and program evaluation, on your own or in partnership with others who have greater skills for research, is an excellent antidote for the negativity syndrome, as well as an excellent way to clarify the power of your work to the stakeholders of your community.

## The Challenges, Meanings, and Opportunities of Connection and Caring

There have also been times in our work that we left sessions feeling our clients' pain in ways that were hard to shake. While this should not overwhelm a child-centered therapist—if it does, you may be off-track in your work—we also would not expect this to ever go away completely. If you are connecting with your clients with deep empathy, you will very likely be affected by your client's life situation and emotional experience. Deepening our understandings of the approach through ongoing study helps us to put our clients' experiences in perspective. Supervision and the support of like-minded friends and colleagues have also helped each of us gain and maintain useful, self-sustaining perspectives as therapists and counselors.

Overall, children in CCPT are most often quite happy—glad to be there. The risk of emotional upset for the child-centered therapist comes not from sitting with clients in pain, which is more common in work with adults, but from realizing all that has not yet been "fixed" or improved in a child's environment. The threat to burnout for child-centered play therapists usually comes from overfocus on children's external worlds.

Remember that CCPT works to strengthen the child for the world that he must live in, and it works to change his way of being and his behavior for the better. The child's change usually has a positive influence on his external world as well. But there are times that this is not or does not seem to be enough. In those moments, we urge you to use your "wrap-around" skills and advocacy skills to improve his external world. And with that said, we caution you not to get so caught up in this work that you convey to him that you think he is not strong enough to master his world. If you have done your work well in CCPT, he will be optimally ready to master his world. Maintain your demonstration of trust in him by staying true to your promise of providing a therapy hour that belongs to him, thereby keeping your focus significantly on his internal world.

# Developing Your "Wrap-Around" Skills

While CCPT is powerful and incredibly helpful in and of itself, no therapy or intervention ought to stand alone. Depending on your setting, a variety of "wrap-around" skills for outside the play sessions may be important, and beneficial.

When serving children, it is almost always supportive to help parents too, whether through brief consultations with attention to the parent–child relationship, parent skill training, or filial therapy. Across settings, it is also often helpful to be well skilled at consulting regarding effective behavior management plans. Especially if a child's mistaken behavior is potentially hurtful, the adult caregivers may have to manage or contain behavior while the child makes lasting progress in counseling.

Counselors in outpatient counseling agencies or private practice settings usually have greater access to parents, since someone has to bring the child to counseling. Counselors in schools may have fewer regular meetings with parents, but school settings offer other opportunities to intervene with teachers, peers, and administrators in systematic ways. Additionally, school counselors often take opportunities to teach inter- and intrapersonal mental health skills designed to help children at all ranges of difficulty, including normal developmental issues. We find that those lessons at times support the work of children whose difficulties warrant greater therapeutic interventions. We have occasionally noticed children in CCPT referencing what we knew to be topics of classroom guidance lessons. We took that to mean that while they were not able to incorporate the skills of the lesson at the time they were taught, after progress in CCPT they sometimes come back to the concepts as they become ready and able to incorporate them.

As you know, CCPT does not stand alone. It rests in a family of therapeutic approaches, stemming from the person-centered approach and extending to filial therapy and other approaches that utilize the power of the therapeutic relationship.

# Self-Care From the Child-Centered Perspective

We encourage you to strive to apply the same kinds of care you provide to your clients to yourself. Please don't take our guidance as a claim that we are able to do this all or even most of the time—but just that we strive to do so, and in difficult times have benefited from reminding one another to do so.

## Self-Empathy

Strive to let yourself feel what you feel, to learn from your feelings at existential levels, but mostly just to feel them. If you are hurt, then you are hurt. The hurt may teach you to avoid a certain situation or behavior, but a lot of intellectualizing and thinking about it may not teach you much more than simply feeling the hurt will. Contrary to feeling the hurt, many people will fear negative feelings, deny them, ignore them, or try to just make them go away, never allowing themselves to feel something that painful. That way of being is quite opposite to the opportunities provided clients in CCPT.

## Self-Acceptance

Strive to accept yourself in the ways you accept your clients. You are who you are at each time in your development. In each moment you make mistakes that you need to be aware of, mistakes that bring about negative feelings, if you let yourself feel them, that will help you grow to avoid the same mistakes again.

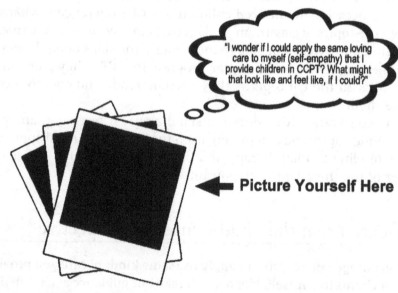

"I wonder if I could apply the same loving care to myself (self-empathy) that I provide children in CCPT? What might that look like and feel like, if I could?"

**◄─ Picture Yourself Here**

Figure 17.2

Similarly, your abilities, talents, and past choices are what they are. While it may be impossible to avoid comparisons to others, the comparisons really do not matter. In the end, each person simply is who he is, and each moment offers the opportunity to change to be who you most want to be.

Carl Rogers wrote that, "When I accept myself as I am, then I change" (Rogers, 1951, p. 17). We have looked at this statement as a paradox (Cochran & Cochran, 2006). If one accepts oneself just as is, why would one change? Part of the answer for us includes that without self-acceptance, one cannot see oneself. If one cannot see oneself, one cannot in reality *choose* the change. Another "Mr. Rogers"—in a book called *Life's Journeys: Things to Remember Along the Way*—is quoted as saying, "The toughest thing is to love somebody who has done something mean to you—especially when that somebody is yourself. Look inside yourself and find that loving part of you. Take good care of that part because it helps you love your neighbor" (Rogers, 2005, p. 99). These words of wisdom on self-acceptance are especially helpful in our self-care, growth, and ability to care for others.

## Using Limits Wisely

Try to think of your own mistakes in terms of a child's encountering a limit in CCPT. With self-empathy and self-acceptance, you will see your mistakes and be able to move on. For instance, we are all likely aware of the self-dialogue that often transpires when we've made a mistake that has hurt another. Afterwards, a common reaction in self-dialogue might go something like, "Oh, ugh! That was really awful of me! I really messed up and hurt that person's feelings." Rather than falling into this common self-chastising mode, next time try to think through an adult-to-self, out-of-session version of the "empathy sandwich." For example, you might say to yourself, "You really wanted to control that situation. In trying to feel in control, you acted in a way that hurt someone else's feelings. And now you feel guilty. One of the things you may not do is take over situations in such a way that you hurt others. Instead, you may . . . (make amends, be and act differently in specific ways, seek a different way of relating). [After a self-reflective pause] So, now you have a plan to move beyond this . . . and you're okay with that." While this "little talk with yourself" might at first seem strange, with use you will find that acceptance of yourself as human—capable of mistakes, and in need of empathy and limits, too—is personally beneficial to you and your work in providing CCPT.

# Seeking Like-Minded Others: Our Alphabet Soup of Favorite Supportive Organizations

A group of former students and developing child-centered play therapists were together by chance at an unrelated event. They were relieved to see and talk to each other, noting that they cannot really express to others outside the profession their joys at the little victories and milestones in CCPT, like when a very hard-to-warm-up child begins to soften and be comfortable in relating, or when a child who so clearly needs it, begins to shift from Warm-up and show some Aggressive/ Regressive Stage play. These students were learning the benefit of keeping regular contact with each other and/or with any like-minded professionals who deeply understand *what they are doing and why* in their sessions. In the following pages, we review (in alphabetical order— not indicating hierarchy) the professional associations that we most recommend for fellowship with and support from like-minded persons.

## Association for the Development of the Person-Centered Approach (ADPCA)

ADPCA is "an international network of individuals who support the development and application of the person-centered approach" (www. adpca.org), including CCPT. We have found its conferences to be exceptionally warm and also filled with genuine, "in the moment," person-to-person interactions. You can meet people there who deeply consider person-centered approaches, and strive to live and develop in person-centered ways. The annual meeting normally includes small and large group interactions, as well as scholarly and practice-based presentations and discussion groups. A list-serve is also provided for ongoing connections.

## Association for Filial and Relationship Enhancement Methods (AFREM)

AFREM is dedicated to the development and support of the methods and persons applying filial therapy (FT) and relationship enhancement (RE) methods. Its mission includes promoting the filial and RE approaches throughout the world "in order to develop healthy relationships, reconciliation, and peace in homes, workplaces, and society" (www.AFREM.org). Among the resources AFREM provides, its annual meeting always features excellent, advanced, and in-depth learning opportunities related to FT and RE.

## Association for Play Therapy (APT)

APT has, of course, done excellent work in promoting play therapy and its uses in the therapeutic care of children and families. APT publishes the *International Journal of Play Therapy*, and its annual conference can be seen as a meeting of the minds of the many good people and great ideas within the family of play therapy approaches.

## Counseling Association of Humanistic Education and Development (C-AHEAD)

C-AHEAD is the humanistic division of the American Counseling Association (ACA). C-AHEAD's logo is, "The Heart and Conscience of the ACA: Helping People Move Mountains" (www.c-ahead.com). C-AHEAD supports and embraces the family of humanistic approaches to counseling within ACA. A sampling of its signature foci and products include advocacy for counselor wellness as an important factor in therapeutic relationships and its wellness; a center providing hands-on growth opportunities for participants at each ACA conference; the *Journal of Humanistic Counseling, Education and Development;* and the Make a Difference Grant.

## National Institute of Relationship Enhancement (NIRE)

NIRE is perhaps the oldest institute training child-centered play thera-pists. It provides workshops, ongoing individualized training, and certi-fications of skill mastery in CCPT, filial therapy, and relationship enhancement therapy. It is a particularly excellent source of supervi-sion and training in the child-centered approach most closely matched to this book.

NIRE was founded in 1992 by Bernard Guerney, Jr. as a nonprofit educational corporation and a branch of its parent organization, the Institute for the Development of Emotional and Life Skills (IDEALS), which Dr. Guerney had previously founded in 1972. Its mission includes contributing to "the advancement of honesty, compassion, and under-standing in relationships by developing, teaching, and disseminating relationship enhancement skills for the benefit of the individual, the family, the community, and the workplace" (www.nire.org).

# World Association of Person-Centered and Experiential Psychotherapy and Counseling (WAPCEPC)

The world association aims "to provide a worldwide forum for professionals in science and practice who:

- have a commitment to the primary importance of the relationship between client and therapist in psychotherapy and counseling;
- hold as central to the therapeutic endeavor the client's actualizing process and phenomenological world;
- embody in their work those conditions and attitudes conducive to therapeutic movement first postulated by Carl Rogers;
- have a commitment to an understanding of both clients and therapists as persons, who are at the same time individuals in relationship with others and [are of] their diverse environments and cultures;
- have an openness to the development and elaboration of person-centered and experiential theory in the light of current and future practice and research (www.pce-world.org)."

Each WAPCEPC conference is held in a different part of the world. Its journal is *Person-Centered and Experiential Psychotherapies* (PCEP).

## Activity for Further Study and Development

This chapter is, of course, all about further study and development. A logical task toward that end is to be concrete and make a plan. Therefore, we suggest you draft and discuss with peers your plan for ongoing development as a child-centered play therapist. What might you read to continue your learning or where might you seek your material? Where, how, and when will you seek your supervision and ongoing training and the support of like-minded persons? How will you avoid burnout, and how will you care for yourself? Be as specific as possible and seek feedback from loved ones as you develop this plan. Write it down, and keep it close for guidance when needed.

## Skills Support Resource A

### From Chapter 5: Preparing Your Setting for Providing Child-Centered Play Therapy

*Some Sample "Solutions" for Setting Challenges Presented for Therapists and Counselors in the Application Focus Issue (Corrine, Maura, Javier, and Aliah)*
*Corrine:* Corrine found that most of her difficulties in her shared space with an adult counselor were easily dealt with through setting limits with empathy. She placed a large area rug with a bright jungle scene in her space, and with the more rambunctious children limited play to the "area on the jungle rug." When children would protest, or limit test by, for example, "accidentally" throwing the Nerf ball over into the more grown-up office space area, and wanting to go retrieve it, she was able to use empathy first, "you really want to throw the ball and go into the office area. In special playtime we stay on the jungle rug, and play over here." Once children learned this structural limit, they focused on their playtime very contented to stay in the designated play area of the office.

*Maura:* After speaking with her supervisor who viewed videotapes of Maura's sessions with children, she was reminded that she "is the best toy in the playroom." Her supervisor pointed out Maura's exceptional use of the CCPT skills necessary to structure and set limits when necessary, and then gave examples of instances when Maura's deep empathy, unconditional positive regard, and genuineness had come shining through! A colleague reminded her that many play therapists remain seated for play sessions in "rolling office chairs"—and that her wheelchair was much like this! Most of Maura's worries were due to some self-consciousness over being in a wheelchair. This was alleviated when she watched videotaped sessions and noticed that though the children had expressed some curiosity about her wheelchair, it did not hinder her ability to be a great child-centered play therapist.

*Javier:* After speaking with his supervisor, Javier tried installing "Parent Feedback Box" on the counter beside the checkout window at his agency. He explained to parents in the initial consultation that he would not be able to speak about their child in the waiting room, but that he would be glad to schedule a time with them at the office or by phone. He empathized with those parents who objected, and still wished to be heard during appointment time, but asked that they fill out a checklist or write down their concerns instead of speaking in front of the child in the waiting room. This worked to help Javier build relationships with the parents, and have a written record of their feedback as well. Some parents even reported that the act of writing it all down was helpful to them!

*Aliah:* Aliah found that in speaking to the school counselors at the schools, and getting to know the speech and language therapists, art and music teachers, and school psychologists serving her schools, she was able to secure and reserve some spaces that she routinely shared with them when they were not there. She made and laminated a "Counseling in Progress Until: *(Fill in Time)*—Please Do Not Disturb" sign to post on the door of whichever space she ended up in. She also purchased a folding screen, rug, and a "white noise" machine which she always had available in her car in case she was moved to a corner of the cafeteria for a day. After building relationships at the schools she served, this rarely happened, and her reserved spaces became more consistently available.

## Skills Support Resource B

## From Chapter 6: Practice Activity for Tracking and Empathic Responding

For the following child experiences, identify which of the five dimensions (feeling, like/dislike/preference, intention/motivation, belief, or desire for relationship) appear to be present. Some statements may have more than one dimension present. Then give a possible empathic response for each.

1. [Child spends 20 seconds aiming the gun toward a target and fires, missing.] Darn! I missed the stupid target.
2. [Child is looking through the crayon box, checking each one out until she spots the green one, smiles, and then starts to use it to color the picture of a frog she drew.]
3. [Child is playing ring toss with the counselor.] You should stand further back because you are bigger than me.
4. [The counselor announces that the play session is over for the day; the child runs and frantically puts her arms around the counselor's legs] [In a whining voice] Our time can't be over yet!

5. [The child sets up a role-play in a dollhouse. He has a mom shout at the baby.] You be quiet and stop your crying right now or you won't get any dinner!

**Answers:**

1. Intention/motivation dimension [Child spends 20 seconds aiming gun.]
1. Feeling dimension [Darn! I missed the stupid target.]
1. Possible empathic response: You were trying so hard to hit it; you are mad you missed.
2. Intention/motivation [Child is looking through the crayon box, checking each one out.]
2. Like/dislike [She spots the green one, smiles, then starts to use it.]
2. Possible empathic response: You are really looking for the right color; green is the one you wanted!
3. Belief.
3. Possible empathic response: You don't believe it would be fair for me to be at the same distance as you when I toss.
4. Feeling; desire for relationship.
4. Possible empathic response: You are sad that *our* time is up; you don't want to leave.
5. Feeling; intention.
5. Possible empathic response: The mom is angry because the child won't stop crying; she wants the baby to stop crying or she is going to punish it.

## Skills Support Resource C

## From Chapter 7: Activities for Structuring and Limit Setting

*Suggested Therapist' Responses to Vignettes from Putting It All Together:
Structuring and Limit Setting Applied*
**Vignette 1: Antonio Doesn't Want to Leave**

> **THERAPIST:** *You need more time! You're going to hide in your fort!*
> **ANTONIO:** *[Pokes his head out] Can't I just pleeease have more time today?*

THERAPIST: *You built your fort, and were ready to play more . . . it's disappointing for you. But Antonio, our time is up now . . . until next week. [Antonio stays in the fort, ignoring the therapist. The therapist gets up and walks over, and bends down to try to make eye contact with Antonio.] Antonio . . . I know you don't want to go, but our time is up until next week.*

ANTONIO: *I wanted to have the big fight!*

THERAPIST: *You wanted to have the big fight. But it's time to go. We have to leave the playroom now.*

The therapist moves toward the door to the playroom and opens it. It is quiet for a few seconds, then she firmly but matter-of-factly and in a gentle tone repeats the message that "our time is up for today, Antonio." After another few repetitions, Antonio comes out from behind his fort, and runs past the therapist, and into the hallway.

ANTONIO: *You better help me build it back next week!*

THERAPIST: *And you're already thinking about next week, you want me to help you build it back!*

### Vignette 2: Sam Is Angry and Reluctant to Come to Therapy

COUNSELOR: *[Reaching out to hold steady the top of the Bobo (bop bag) and making eye contact with Sam] Whoa—just a minute there. Sam! You want to kick that Bobo toward me . . . but one of the things you may not do is kick the Bobo right toward me.*

SAM: *[Smirking, but making eye contact with his counselor briefly] Bobo . . . what's a Bobo? That's a stupid name for it!*

COUNSELOR: *You don't like that name I use for it—you think it's stupid!*

SAM: *[Pulls the Bobo off to the side and smacks it toward the wall.]*

COUNSELOR: *And you pulled it over and smacked it down again!*

SAM: *Yep—it's a stupid guy and I'm gonna smack him down again and again!*

### Vignette 3: Taneesha Warms Up at the "Beach"

THERAPIST: *[Moving in closer, to get Taneesha's attention] Taneesha, that's fun for you . . . but one of the things you may not do is throw the sand over your head.*

TANEESHA: *[Stops throwing the sand, and frowns] But it's fun at the beach. I wanna throw it more!*

THERAPIST: *You were having fun . . . and you want to throw it more. But that's one of the things you may not do in here.*

TANEESHA: *[Lifts the sand up, but not over her head now, and lets it sift gently through her fingers.]*

THERAPIST: *You are letting the sand fall softly between your fingers now.*

TANEESHA: *It's like raining sand . . . [She begins a song] . . . rainy sand, rainy sand . . . I love rainy sand.*

THERAPIST: *It's like . . . raining sand. You like that.*

## Vignette 4: Anxious Krista Plays a Game of "Catch"

COUNSELOR: *[Dodges the ball coming toward his face. It hits and bounces off the wall behind him.] You threw that ball hard and right at my head . . . [The counselor pauses, and picks up the ball, and slowly sits down on the edge of the table. He looks for eye contact, and silently waits until Krista looks at him].*

KRISTA: *Yep . . . now throw it back!*

COUNSELOR: *You want to keep throwing the ball . . . but Krista . . . remember when I said I'd let you know if there is something you may not do in here?*

KRISTA: *I guess so . . . what, we can't play catch anymore or what?*

COUNSELOR: *We can play catch . . . but you may not throw the ball so hard and fast toward my head.*

KRISTA: *It wasn't on purpose . . . I was just messing with you, that's all!*

COUNSELOR: *And you want me to know that it wasn't on purpose.*

KRISTA: *And that I don't wanna hurt you . . . or nothing like that.*

COUNSELOR: *You want me to know that about you . . . that you wouldn't want to hurt me.*

KRISTA: *Sometimes I'm just acting up . . . I don't know why it happens.*

COUNSELOR: *Sometimes it's hard for you to know why you do some things. . . .*

## Vignette 5: Corey Puts His Favorite Power Figures in His Pocket

THERAPIST: *Hey . . . Corey. I think Slasher and Highjumper are still in your pocket. You remember that the toys always stay here in the playroom, right?*

> **COREY:** *[Smiling broadly] Oh, man! How'd you guys get in there? [Corey takes them out, hugs them, and puts them in the toy bin.] See you guys next week!*
> **THERAPIST:** *You are looking forward to playing with them next week.*

# Skills Support Resource D

## From Chapter 8: Activities for Responding to Questions, Requests, and Commands

*Answers for Activity A*

1. "What is your favorite football team?"
   Category: Informational Subtype: Personal information
2. "Let's play cards. Which card game do you want to play?"
   Category: Structuring Subtype: Request for direction
3. "Can I come back again tomorrow?"
   Category: Structuring Subtype: Parameters of therapy
4. "Let's see who won. How much is 12 plus 9?"
   Category: Informational Subtype: Factual information
5. "Does your husband hit your kids?"
   Category: Informational Subtype: Personal information
6. "How many legs does a spider have?"
   Category: Informational Subtype: Factual information
7. "What is your favorite type of pizza?"
   Category: Informational Subtype: Personal information
8. "What color should I make this doggy?"
   Category: Structuring Subtype: Request for direction
9. "Will you tell my mom that I created a mess in here?"
   Category: Structuring Subtype: Parameters of therapy

*Answers for Activity B*

1. "What is your favorite football team?"

   Empathy followed by providing of requested information

   > **THERAPIST:** *You would like to know what football team I like. I like the Steelers.*

2. "Let's play cards. Which card game do you want to play?"

Empathy followed by clarification of child's freedom to make decisions

> **THERAPIST:** *You would like me to choose what game we play, but in here you get to make that decision.*

3. "Can I come back again tomorrow?"

Empathy followed by providing of requested information

> **THERAPIST:** *You would really like to come back and play again tomorrow, but we will not meet again until next week.*

4. "Let's see who won. How much is 12 plus 9?"

Empathy followed by providing of requested information

> **THERAPIST:** *You are not quite sure what those two numbers add up to be. They add to 21.*

5. "Does your husband hit your kids?"

Empathy followed by the setting of a boundary/personal limit

> **THERAPIST:** *You wonder about my husband and how he treats our kids. But in your special time it is your life and family that is important, not mine.*

6. "How many legs does a spider have?"

Empathy followed by providing of requested information

> **THERAPIST:** *You are not sure how many legs they have. 8.*

7. "What is your favorite type of pizza?"

Empathy followed by providing of requested information

> THERAPIST: *You are wondering what kind of pizza I like. I like green pepper and onion.*

8. "What color should I make this doggy?"

Empathy followed by clarification of child's freedom to make decisions

> THERAPIST: *You would like me to decide what color it will be, but in here you get to make that decision.*

9. "Will you tell my mom that I created a mess in here?"

Empathy followed by providing of requested information

> THERAPIST: *You are worried that I might tell your mom about what you do in the playroom. I will not tell your mom what you do in here. You may tell her, but I will not.*

## Answers for Activity C

1. (a) comply with request

This is a request with possible underlying theme of control. No limit is necessary, unless you become fatigued, at which time a personal limit might need to be set.

2. (b) set a limit

This request would require you to you set a limit to maintain proper therapeutic boundaries. You might be able to still allow the role-play to continue by limiting the actions of the child and "pretending" the role of taking off your shirt for the doctor exam.

3. (a) comply with request

This is a request with a possible dependency or nurturance themes. No limit is necessary. In helping the child you would be careful to provide such help slowly and be ready for the child to take over the reconstruction of the tower if the child desired.

4. (b) set a limit

This request is requiring you to violate Axline's principles of letting the child lead the way and establishing an atmosphere of permissiveness, and so a limit must be set.

5. Likely (b) set a limit

This request would likely require you to set a personal limit since it is likely that you could not physically comply with the request, or if you tried it would be quite aversive and affect the quality of your unconditional positive regard for the child. However, if you were skilled at standing on your head, and it would not be aversive, you could comply with the request, and it would likely send a powerful message to the child about your ability to make decisions in the playroom.

## Skills Support Resource E

### From Chapter 10: Activities for Practice and Review on Stages of CCPT

*Activity A: Identifying Stages of CCPT*

1. **Answer:** Warm-up Stage: Although Kenesha is participating in a variety of different types of play, none of them predominate and none of them rise to the level of a sustained theme and are part of an exploratory process where she is checking out the possibilities of the playroom and discovering what limits may exist.

2. **Answer:** Aggressive Stage: Kenesha is working on issues related to control, dominance, and feeling more powerful than others.

3. **Answer:** Aggressive Stage: Although Kenesha switches between two role-plays, they both contain themes of control—in one case Kenesha exerts control, in the other she deals with accepting controls placed on her.

4. **Answer:** Transitional (Aggressive/Regressive) Stage: Kenesha is spending roughly equal time in themes of control/dominance and nurturance. Although even some of the time during the more nurturing role-play contains some control/hostility (e.g., occasionally some of the maid's favorite meals are taken away before

she can eat them), clearly both sets of themes are given significant attention in the session.

5. **Answer:** Regressive Stage: Both parts of the session focus on regressive themes, first separation/attachment issues and second nurturance issues.

6. **Answer:** Transitional Stage (Regressive/Mastery): This is a bit of a tricky one. Although the theme of the early part of the play is Regressive in nature, the ending is one that emphasizes both attachment issues (protection of the princess) but also has a somewhat Mastery quality in that the queen successfully protects the princess and thus represents a resolution of the Regressive Stage issue. The second half of the activity has a pure Mastery theme of competence to it.

7. **Answer:** Mastery Stage: Kenesha is trying challenging activities where she is trying to demonstrate her competence and skillfulness. When she does not succeed she does not change the rules, complain, or resort to "cheating" in order to defeat the therapist. She is showing good frustration tolerance.

## Skills Support Resource F

## From Chapter 11: Responses to Application Focus Activity Impasses

*Response to Application Focus Activity A*

Carlos seemed all ready to go along with whatever the therapist recommended, but the therapist had not built a relationship with him. She had not helped him tell his story through connecting with empathy. Therefore, she did not yet understand his and Nita's situation from his perspective, and thus has not conveyed that she understood. She has not been able to convey her caring, has not addressed the underlying positive, and has not conveyed that she has a plan, that she knows what she is doing and can follow procedures known to work.

To make it work from the point of impasse, she can and will have to go back and address these tasks. She may have to begin by admitting to Carlos, "Carlos, I think that in my desire to help and in seeing how ready you are to make progress, I skipped a number of steps in our getting ready to work together. So, first let me explain more, and then I think I need to hear more of your reservations and concerns. First, we will need to be in regular contact—you will not be turning Nita over to me—we will be working together. What I recommend is that we meet monthly to exchange feedback; you let me know what changes you see for Nita at home and school, and I can keep you up to date regarding her progress in sessions." As he appears to begin to express continued reluctance, she continues, "I also want us to establish goals for Nita together on which I'd like you to give me weekly reviews. And if you would like us to meet for this feedback more often, we can even meet each week following Nita's session." At this point, the therapist must stop to hear his reactions and help him process his response in empathy. She may then have to go further than usual in explaining a child's need to express things in play therapy that she cannot yet express to her parent, who she likely loves and longs to please the most. Most importantly, however, she restarts Carlos's communication to her; the most important thing she can do is backtrack in responding to him with empathy. This will build their connection as well as lead them to discuss the key areas to his reservations.

*Response to Application Focus Activity B*
In this case, the counselor has not tried to connect with the teacher at all. She has taken for granted the readiness to work together without any connection, input, or alliance. In many cases, professional teachers stand always ready for such supportive relationships, but teachers are human, too. They can get frustrated, burnt out, and see themselves as overworked and devalued (which they all too often are in society). A connection developed through providing empathy and respectful requests for input and alliance can go a long way in countering the burnout and frustration that sometimes inhibits teacher's work.

# Skills Support Resource G

## From Chapter 12: Incremental Projections of Progress for Detailed Treatment Plan

The following detailed charting is provided as an example of how goals and objectives can be charted, if needed. For such detailed charting to be necessary, you may assume a residential treatment center where the misbehaviors are expected to be severe and the therapies are expected to be long, with setbacks experienced due to such environmental factors. Items 1(b)–(d) use Teacher Rating Form—Child Behavior

Checklist (Achenbach & Rescorla, 2001) numbers from a recent client served with CCPT. Benchmarks for item 1(a) are more frequent, as they can be derived from weekly averages of teacher ratings.

> **Goal 1:** *[child name] will be on task comparably to peers*
> Objectives and benchmarks:

(a)   Increase on task ratings in key learning periods from 25% at baseline to 85% (which is within the estimated class average), with benchmarks averaging 45% rating after 2 months, 65% rating after 4 months, 85% rating after 6 months.

(b)   Increase teacher ratings of adaptive functioning from current baseline of sum of 5 (clinical range) to more than 10 (border-line range) after 3 months, and 15 (normal range) after 6 months.

(c)   (Assuming from case conceptualization that much of client's attention difficulties result from anxiety and hypervigilance.) Reduce baseline attention problems score from baseline of 45 (clinical range) to 35 (borderline range) after 3 months, and 25 (normal range) after 6 months.

(d)   (Note that most aggressive behavior is impossible during on-task learning time.) Reduce aggressive behavior ratings from current baseline of 27 (clinical range) to 20 after 3 months, and 13 (normal range) after 6 months.

## Skills Support Resource H

## From Chapter 15: Activity for Novice Play Therapists' Likely Inhibitions or Errors

*Our Thoughts on Novice Play Therapists' Likely Inhibitions or Thought Errors from Scenario 1: "Ibrahim"*
Ibrahim's counselor might understandably be inhibited by his lack of proficient English. Certainly, with other modes of counseling his lack of English proficiency could be an insurmountable barrier.

Also, he feels culturally disconnected. Very likely, many of the people in his current situation are inhibited by his differences and make mistakes such as treating him like he is wounded or fragile. Quite likely, he is deeply wounded, but treating him "with kid gloves," treating him like he is such an exception to the norm, can inhibit connections, keeping him disoriented, disconnected, and separate when what he needs most is a person to connect with in order to orient himself.

Also, Ibrahim's somewhat unusual scoffing and humorous (teasing) scolding about "toys at school" might also push some novice play therapists' buttons, causing the novice play therapist to be inhibited by the panicked thought, "Oh no, he's rejecting play therapy. This isn't going to work. . . . " Our advice is "stay steady." By reacting, Ibrahim has given his counselor his first reaction, and his counselor is in communication. The next step is to follow Ibrahim's lead. CCPT can and has worked across many situations like Ibrahim's.

### Our Thoughts on Novice Play Therapists' Likely Inhibitions or Thought Errors from Scenario 2: "Gavin"

For Gavin, the inhibition that we might expect is a worry that because of his diagnosis and unusual behavior, a specialized treatment is needed. If his diagnosis is correct, which it seems to be, then by definition he will have difficulty connecting. But we see this as a reason *for* CCPT, rather than a reason to stray from CCPT. CCPT will give him an opportunity to connect in which he cannot fail. It will let him approach connection as slowly as he needs to. And in allowing this slow approach, you will likely be surprised, if you hold steady, just how quickly he does connect and then how quickly his behavior improves with others following his connection to you.

We would encourage you not to be inhibited by his diagnosis. While you might remind yourself from understanding his diagnosis to expect slower progress, you can and should expect his progress through CCPT. The child-centered approach has helped many similar children.

As a side note, if his diagnosis is correct, some of his aggressive behavior may be inadvertently caused by caregivers trying to force him to connect when he is not ready and able. If you have expertise in understanding this situation related to his Asperger's syndrome, you may be able to provide a helpful wrap-around service in sharing understandings with caregivers regarding slower, more facilitative guidance through the structures of his day vs. trying so hard to have him succeed at social levels that he is not yet ready for.

### Our Thoughts on Novice Play Therapists' Likely Inhibitions or Thought Errors from Scenario 3: "Destiny"

It seems to us that a novice therapist might fall into the trap of assumed cultural and context problems based on Destiny's unusual family arrangements. One might assume a base of difficulties stemming from her mixed racial identity, and/or might assume some sort of confusion on her part based on her shared housing with three grandparents. Considering background information, another might guess the possibility of abandonment issues related to her biological mother's having started a new family without her, or due to her biological father's minimal involvement in her life. But later, with greater connection, listening to, and understanding of her grandparents, you may learn that none of the above assumptions were true. It may be that her anxieties are arising at this time as she has simply hit a stage in her school and life development that taxes her resilience in ways she has not been stressed before; or perhaps you may find that she is reacting strongly to an illness of one grandparent; or perhaps you find that she is caught up in, and reacting strongly to, some of her grandparents' very vocal worry for her father's possibly going off to war. It may be that this current reaction is made worse for her due to early attachment or security issues. There are *many* possibilities.

Fortunately, while figuring these things out could be helpful *outside* of her play sessions, it is important to remember that *you do not need to know the why's of her difficulties in order to help her in CCPT.* You know enough to know that her behaviors warrant therapy and that her custodial parents are concerned and supportive of that. So, what is important is that she has a chance to process what she is experiencing. It doesn't really help her process her unique experience and come to new decisions for how to make meaning of, and respond to her current situation for you to know *why* she is having her current difficulties. In fact, if you thought you knew, and then made assumptions within her session that led you to be overly analytic and interpretive in your responses, your well-intentioned efforts may only serve to slow her process and movement past the current roadblock to her development. It isn't that her context doesn't matter—every person's context matters. But, in the end, her therapy hour needs to be *her hour*, the hour when you and she are focused on her "here-and-now" and which includes her culture from without and from within. In the end, she needs to understand her culture, and she will, although it may be in ways inexpressible in words. After all, that is part of the point of play therapy (i.e., experiencing and expressing what cannot be experienced and expressed in words). As always, the key goals are for her to experience, express, and understand herself and her experiences in the modes that she can access, and for you to "be right there with her"—whether you also fully understand her internal world or not.

# Special Reference List
# for Chapter Opening Quotes

## Chapter 1

Axline, V. M.(1969). *Play therapy* (p.9). New York: Ballantine Books.

## Chapter 2

Hatch, E. J., & Guerney, B. (1975). A pupil relationship enhancement program. *Personnel and Guidance Journal, 54,* 103.

Landreth, G. (2002). *Play therapy: The art of the relationship* (p.109). New York: Brunner-Routledge.

Oaklander, V. (1978). *Windows to our children* (p. 160). Moab, UT: Real People Press.

Rogers, C. R. (1961). *On becoming a person* (p. 33). Boston: Houghton Mifflin.

## Chapter 3

Axline, V. M. (1969). *Play therapy* (p. 62). New York: Ballantine Books.

Landreth, G. (2002). *Play therapy: The art of the relationship* (p. 97). New York: Brunner-Routledge.

Moustakas, C. (1997). *Relationship play therapy* (p. 18). Northvale, NJ: Jason Aronson.

## Chapter 4

Axline, V. M. (1969). *Play therapy* (p. 73). New York: Ballantine Books.

## Chapter 5

Axline, V. M. (1969). *Play therapy* (p. 16). New York: Ballantine Books.

Landreth, G. (2002). *Play therapy: The art of the relationship* (p. 125). New York: Brunner-Routledge.

Moustakas, C. (1953). *Children in play therapy: A key to understanding normal and disturbed emotions* (p. 4). New York: McGraw-Hill.

## Chapter 6

Ginott, H. G. (1969). *Between parent and child* (p. 26). New York: Avon Books.

## Chapter 7

Rogers, F. (2006). *Many ways to say I love you* (p. 108). New York: Hyperion Books.

## Chapter 8

Landreth, G. (2002). *Play therapy: The art of the relationship* (p. 221). New York: Brunner-Routledge.

## Chapter 9

Allen, F. H. (1942). *Psychotherapy with children* (p. 265). New York: Norton.
Singer, D., & Singer, J. (1990). *The house of make believe* (p. 152). Cambridge, MA: Harvard University Press.

## Chapter 10

Axline, V. (1964). *Dibs: In search of self* (pp.188, 214). Boston: Houghton Mifflin.

## Chapter 11

Axline, V. (1964). *Dibs: In search of self* (p. 93). Boston: Houghton Mifflin.

## Chapter 12

Rogers, C. R. (1961). *On becoming a person* (p. 25). Boston: Houghton Mifflin.

## Chapter 13

Ginott, H. G. (1969). *Between parent and child.* New York: Avon Books. (p. 157).

## Chapter 14

Allen, F. H. (1942). *Psychotherapy with children* (p. 265). New York: Norton.

## Chapter 15

Boy, A. V., & Pine, G. J. (1995). *Child-centered counseling and psychotherapy* (p. 211). Springfield, IL: Thomas.
Landreth, G. L., & Sweeney, D. S. (1997). Child-centered play therapy. In K. O'Conner & L. M. Braverman (Eds.), *Play therapy: Theory and practice: A comparative presentation* (p. 25). New York: Wiley.

Mead, M. (1935). Sex and temperament in three primitive societies, concluding remarks. As quoted in E. M. Beck (Ed.), J. Bartlett (compiler), *Familiar quotations* (15th ed.; p. 853) (1980). Boston: Little, Brown.

## Chapter 16

Boy, A. V., & Pine, G. J. (1995). *Child-centered counseling and psychotherapy* (p. 196). Springfield, IL: Charles C. Thomas.

## Chapter 17

Moustakas, C. (1997). *Relationship play therapy* (p. 17). Northvale, NJ: Jason Aronson.

# References

Achenbach, T., & Rescorla, L. (2001). *Manual for the ASEBA school-age forms and profiles.* Burlington, VT: University of Vermont, Research Center for Children, Youth, and Families.

Adler, A. (1926/1972). *The neurotic constitution.* Freeport, NY: Books for Libraries Press.

Adler, A. (1931/1958). *What life should mean to you.* New York: Capricorn Books.

Adler, A. (1964). *Problems on neurosis.* New York: Harper & Row.

Ainsworth, M. D. S., Blehar, M. C., Waters, E., & Wall, S. (1978). *Patterns of attachment: A psychological study of the strange situation.* Hillsdale, NJ: Erlbaum.

Alexander, D. W. (1992). *''It happened to me''—A story for child victims of crime or trauma.* Huntington, NY: Bureau for At-Risk Youth.

Allen, F. H. (1942). *Psychotherapy with children.* New York: Norton.

American Association of Marriage and Family Therapists. (2001). *AAMFT Code of ethics.* Alexandria, VA: Author.

American Counseling Association. (2005). *ACA Code of ethics.* Alexandria, VA: Author.

American Psychiatric Association. (1994). *Diagnostic and statistical manual of mental disorders* (4th ed.). Washington, DC: Author.

American Psychiatric Association. (2000). *Diagnostic and statistical manual of mental disorders* (4th ed., Text Revision). Washington, DC: Author.

American Psychological Association. (2002). *APA ethical principles of psychologists and code of conduct.* Washington, DC: American Psychological Association.

Ames, L. B., & Haber, C. C. (1991). *Your nine year old: Thoughtful and mysterious.* New York: Dell.

Ames, L. B., & Ilg, F. L. (1991). *Your one year old: The fun loving and fussy 12- to 24-month-old.* New York: Dell.

Andronico, M. (1983). Filial therapy: A group for parents of children with emotional problems. In M. Rosenbau (Ed.), *Handbook of short-term therapy groups.* New York: McGraw-Hill.

Andronico, M., Fidler, J., Guerney, B., & Guerney, L. (1969). The combination of didactic and dynamic elements in filial therapy. In B. Guerney, Jr. (Ed.), *Psychotherapeutic agents: New roles for non-professionals, parents and teachers.* New York: Holt, Rinehart, & Winston.

Arend, R., Gove, F. L., & Sroufe, L. A. (1979). Continuity of individual adaptation from infancy to kindergarten: A predictive study of ego-resiliency and curiosity in preschoolers. *Child Development, 50,* 950–959.

Ash, C. L., Askew, R. G., & Kopp, D. D. (1996). House plants: Proper care and problem solving. Retrieved November 22, 2009, from North Dakota State University, Agriculture and University Extensions web site: www.ag.ndsu.edu/pubs/plantsci/landscap/pp744w.htm.

Association for Play Therapy. (2009a). *APT Play therapy best practices.* Fresno, CA: Author.

Association for Play Therapy. (2009b). *APT Paper on touch*. Fresno, CA: Author.

Axline, V. M. (1947). Nondirective play therapy for poor readers. *Journal of Consulting Psychology, 11*, 61–69.

Axline, V. M. (1947). *Play therapy: The inner dynamics of childhood*. Boston: Houghton Mifflin.

Axline, V. M. (1948). Play therapy: Race and conflict in young children. *Journal of Abnormal and Social Psychology, 43*, 300–310.

Axline, V. M. (1949). Play therapy: A way of understanding and helping reading problems. *Childhood Education, 26*, 156–161.

Axline, V. M. (1964). *Dibs: In search of self*. Boston: Houghton Mifflin.

Axline, V. M. (1969). *Play therapy*. New York: Ballantine Books.

Axline, V. M., & Rogers, C. R. (1945). A teacher-therapist deals with a handicapped child. *Journal of Abnormal and Social Psychology, 40*, 119–142.

Baggerly, J. (2004). The effects of child-centered group play therapy on self-concept, depression, and anxiety of children who are homeless. *International Journal of Play Therapy, 13*, 31–51.

Baggerly, J., & Jenkins, W.W. (2009). The effects of child-centered play therapy on developmental and diagnostic factors in children who are harmless. *International Journal of Play Therapy, 18*, 45–55.

Bandura, A. (1986). *Social foundations of thought and action: A social cognitive theory*. Englewood Cliffs, NJ: Prentice Hall.

Barlow, K., Strother, J., & Landreth, G. (1986). Sibling group play therapy: An effective alternative with an elective mute child. *The School Counselor, 34*, 44–50.

Barlow, K., Strother, J., & Landreth, G. (1985). Child-centered play therapy: Nancy from baldness to curls. *The School Counselor, 32*, 347–356.

Beck, A. T., Rush, A. J., Shaw, B. F., & Emery, G. (1979). *Cognitive therapy of depression*. New York: Guilford Press.

Beck, A. T., & Weishaar, M. E. (2008). Cognitive therapy. In R. J. Corsini & D. Wedding (Eds.), *Current psychotherapies* (8th ed., pp. 263–294). Belmont, CA: Thomson Brooks/Cole.

Beck, J. S. (1995). *Cognitive therapy: Basics and beyond*. New York: Guilford Press.

Bennett, B., Bricklin, P., Harris, E., Knapp, S., VandeCreek, L., & Younggren, J. (2006). *Assessing and managing risk in psychological practice*. Rockville, MD: The Trust Publishers.

Bergin, A. E., & Lambert, M. J. (1978). The evaluation of therapeutic outcomes. In S. L. Garfield and A. E. Bergin (Eds.), *Handbook of psychotherapy and behavior change* (2nd ed., pp. 139–189). New York: Wiley.

Bersoff, D. (2008). *Ethical conflicts in psychology* (4th ed.). Washington, DC: American Psychological Association.

Beutler, L. E. (1989). Differential treatment selection: The role of diagnosis in psychotherapy. *Psychotherapy, 26*, 271–281.

Bills, R. (1950). Nondirective play therapy with retarded readers. *Journal of Consulting Psychology, 14*, 140–149.

Bixler, R. (1945). Treatment of a reading problem through nondirective play therapy. *Journal of Consulting Psychology, 9*, 105–118.

Bohart, A. C., Elliot, R., Greenberg, L. S., & Watson, J. C. (2002). *Empathy*. In J. C. Norcross (Ed.), *Psychotherapy relationships that work* (pp. 89–108). New York: Oxford Press.

Bowlby, J. (1969). *Attachment and loss: Vol. 1. Attachment*. New York: Basic Books.

Bowlby, J. (1973). *Attachment and loss. Vol. 2. Separation: Anxiety and anger.* New York: Basic Books.

Boy, A. V., & Pine, G. J. (1995). *Child-centered counseling and psychotherapy.* Springfield, IL: Thomas.

Bozarth, J. (1998). *Person-centered therapy: A revolutionary paradigm.* Ross-on-Wye, UK: PCCS Books.

Bratton, S., & Landreth, G. (1995). Filial therapy with single parents: Effects on parental acceptance, empathy, and stress. *International Journal of Play Therapy, 4,* 61–80.

Bratton, S., Landreth, G., Kellam, T., & Blackard, S. R. (2006). *Child–parent relationship therapy (CPRT) treatment manual: A 10-session filial therapy model for training parents.* New York: Routledge/Taylor and Francis Group.

Bratton, S., & Ray, D. (2000). What research shows about play therapy. *International Journal of Play Therapy, 9,* 47–88.

Bratton, S., Ray, D., & Moffit, K. (1998). Filial/family play therapy. An intervention for custodial grandparents and their grandchildren. *Educational Gerontology, 24,* 391–406.

Bratton, S., Ray, D., Rhine, T., & Jones, L. (2005). The efficacy of play therapy with children: A meta-analytic review of the outcome research. *Professional Psychology: Research and Practice, 36,* 375–390.

Buber, M. (1955). *Between man and man.* ( R. G. Smith,Trans.). Boston: Beacon.

Bugental, J. F. T. (1978). *Psychotherapy and process: The fundamentals of an existential-humanistic approach.* New York: McGraw-Hill.

Bukatko, D., & Daehler, M. W. (2004). *Child development* (5th ed.). New York: Houghton Mifflin.

Cairns, R. B., & Ornstein, P. A. (1979). Developmental psychology. In E. Heart (Ed.), *The first century of experimental psychology.* Hillsdale, NJ: Erlbaum.

Caplin, W., Pernet, K., & VanFleet, R.(in progress). *Short-term group filial therapy for disadvantaged families* (working title). Boiling Springs, PA: Play Therapy Press.

Carmichael, K. (1994). Play therapy for children with physical disabilities. *Journal of Rehabilitation, 60,* 50–53.

Ceballos, P. (2008). *School-based Child Parent Relationship Therapy (CPRT) with low income first generation immigrant Hispanic parents: Effects on child behavior and parent child relationship stress.* Ann Arbor: Proquest, LLC.

Celaya, E. (2002). *A preventative program: Filial therapy for teen mothers in foster care.* Ann Arbor: Proquest.

Chau, I., & Landreth, G. (1997). Filial therapy with Chinese parents: Effects on parental empathic interactions, parental acceptance of child and parental stress. *International Journal of Play Therapy, 6,* 75–92.

Cochran, J.L. (1996). Using play and art therapy to help culturally diverse students overcome barriers to school success. *The School Counselor, 43,* 287–298.

Cochran, J. L., & Cochran, N. H. (1999). Using the counseling relationship to facilitate change in elementary school students with conduct disorder. *Professional School Counseling, 2,* 395–403.

Cochran, J. L., & Cochran, N. H. (2006). *The heart of counseling: A guide to developing therapeutic relationships.* Belmont, CA: Thomson Brooks/Cole.

Cochran, J. L., Cochran, N. H., Fuss, A., Nordling, W. (in press). Outcomes and process through stages of child-centered play therapy for a boy with highly disruptive behavior driven by self-concept issues. *Journal of Humanistic Counseling, Education & Development.*

Cochran, J. L., Cochran, N. H., & Hatch, E. J. (2002). Empathic communication for conflict resolution among children. *Person-Centered Journal, 9*, 101–112.

Cochran, J. L., Cochran, N. H., Nordling, W., McAdam, A., & Miller, D. (in press). Two case studies of child-centered play therapy for children referred with highly disruptive behavior. *International Journal of Play Therapy.*

Cochran, J. L., Fauth, D. J., Cochran, N. H., Spurgeon, S. L, & Pierce, L. M. (in press). Growing play therapy up: Extending child-centered play therapy for highly aggressive teenage boys. *Person-Centered and Experiential Psychotherapies.*

Cochran, J. L., Fauth, D. J., Cochran, N. H., Spurgeon, S. L, & Pierce, L. M. (in press). Reaching the "unreachable": Outcomes from a person-centered experiential approach for highly aggressive youth. *Person-Centered and Experiential Psychotherapies.*

Conners, C. K. (1997). *Conners' rating scales—revised: User's manual.* Tonawanda, NY: Multi-Health Systems.

Cooper, M. L., Shaver, P. R., & Collins, N. L. (1998). Attachment styles, emotion regulation, and adjustment in adolescence. *Journal of Personality and Social Psychology, 74*, 1380–1397.

Costas, M., & Landreth, G. (1999). Filial therapy with non-offending parents of children who have been sexually abused. *International Journal of Play Therapy, 8*, 43–66.

Danger, S., & Landreth, G. (2005). Child-centered group play therapy with children with speech difficulties. *International Journal of Play Therapy, 14*, 81–102.

de Shazer, S. (1988). *Clues: Investigating solutions in brief therapy.* New York: Norton.

Deci, E. L. (1975). *Intrinsic motivation.* New York: Plenum Press.

Deci, E. L., & Ryan, R. M. (1980). The empirical exploration of intrinsic motivational processes. In L. Berkowitz (Ed.), *Advances in experimental social psychology* (Vol. 13, pp. 39–80). New York: Academic Press.

Demanchick, S. P., Cochran, N. H., & Cochran, J. L. (2003). Person-centered play therapy for adults with developmental disabilities. *International Journal of Play Therapy, 12*, 47–65.

Dematatis, C. (1981). *A comparison of traditional filial therapy program to an integrated Filial–IPR program.* Ann Arbor: UMI Company.

DeMulder, E. K., Denham, S., Schmidt, M., & Mitchell, J. (2000). Q-sort assessment of attachment security during the preschool years: Links from home to school. *Developmental Psychology, 36*, 274–282.

Dupent, J., Landsman, T., & Valentine, M. (1953). The treatment of delayed speech by client-centered therapy. *Journal of Consulting Psychology, 18*, 122–125.

Edwards, N. A., Ladner, J., & White, J. (2007). Perceived effectiveness of filial therapy for a Jamaican mother: A qualitative case study. *International Journal of Play Therapy, 16*, 36–53.

Ellis, A. (2008). Rational emotive behavior therapy. In R. J. Corsini & D. Wedding (Eds.), *Current psychotherapies* (8th ed.) (pp. 187–222). Belmont, CA: Brooks/Cole.

Ellis, A., & Dryden, W. (1997). *The practice of rational emotive behavior therapy.* New York: Springer.

Erikson, E. H. (1950). *Childhood and society.* New York: Norton.

Erikson, E. H. (1964). *Insight and responsibility.* New York: Norton.

Fairbairn, W. R. D. (1954). *An object relations theory of the personality.* New York: Basic Books.

Fall, M. (1999). A play therapy intervention and its relationship to self-efficacy and learning behaviors. *Professional School Counseling, 2*, 194–205.

Fall, M., & McLeod, E. (2001). Identifying and assisting children with low self-efficacy. *Professional School Counseling, 4*, 334–341.

Farber, B. A., & Lane, J. S. (2002). Positive regard. In J. C. Norcross (Ed.), *Psychotherapy relationships that work* (pp. 175–194). New York: Oxford Press.

Fish, J.M. (1996). Prevention, solution-focused therapy, and the illusion of mental disorders. *Applied & Preventive Psychology, 5,* 37–40.

Freud, S. (1915-1917). *Introductory lectures on psychoanalysis.* London: Hogarth Press.

Friedman, M. (1995). The case of Dawn. In K. J. Schneider, & R. May (Eds.), *The psychology of existence: An integrative, clinical perspective* (pp. 308–315). New York: McGraw-Hill.

Friedman, M. (2001). Expanding the boundaries of theory. In K. J. Schneider, J. F. T. Bugental, & J. F. Pierson (Eds.), *The handbook of humanistic psychology: Leading edges in theory, practice, and research* (pp. 343–348). Thousand Oaks, CA: Sage.

Frost, J. L., Wortham, S. C., & Reifel, S. (2005). *Play and child development,* 2nd ed. Upper Saddle River, NJ: Pearson Education.

Garza, Y., & Bratton, S. (2005). School-based child-centered play therapy with Hispanic children: Outcomes and cultural considerations. *International Journal of Play Therapy, 14,* 51–80.

Ginott, H.G. (1969). *Between parent and child.* New York: Avon Books.

Ginsberg, B.G. (1997). *Relationship enhancement family therapy.* New York: Wiley.

Glass, N. (1986). *Parents as therapeutic agents: A study of the effects of filial therapy.* Ann Arbor: UMI Company.

Glauser, A. S., & Bozarth, J. D. (2001). Person-centered counseling: The culture within. *Journal of Counseling and Development, 79,* 142–147.

Glazer-Waldman, H., Zimmerman, J., Landreth, G., & Norton, D. (1992). Filial therapy: An intervention for parents of children with chronic illness. *International Journal of Play Therapy, 1,* 31–42.

Glover, G. (2001). Cultural considerations in play therapy. In G. Landreth (Ed.), *Innovations in play therapy: Issues, process, and special populations* (pp. 31–41). Philadelphia, PA: Brunner-Routledge.

Glover, G., & Landreth, G. (2000). Filial therapy with Native Americans on the Flathead Reservation. *International Journal of Play Therapy, 9,* 57–80.

Goldstein, K. (1934/1959). *The organism: A holistic approach to biology derived from psychological data in man.* New York: American Book. (Originally published in 1934.)

Graves, J., & Robinson, J. (1976). Proxemic behavior as a function of inconsistent verbal and nonverbal messages. *Journal of Counseling Psychology, 23,* 333–338.

Grigsby, A. (2007, June 18). Finding a new home: An injured bald eagle rescued last year is released back into the wild. *The Missourian.* Retrieved November 22, 2009, from www.columbiamissourian.com/stories/2007/06/18/finding-new-home/.

Grskovic, J., & Goetze, H. (2008). Short-term filial therapy with German mothers: Findings from a controlled study. *International Journal of Play Therapy, 17,* 39–51.

Guerney, B., Jr. (1964). Filial therapy: Description and rationale. *Journal of Consulting Psychology, 28,* 304–310.

Guerney, L. (1976). Filial therapy program. In D. Ohlson (Ed.), *Treating relationships.* Lake Mills, IA: Graphic.

Guerney, L. (1979). Play therapy with learning disabled children. *Journal of Clinical Child Psychology,* 242–246.

Guerney, L. (1980a). Filial therapy. In R. Herink (Ed.), *The psychotherapy handbook.* New York: New American Library.

Guerney, L. (1980b). *Parenting: A skills training manual.* State College, PA: Ideals.

Guerney, L. (1983a). Introduction to filial therapy: Training parents as therapists. In P. Keller & L. Ritt, *Innovations in clinical practice: A source book*: Sarasota, FL: Professional Resource Press.

Guerney, L. (1983b). Client-centered (non-directive) play therapy. In C. Schaefer & K. O'Conner (Eds.), *Handbook of play therapy* (pp. 21–64). New York: Wiley.

Guerney, L. (1983c). Play therapy with learning disabled children. In C. Schaefer & K. O'Conner (Eds.), *Handbook of play therapy* (pp. 419–435), New York: Wiley.

Guerney, L. (1995). *Parenting: A skills training manual* (5th ed.). Silver Spring, MD: Ideals.

Guerney, L. (1997). Filial therapy. In K. O'Connor & L. Braverman (Eds.). *Play therapy: Theory and practice*. New York: Wiley.

Guerney, L. (2000). Filial therapy into the 21st century. *International Journal of Play Therapy, 9*, 1–17.

Guerney, L. (2001). Child centered play therapy. *International Journal of Play Therapy, 10*, 13–31.

Guerney, L. (2008). Supervising filial therapy. In A. Drewes & A. Mullen, *Supervision can be playful: Techniques for child and play therapist supervisors*. Lanham, MD: Rowman & Littlefield.

Guerney, L., & Ryan, V. (in progress). *Group filial therapy: An enriched guide to working with children and parents* (working title).

Guerney, B. & Stover, L. (1971). Filial therapy: Final report on MH 18254-01. University Park: Pennsylvania State University.

Guo, Y. (2005). Filial therapy for children's behavioral and emotional problems in mainland China. *Journal of Child and Adolescent Psychiatric Nursing, 18*, 171–180.

Haase, R., & Trepper, D. (1972). Nonverbal components of empathic communication. *Journal of Counseling Psychology, 19*, 417–424.

Harris, Z., & Landreth, G. (1997). Filial therapy with incarcerated mothers: A five week model. *International Journal of Play Therapy, 6*, 53–73.

Hatch, E. J. and Guerney, B. (1975). A pupil relationship enhancement program. *Personnel and Guidance Journal, 54*, 102–105.

Havighurst, R. J. (1972). *Developmental tasks and education* (3rd ed.). New York: Longman.

Hawkes, D., Marsh, T. L., & Wilgosh, R. (1998). *Solution-focused therapy*. Boston: Butterworth Heinemann.

Hendricks, S. (1971). A descriptive analysis of the process of client-centered therapy. (Doctoral dissertation, North Texas State University, 1971.) *Dissertation Abstracts International, 32*, 3689A.

Hycner, R., & Jacobs, L. (1995). *The healing relationship in gestalt therapy: A dialogic, self psychology approach*. Highland, NY: Gestalt Journal Press.

Jang, M. (2000). Effectiveness of filial therapy for Korean parents. *International Journal of Play Therapy, 9*, 21–38.

Jones, E., & Landreth, G. (2002). The efficacy of intensive individual play therapy for chronically ill children. *International Journal of Play Therapy, 11*, 117–140.

Kale, A., & Landreth, G. (1999). Filial therapy with parents of children experiencing learning difficulties. *International Journal of Play Therapy, 8*, 35–56.

Kalichman, S. (1999). *Mandated reporting of suspected child abuse: Ethics, law, and policy* (2nd ed.). Washington, DC: American Psychological Association.

Kernberg, O. F. (1975). *Borderline conditions and pathological narcissism*. Northvale, NJ: Jason Aronson.

Kidron, M. (2004). Filial therapy with Israeli parents. *Dissertation Abstracts International: Section A: Humanities and Social Sciences, 64*(12-A), 4327.

Kochanska, G. (2001). Emotional development in children with different attachment histories: The first three years. *Child Development, 72*, 474–490.

Koocher, G., & Keith-Spiegel, P. (2008). *Ethics in psychology and the mental health professions: Standards and cases.* New York: Oxford Press.

Kot, S., Landreth, G., & Giordano, M. (1998). Intensive child-centered play therapy with child witnesses of domestic violence. *International Journal of Play Therapy, 2*, 17–36.

Krumboltz, J. D., Becker-Haven, J. F., & Burnett, K. F. (1979). Counseling psychology. *Annual Review of Psychology, 30*, 555–602.

Laible, D. J., & Thompson, R. A. (2000). Mother–child discourse, attachment security, shared positive affect, and early conscience development. *Child Development, 71*, 1424–1440.

Lambert, M. J. (1992). Psychotherapy outcome research: Implications for integrative and eclectic theories. In J. C. Norcross & M. R. Goldfried (Eds.), *Handbook of psychotherapy integration.* New York: Basic.

Landreth, G. (1991). *Play therapy: The art of the relationship.* Muncie, IN: Accelerated Development.

Landreth, G. (2001). *Innovations in play therapy: Issues, process, and special populations.* Philadelphia: Brunner-Routledge.

Landreth, G. (2002). *Play Therapy: The art of the relationship.* New York: Brunner-Routledge.

Landreth, G., & Bratton, S. (2006). *Child parent relationship therapy CPRT): A 10-session filial therapy model.* New York: Brunner-Routledge.

Landreth, G., Homeyer, L., Bratton, S., Kale, A., & Hilpl, K. (2000). *The world of play therapy literature* (3rd ed.). Denton, TX: University of North Texas Center for Play Therapy.

Landreth, G., & Lobaugh, A. (1998). Filial therapy with incarcerated fathers: Effects on parental acceptance of child, parental stress and child adjustment. *Journal of Counseling and Development, 76*, 157–165.

Landreth, G., & Sweeney, D. S. (1997). Child-centered play therapy. In K. O'Conner & L. M. Braverman (Eds), *Play therapy: Theory and practice: A comparative presentation* (pp. 17–45). New York: Wiley.

Lau, K., Kraus, K., & Morse, R. (2008). *Mandated reporting of child abuse and neglect: A practical guide for social workers.* New York: Springer.

Ledyard, P. (1999). Play therapy with the elderly: A case study. *International Journal of Play Therapy, 8*, 57–75.

Lee, M. & Landreth, G. (2003). Filial therapy with immigrant Korean parents in the United States. *International Journal of Play Therapy, 12*, 67–85.

Locke, J. (1964). Some thoughts on education. In P. Gay (Ed.), *John Locke on education.* New York: Teacher's College. (Original work published 1693)

Lowenfield, M. (1935). *Play in childhood.* London: Gollanez.

Luborsky, E. B., O'Reilly-Landry, M., & Arlow, J. A. (2008). Psychoanalysis. In R. J. Corsini & D. Wedding (Eds.), *Current psychotherapies* (8th ed., pp. 15–62). Belmont, CA: Brooks/Cole.

May, R. (1967). *Psychology and the human dilemma.* New York: Norton.

McGoldrick, M., Giordano, J., & Garcia-Preto, N. (Eds.) (2005). *Ethnicity and family therapy* (3rd ed.). New York: Guilford Press.

Mendelowitz, E., & Schneider, K. (2008). Existential psychotherapy. In R.J. Corsini & D. Wedding (Eds.), *Current psychotherapies* (8th ed., pp. 295–327). Belmont, CA: Brooks/Cole.

Mosak, H. H., & Maniacci, M. (2008). Adlerian psychotherapy. In R. J. Corsini & D. Wedding (Eds.), *Current psychotherapies*, (8th ed., pp. 63–106). Belmont, CA: Thomson Brooks/Cole.

Moustakas, C. (1997). *Relationship play therapy*. Northvale, NJ: Jason Aronson.

Moyles, J. (2005). *The excellence of play*. Maidenhead, Berkshire, UK: Open University Press.

Murch, S. J., & Saxena, P. K. (2005). *Journey of a single cell to plant*. Enfield, NH: Science Publishers.

Muro, J., Ray, D.C, Schottelkorb, A., Smith, M.R., & Blanco, P.J. (2006). Qualitative analysis of long-term child-centered play therapy. *International Journal of Play Therapy, 15*, 35–58.

National Association of Social Workers. (2008). *NASW Code of ethics*. Washington, DC: National Association of Social Workers.

Norcross, J. C. (Ed.) (2002). *Psychotherapy relationship that works*. New York: Oxford Press.

Nordling, W., & Guerney, L. (1999). Typical stages in the child-centered play therapy process. *The Journal for the Professional Counselor, 14*, 17–23.

Nordling, W. (2009, September). *Child-centered play therapy*. Workshop sponsored by the National Institute for Relationship Enhancement, Bethesda, MD.

Oaklander, V. (1978). *Windows to our children*. Moab, UT: Real People Press.

Orlinsky, D. E., & Howard, K. I. (1978). The relation of process to outcome in psychotherapy. In S. L. Garfield and A. E. Bergin (Eds.), *Handbook of psychotherapy and behavior change* (2nd ed.; pp. 283–330). New York: Wiley.

Oxman, L. K. (1972). The effectiveness of filial therapy: A controlled study (doctoral dissertation, Rutgers State University, 1972). *Dissertation Abstracts International, 32*, 6656.

Patterson, C. H. (1984). Empathy, warmth and genuineness: A review of reviews. *Psychotherapy, 21*, 431–438.

Patterson, C. H. (1996). Multicultural counseling: From diversity to universality. *Journal of Counseling and Development, 74*, 227–321.

Patterson, C. H. (2004). Do we need multicultural counseling competencies? *Journal of Mental Health Counseling, 26*, 67–73.

Perls, F., Hefferline, R., & Goodman, P. (1951/1994). *Gestalt therapy: Excitement and growth in the human personality*. New York: Gestalt Journal Press.

Peschken, W. E., & Johnson, M. E. (1997). Therapist and client trust in therapeutic relationship. *Psychotherapy Research, 7*, 439–447.

Piaget, J. (1929). *The child's conception of the world*. London: Routledge & Kegan Paul.

Piaget, J. (1951). *Play, dreams, and imitation in childhood*. London: Routledge.

Piaget, J. (1954). *The construction of reality in the child*. New York: Basic Books.

Piaget, J. (1971). *Biology and knowledge: An essay on the relationship between organic regulations and cognitive processes*. Chicago: University of Chicago Press.

Rank, O. (1936). *Will therapy*. (J. Taft, Trans.). New York: Knopf.

Ray, D., Bratton, S., Rhine, T., & Jones, L. (2001). The effectiveness of play therapy: Responding to critics. *International Journal of Play Therapy, 10*, 85–108.

Ray, D., Blanco, P. J., Sullivan, J. M., & Holliman, R. (2009). An exploratory study of child-centered play therapy with aggressive children. *International Journal of Play Therapy, 18*, 162–175.

Ray, D., Schottelkorb, A., & Tsai, M. (2007). Play therapy with children exhibiting symptoms of attention deficit hyperactivity disorder. *International Journal of Play Therapy, 16,* 95–111.

Rogers, C. R. (1951). *Client-centered therapy: Its current practice, implications, and theory.* Boston: Houghton Mifflin.

Rogers, C. R. (1961). *On becoming a person.* Boston: Houghton Mifflin.

Rogers, C. R. (1957). The necessary and sufficient conditions for therapeutic personality change. *Journal of Consulting Psychology, 21,* 95–103.

Rogers, C. R. (1967). Toward a modern approach to values: The valuing process in the mature person. In C. R. Rogers & B. Stevens (Eds.), *Person to person: The problem of being human* (pp. 13–28). New York: Real People Press.

Rogers, C. R. (1977). *Carl Rogers on personal power.* New York: Delacrote Press.

Rogers, C. R. (1980). *A way of being.* Boston: Houghton Mifflin.

Rogers, C. R. (1987). The underlying theory: Drawn from experience with individuals and groups. *Counseling and Values, 32,* 38–46.

Rogers, F. (2006). *Many ways to say I love you.* New York: Hyperion Books.

Rousseau, J. J.(1895). Émile, or on education (W. H. Payne, Trans.). New York: Appleton. (Original work published 1762)

Ryan, S., & Nordling, W. (2003). Adapting filial therapy in the face of adversity: The case of an inner-city family. In R. Van Fleet & L. Guerney (Eds.), *Casebook of filial play therapy,* (pp. 399–416). Boiling Springs, PA: Play Therapy Press.

Ryan, V. (2007). Filial therapy: Helping children and new carers from secure attachment relationships. *The British Journal of Social Work, 37,* 643–657.

Scuka, R.F. (2005). *Relationship enhancement therapy: Healing through deep empathy and intimate dialog.* New York: Routledge.

Sensue, M. E. (1981). Filial therapy follow-up study: Effects on parental acceptance and child adjustment. *Dissertation Abstracts International, A 42*(01).

Shapiro, D. A., & Shapiro, D. (1982). Meta-analysis of comparative therapy outcome studies: A replication and refinement. *Psychological Bulletin, 92,* 581–604.

Sheely, A. (2008). *School-based child-parent relationship therapy (CPRT) with low income black American parents: Effects on children's behaviors and parent-child relationship stress, a pilot study.* Ann Arbor: Proquest.

Sherer, M., & Rogers, R. (1980). Effects of therapist's nonverbal communication on rated skill and effectiveness. *Journal of Clinical Psychology, 36,* 696–700.

Shen, Y. (2002). Short-term group play therapy with Chinese earthquake victims: Effects of anxiety, depression, and adjustment. *International Journal of Play Therapy, 11,* 43–63.

Singer, D. and Singer, J. (1990). *The house of make believe.* Cambridge, MA: Harvard University Press.

Singer, J. (1973). *The child's world of make believe: Experimental studies of imaginative play.* London: Academic Press.

Skinner, B. F. (1953). *Science and human behavior.* New York: Macmillan.

Skinner, B. F. (1974). *About behaviorism.* New York: Knopf.

Solis, C. M., Meyers, J., & Varjas, K. M. (2004). A qualitative case study of the process and impact of filial therapy with an African-American parent. *International Journal of Play Therapy, 13,* 99–118.

Stover, L., & Guerney, Jr., B. (1967). The efficacy of training procedures for mothers in filial therapy. *Psychotherapy Research and Practice, 4,* 110–115.

Sywulak, A. E. (1977). *The effects of filial therapy on parental acceptance and child adjustment.* Unpublished doctoral dissertation. Pennsylvania State University.

Tew, K., Landreth, G., Joiner, K., & Solt, M. (2002). Filial therapy with parents of chronically ill children. *International Journal of Play Therapy, 11,* 79–100.

VanFleet, R. (1992). Using filial therapy to strengthen families with chronically ill children. In L. VandeCreek, S. Knapp, & T. Jackson (Eds.), *Innovations in clinical practice: A source book, Vol. 11,* (pp. 87–97). Sarasota, FL: Professional Resource Exchange.

VanFleet, R. (2005). *Filial therapy: Strengthening parent–child relationships through play.* Sarasota, FL: Practitioner's Resource Press.

Vygotsky, L. (1978). *Mind in society: The development of higher psychological processes.* Cambridge, MA: Harvard University Press.

Walker, K.F. (2008). Filial therapy with parents court-referred for child maltreatment. *Dissertation Abstracts International Section A: Humanities and Social Sciences, 68*(8A), 3300.

Wampold, B. E. (2001). *The great psychotherapy debate: Models, methods, and findings.* Mahwah, NJ: Erlbaum.

Warren, S. L., Huston, L., Egeland, B., & Sroufe, L. A. (1997). Child and adolescent anxiety disorders and early attachment. *Journal of the American Academy of Child and Adolescent Psychiatry, 36,* 637–644.

Wilkins, P. (2000). Unconditional positive regard reconsidered. *British Journal of Guidance and Counselling, 28,* 23–36.

Williams, W. & Lair, G. (1991). Using a person-centered approach with children who have a disability. *Elementary School Guidance & Counseling, 25,* 194–203.

Withee, K. (1975). A descriptive analysis of the process of play therapy. Unpublished doctoral dissertation, North Texas State, Denton, TX.

Wubbolding, R.E. (2000). *Reality therapy for the 21st century.* Philadelphia: Brunner-Routledge.

Yolum, I. (1980). *Existential psychotherapy.* New York: Basic Books.

Yontef, G., & Jacobs, L. (2008). Gestalt therapy. In R. J. Corsini & D. Wedding (Eds.), *Current psychotherapies* (8th ed.; pp. 328–367). Belmont, CA: Brooks/Cole.

Yuen, T., Landreth, G., & Baggerly, J. (2002). Filial therapy with immigrant Chinese families. *International Journal of Play Therapy, 1,* 63–90.

# NAME INDEX